PIG DISEASES

Eighth edition

2006

© D. J. Taylor 2006

ISBN 0 9506932 7 8

First edition 1979
Second edition 1981
Third edition 1983
Fourth edition 1986
Reprinted November 1986
Fifth edition 1989
Sixth edition 1995
Reprinted January 1997
Seventh edition 1999
Eighth edition 2006

Published by and copies obtainable from the author:

Dr. D. J. Taylor
31 North Birbiston Road
Lennoxtown
Glasgow
G66 7LZ

www.pigdiseases.co.uk

Design and production in association with
Book Production Consultants Ltd, Cambridge

Printed in Great Britain by
St Edmundsbury Press Ltd, Bury St Edmunds, Suffolk

CONTENTS

FOREWORD

The first edition of this book was written as student notes, but demand from veterinarians, veterinary students and farmers led to its publication. It is intended primarily to describe diseases of pigs present in the UK and Europe, those that threaten the European pig industry or those which may yet be identified here. It deals mainly with conditions found in intensive units and can, therefore, be used worldwide. Conditions which are uncommon in such intensive units may be dealt with in less detail.

Treatment is only described in general as the book is intended for the use of Veterinary Surgeons who, in the UK, are supplied annually with the NOAH Compendium of Data Sheets for Veterinary Products. These data sheets give details of the veterinary products cited. In other countries, similar books exist and provide local trade names for the therapeutic agents and vaccines described. Prescribing practice and the availability of medicines and vaccines differ from country to country and those using the book should take account of this and adhere to local requirements, particularly with regard to withdrawal times and legislation. The Veterinary Formulary (Pharmaceutical Press), which describes prescription medicines worldwide may be of assistance. Feeding, housing and management techniques are adequately described in existing books such as those published by Farming Press, Ipswich, UK. Further information about disease may be found in 'Diseases of Swine' edited by B.E.Straw and others and the other books listed in the Introduction. Information is increasingly available on the Internet and some addresses of important sites are included.

The descriptions of diseases and the measures adopted for their control are based on a mixture of personal experience, review of the literature and, in the case of the newer syndromes, word of mouth or case reports. This edition reflects the increasing concern of the veterinary profession and public in the UK about welfare, meat quality and general safety. The account of each disease is supplemented with an opinion on the humane endpoint for slaughter, and on risks to man to be expected from each disease and its therapy.

The normal nutritional requirements of the pig given on pages 298-300 are reproduced with some amendments from Tables 5:1, 5:3 and 11:8 in "Practical Pig Nutrition" by C.T. Whittemore and F.W. Elsey with kind permission of the publishers, Farming Press Ltd of Ipswich. I would like to thank the colleagues who commented on the previous editions of this book and, in particular, those who wrote to provide further information and my daughter, Claire for editing assistance.

D.J. Taylor, MA, PhD, Vet.MB,
Dip.ECVPH, DipECPHM, MRCVS.
31 North Birbiston Road
Lennoxtown
Glasgow
G66 7LZ

davidtaylor@pigdiseases.co.uk
www.pigdiseases.co.uk
June 2006

INTRODUCTION

The UK pig industry with 470,000 sows,(2005), 554,000 breeding stock and 4,864,000 (2005) pigs (approximately 8,600,000 slaughter pigs 2005, 9,367,000, 2004) is small when compared with the total pig populations of the E.C. 25 (134,054,000 2004, estimate). The price of grain within the E.C. has recently declined, but, for the moment, the strength of the pound sterling and the over-supply of pigmeat in the EU means that margins for UK pig producers are poor and the UK industry contracted by 5.8%% in the year to June 2005. Pigmeat consumption in the UK was around 1,500,000 tonnes in 2005 of which 858,000 tonnes was imported. Costs in the UK are higher than those elsewhere in the EU at present because of the ban on sow stalls and tethers for welfare reasons. UK farmers were also affected by the Classical Swine Fever outbreak in 2000, the Foot and Mouth outbreak in 2001 and the continuing effects of the Postweaning Multisystemic Wasting Syndrome (PMWS) which began in 1999. Other factors such as the disposal of offal to landfill, the ban on the use of meat and bone meal consequent on the BSE crisis, the withdrawal of antimicrobial growth promoters, the environmental, food safety, and new welfare legislation have affected management techniques and the spectrum of enteric disease throughout the Community.

The past freedom of the UK from diseases such as swine fever and Aujeszky's Disease, coupled with the development of hybrid breeding stock, led to a flourishing export trade in British pigs with Europe and with other parts of the world. Specialisation in the pig industry and the requirements of exporters and purchasers of pigmeat demand an ever increasing degree of technical knowledge from the veterinarian. This book is intended to form a foundation for such expertise.

Structure of the industry in the UK

Herd sizes in Britain may now be stable. The total number of holdings has fallen dramatically in recent years and numbered 10,1000 in 2003 of which 5,500 had over 50 pigs. The concentration of pigs in large herds is reflected in the trade in breeding stock; 75% of all gilts and 65% of all boars sold are supplied by 4-8 large breeding companies.

In some areas of the country the pig herds are now large and scattered particularly where there have been closures of slaughterhouses. In future, however, the industry will be organised much as at present but with fewer small scale producers and still fewer units. The organisation of the industry and the type of units and enterprises found are important factors in the diseases which occur. Traditional patterns of husbandry - the single fattening pig or breeding sow, the mixed farm with a few sows and a boar producing weaners for sale or to fatten on the farm, still persist. Organic farming, wild boar farming, the maintenance of rare breeds, the pet pig, transgenic pigs for xenotransplantation and the experimental pigs used in veterinary and biomedical science all represent new challenges for the pig veterinarian.

The use of adapted or old-fashioned buildings and the practice of home mixing rations still give rise to the husbandry, nutritional and parasitic problems which have often disappeared from the larger units. The larger enterprises may be divided into several groups from a health stand-point. The larger breeder-weaner or producer/finisher may run a closed herd apart from purchases of boars or operate using artificial insemination alone and has a variable incidence of disease.

Breeding companies are organised in a pyramid with a nucleus herd supplying multipliers with grand-parent stock and these then produce the parents of the slaughter generation which are sold to the farmer. Constant genetic turnover in the nucleus herd results in the use of young boars and gilts with and the movement of animals from nucleus to multiplier to farm creates a channel by which disease in the nucleus or in a multiplier can rapidly spread to a large number of farms. Finishing may be run on a large scale by feeding companies which own pigs, rent buildings and labour from farmers and supply their own feed. They frequently populate sites on an all-in, all-out basis but may purchase their weaners from a number of sources and mix them, a practice which frequently results in disease. A few farms feed byproducts, many purchase stock from a number of sources and disease can result from this practice. The difficulty of balancing byproducts of varying quality and the destruction of nutrients by heating may result in nutritional problems not seen elsewhere. Both in-feed and water medication is difficult to administer on such farms. The husbandry system within a farm also affects the disease pattern and the productivity of the unit. The age at which pigs are weaned is the most important factor. Traditional 8-week weaning is uncommon except on organic farms. Six week, and 5-week weaning occur but 4 week weaning is the rule. Weaning at 5 days of age may be recommended in some disease control programmes, but weaning at this age is not allowed on welfare grounds and the 14-16 day weaning practised in Segregated Early Weaning programmes in the US cannot be carried out in the EU. After 4-week weaning, housing in large groups in flat decks or kennels, sometimes on a separate farm, is common with attendant respiratory and behavioural problems. The size of subsequent groups of weaned pigs and the nature of the floors and dung disposal (slats, continuous dunging channel, deep straw) also affects the incidence and nature of disease. Airspace, its size and the type of nutrition - floor fed meal, skim milk, liquid feed, trough feeding are also important. The vaccines and additives used may also have a bearing on the diseases seen. Finally, the way in which breeding stock are housed and handled is important when considering reproductive problems.

Health programmes and health status in the Pig Industry

Pigs may have "conventional" health status i.e. are normal farm stock although perhaps free from some diseases or they may be hysterectomy-derived (primary S.P.F.) or bred from such animals (secondary S.P.F.). The latter class of animal is normally maintained behind some type of barrier and is known as "S.P.F.", "Minimal Disease" (M.D.) or "High Health Status" in advertisements. Some pure bred herds are descendants of hysterectomy-derived pigs and the nucleus herds and multipliers of most breeding companies are of this type. Health schemes include single farm programmes (Farm Health Plans) and those applied to all the farms belonging to one breeding or feeding company, Quality Assurance organisation or supermarket chain. The recent development of slaughterhouse monitoring for salmonella antibody is National, as is the carcase monitoring for the organism, but slaughterhouse monitoring for production diseases is carried out on a devolved basis for the 4 regional industry levy organisations of which BPEX (England) is the largest. This monitoring programme started in June 2005 in England and will provide individual farm information and some National figures for these diseases will then become available

3

Disease and its investigation

Two diseases or infections have dominated day to day farm management in recent years, firstly the widespread presence of the virus of the porcine respiratory and reproductive syndromes (PRRS, PEARS, SIRS) and the variable effect of the infection on individuals herds (from 1991) and PMWS/Porcine Dermatitis and Nephropathy Syndrome (PDNS) (1999). This last complex has had a devastating effect on the industry and was responsible for some of the contraction noted above.

The application of molecular biology, genetics and immunology has revolutionised many aspects of the study of pig diseases. The production of DNA probes and the polymerase chain reaction (PCR) enable the frequency of single genes to be determined in pig populations and will allow the selection of disease-resistant stock. Similar methods and user-friendly peroxidase-linked immunoassays such as ELISA tests, have allowed a new sensitivity and specificity in diagnosis. This in turn has been reflected in an extension of the veterinarian's ability to study the pathogenesis and epidemiology of disease. The application of molecular techniques has created new vaccines and treatments which are currently being introduced. Their specificity is often high and they are often very effective against the target agent. Diseases such as *E.coli* enteritis, Oedema Disease, enzootic pneumonia, Glasser's Disease, swine dysentery and pleuropneumonia may all be controllable as a result of these novel vaccines.

Herd medication and disease eradication procedures

The advances in the understanding of disease and the ability to detect and control it have consolidated the ability of the veterinary profession to eradicate disease from individual herds, pyramids or areas. Combined programmes of treatment and or vaccination, disinfection and restriction of movement or isolation, have been developed for the eradication of Aujeszky's Disease, Oedema Disease, swine dysentery, enzootic pneumonia, mange, atrophic rhinitis and pleuropneumonia. The widespread availability of artificial Insemination (AI) and of disease-free breeding stock (from the high health nucleus and multiplier herds of major companies) has meant that disease-free status can be maintained, particularly where herds are scattered.

The free movement of livestock across national borders within the E.C. has had some dramatic effects on the disease status of individual herds and countries . The outbreak of classical swine fever which spread from Germany to The Netherlands and then on to other countries in traded pigs is an example of international spread of disease through trade. In general, those purchasing stock from distant units should satisfy themselves (where the requirements are not enforced by Government) that the testing programme carried out prior to certification is adequate and that animals are transported in such a way that they are not exposed to disease en route. Incoming stock should always be quarantined. Where production animals are brought from a distance, vaccination programmes for disease such as Aujeszky's Disease in the herd of origin should be continued in the herd of destination.

Computer programmes for monitoring productivity

Recording of herds by commercially-available computer programmes has been widespread, but recording in the feeding herd was discontinued on some farms during the PMWS/PDNS epidemic but is now being resumed. Many large farms now produce figures for their days to slaughter, weaning to service intervals, numbers born, born dead or alive, feed conversion rates and mortality rates. Individual or group growth rates may be available where on-farm performance testing or automatic pen weighing is carried out. These records can be used to interpret at a glance the recent reproductive and growth performance of a herd and to identify problem areas in production. They are now giving information about the performance of finishing herds and are able to provide individual sow health records. They should always be consulted before assessing a production problem.

Welfare

The welfare of pigs continues to be a matter of considerable concern to the Veterinary Profession, the farmer, Parliament, the E.C., the Press and the Public. Pressure to replace intensive systems of management is continuing in the U.K. and some other countries in Europe.

There is particular concern over the behavioural requirements of piglets in flat deck systems, especially after early weaning (3 weeks) and of the sow confined at farrowing. The question of comfort for all classes of stock has been studied and the Welfare Code amended to give certain recommendations for the humane housing of livestock. The castration of piglets is considered unnecessary on both economic and welfare grounds provided they reach slaughter within 160 days. The handling of pigs in transit and at abattoirs is also the subject for new transport legislation and public pressure affects husbandry practices on the farm. The introduction of loose housing for sows and the ban on stalls or tethers introduced welfare problems of its own because of fighting on batching, difficulties with individual feeding and difficulties in detecting and managing sick animals. Studies of sow behaviour have provided guidance on their requirements and new, economical loose housing systems are being developed and installed which allow individual feeding, adequate comfort, exercise and proper inspection. The limitations of electronic sow feeders and single space feeders are now more clearly understood.

Welfare criteria are now being applied more objectively to outdoor sows which represent around 30% of the UK sow herd. This trend to outdoor pig husbandry has re-introduced problems of foxes and parasitism not seen for many years. The release of wild boar/feral pigs into the countryside and the establishment of breeding populations has introduced a new factor into health control on outdoor units.

A general increase in slaughter weights or the effects of disease and reduced growth rate can lead to over-crowding and increase welfare problems.

Improvements in welfare have arisen from the stricter application of antemortem inspections at abattoir for Food Safety reasons, the imminent introduction of Food Chain Information and the requirements of purchasers that only clean, healthy pigs be presented for slaughter. The criteria for humane endpoints and the best methods for humane slaughter have reduced suffering. Training of farm staff in nursing and techniques for humane slaughter has also helped and is becoming increasingly important.

Meat quality

Recent attention to meat quality has introduced meatier pigs growing to higher slaughter weight and using Duroc components to improve marbled fat content. The requirements by supermarkets purchasing in the UK has influenced breeding, husbandry, medication and slaughter policy considerably. Recent concern about residues of antimicrobials and other therapeutic substances in meat has improved the strict observance of withdrawal times. Monitoring for carcase residues is widely practised in the U.K. and in other E.C. countries. The use of antimicrobials in feed is strictly controlled in the U.K. and E.C. Regulations on prescribing, particularly the Medicated Feedstuffs Prescription and the licensing of units allowed to incorporate medication into feedstuffs are in place . These controls, coupled with the maintenance of Treatment Records on farms in the U.K. have reduced the likelihood of residues reaching meat. The recent ban on antimicrobial growth promoters throughout the EU had implications for production and for the physical welfare of pigs in E.C. countries, but has largely (June 2006) been adopted without major disease consequences.

Veterinarians in the Pig Industry

(a) Private Practice

A few veterinarians specialise entirely in pigs but the economics of the pig industry mean that few U.K. practices deal solely with pigs. Many practices, particularly in East Anglia and Yorkshire have several members with an interest in pigs. These members may act as consultants to feed firms and other organisations owning pigs. Some practices have their own diagnostic laboratories. The keeping of pet pigs has stimulated interest in pigs in urban areas. A specialist diploma and certificate course is run by the Royal College of Veterinary Surgeons, Belgravia House, Horseferry Road, London and the European College of Pig Health Management was founded in 2005 and offers Diplomate status.

(b) Industry

Veterinarians are employed by feed firms to service their pig enterprises and by pharmaceutical companies concerned with products for the pig industry. Some breeding companies also employ their own veterinarians to handle health problems both in the U.K. and worldwide. Other veterinarians based in practice or University offer consultations on a part-time basis for these companies and for the Profession. Increasing numbers of veterinarians are being employed in public health, food hygiene and by Quality Assurance Schemes in the food industry. Veterinarians now advise companies producing transgenic pigs for xeno transplantation.

(c) State Veterinary Service, related bodies and Meat Hygiene Service)

Veterinarians specialising in pigs are to be found in the State Veterinary Service, in the Veterinary Laboratory Agency, Weybridge and its regional laboratories, the Lasswade laboratory and the Veterinary Research Laboratories, Stormont. The requirement for laboratory methods in diagnosis or for the confirmation of diagnosis in many pig diseases means that a number of these people are in the Investigation Service, particularly in Centres at Thirsk, Bury St. Edmunds and Winchester, and the Scottish Agricultural College V.I. Centres at Aberdeen and Edinburgh, serving the pig rearing areas. In addition, veterinarians with pig expertise may be employed by the Meat and Livestock Commission and other Government sponsored bodies.

6

(d) Research

Research Institutes including those of the BBSRC, Industry and the Universities provide most opportunities for research into pigs in this country and a few posts exist in Universities for teaching pig diseases. The use of pigs in biomedical research is increasing and may offer opportunities for the veterinarian particularly as a named veterinary surgeon.

Information about pigs and the pig industry (Bibliography)

Many pig farmers in the U.K. read the following journals:-

- Pig International, Watt Publishing, Illinois, a monthly
- Pig Progress, Elsevier International, a bi-monthly.
- International Pig Topics.
and pig articles which appear in less specialised journals.

Information about pig management and husbandry can be found in the following:

- A Quantitative Biology of the Pig (1998), Kyriazakis, I. (Ed). CAB, Wallingford.
- The Genetics of the Pig. (1998). Rothschild, M.F. (Ed) CAB, Wallingford. Controlled Reproduction in Pigs (1997). Gordon, I. CAB, Wallingford.
- The Neonatal Pig: Development and Survival. (1995). Varley, M.A. (Ed). CAB Wallingford.
- Nutrient Requirements of Swine, 10th Ed. National Research Council, CAB, Wallingford. (In the US, National Academy Press).
- Swine Science. (1997). Ensminger, M.E., Parker, R.O. (1997). Interstate Publishers, Inc
- The weaner pig, nutrition and management. M.Varley and J. Wiseman, (2002) CABI Publishing 355pp, ISBN 0851995322
- Pig Husbandry in the Tropics. (5th Ed 1995). Muys, D., Westenbrink, G. Agromisa, Wageningen.
- Pig Health Recording Production and Finance - A Producers' Guide. Pig Veterinary Society, c/o Grove House, Corsham, Malmesbury, Wilts.
- Pig Yearbook 2005 British Pig Executive (Annual).
- The Science and Practice of Pig Production, I. Kyriazakis and C.T. Whittemore , 3rd Edition (2006), Blackwell Science ISBN: 1405124482.
- CABI Index of Current Research on Pigs (Annual) lists papers published worldwide and current research topics

Further information about pig diseases may be obtained from:

- Diseases of Swine, (9th edition 2006). Edited by B.E. Straw B.E., Zimmerman, J.J. D'Allaire, and D.J. Taylor. Blackwell Publishing.
- A Colour Atlas of Diseases and Disorders of the Pig. W. Smith, D.J. Taylor and R.H.C. Penny. (1989). Wolfe Medical. (out of print but useful)
- Managing Pig Health and the treatment of disease, Muirhead, M.R. and Alexander, T.J.L. (1997), 5M Enterprises, Sheffield.
- Lehrbuch der Schweine-krankheiten 2nd Edition (1997) Plonait, H. and Bickhardt, K. Parey, Berlin.

- Pathology of the pig, a diagnostic guide (1996) Sims, L.D., Glastonbury, J.R.W. (Eds) Pig Research and Development Corporation and Agriculture Victoria, 456pp, !SBN 0 7306 65372
- Pig News and Information (Quarterly), Commonwealth Agricultural Bureau lists papers on porcine subjects and these are also available on CD ROM.
- The Pig Disease Information Centre (http://www.pighealth.com) carries topical information and book lists.
- The Pig Site (www.thepigsite.com/-) Hosts a number of pig items, including links to the Pig Journal and Pig Veterinary Society.

The UK Pig Veterinary Society meets twice a year and publishes proceedings currently The Pig Journal, twice a year. Editorial Committee, c/o Southview, East Tytherton, Chippenham, Wilts. SN15 4LX. (http://www.pigjournal.co.uk) Members are informed about International Pig Veterinary Society meetings which are held biennially. The next meeting (IPVS 19) is in Copenhagen in July 2006. The Proceedings, (Proc IPVS 1-18 in this book), are a major source of information

The Pig: Some Basic Information

Native Breeds UK   Large White, Landrace, rarely Saddleback Tamworth, Berkshire, Middle White and Gloucester Old Spot.
Imported: Pietrain, Hampshire, Duroc, Meishan and others from time to time.

Clinical Information

Body temperature : 39°C (102°F)

Lower critical point 38.4°C (101.2°F).
Upper critical point 40°C (103.5°F).
Respiratory rate, resting, 18°C· 20-30 per minute, more in young (up to 50), less in old (to 13-15) in sows.

Pulse (resting) :70-80 per minute, more in young (200-280, newborn).

Packed Cell Volume (PCV)	0.42	(0.37-0.46)		1/1
Red Blood Cells (rbc)	7.0	(6.5-8.0)	x 10^{12}	/1
White Blood Cells (wbc)	18.0	(10.0-23.0)	x 10^9	/1
Platelets	400.0	(250.0-700.0)	10^9	/1
Haemoglobin (Hb)	140	(110-142)		g/l

For blood levels of ions or plasma enzymes, see appropriate section. All blood parameters may change with age. These are adult figures.

Husbandry factors

(a)   Minimum temperature requirements:-

Adults: In service areas,
dry sow houses and yards.   15-20°C, 59-68°F
In farrowing houses   15-18°C, 59-64°F

Piglets to 5 kg.   25-30°C, 77-84°F

Early weaned, 3 weeks and over (5-18kg)	27-32°C,	81-90°F
Weaned pigs (6 weeks and over)	21-24°C,	70-75°F
Growers (19-45kg)	15-21°C,	59-70°F
Finishing pigs (45-95kg)	13-18°C,	55-64°F
Heavy hogs (90-115kg)	10-15°C,	50-59°F

These temperatures should not fluctuate.

(b)   Productivity data

Sexual maturity*:   8-9 months male, 7 months female
Oestrus period   21 days
Gestation length   112-116 days, usually 114 days
* may be younger for Meishan crosses

Levels for some commonly recorded productivity parameters are given below. The values given here may be low when compared with the actual results achieved by top herds in the U.K., using some of the most prolific sow lines and the most recent hybrid stock. Current figures of 13 pigs weaned per litter and 17 born alive in Denmark suggest that all targets should be revised upwards.

Additional parameters may be found in the BPEX Pig Yearbooks and Pig Health, Recording and Finance - A Producers' Guide.

Parameter	Liveweight	Target Level	Interference level
Weaning: Service Interval:		7 days	9 days
Farrowing to first service		87%	80 %
Returns to service		6%	12%
Abortions		1%	2.5%
Failure to farrow		2%	3%
Sow mortality		2.2%	3%
Sow culls/100 sows/yr		30	35%
Total mean numbers born		14.0	11.0
Mean numbers born alive		13.5	11.0
Mean numbers born dead		4%	6%
Litter scatter		10%	18%
Mean numbers weaned/litter		11.0	10.5
Pre-weaning mortality		8%	12%
Weaning weight 28 days		7.0kg	5.0kg
35 days		10.0kg	
42 days		11.0kg	
Litter/sow/yr		2.4	2.3
Piglets/sow/yr		26.0	22
Days to slaughter (Bacon)	86-93 (89)	147	
Heavy (current bacon weight)	105 kg		
Feed conversion efficiency	6.2-68 kg	2.04	
	6.2-76 kg	2.08	
	6.7-90 kg	2.3	
Daily liveweight gain (g)	6.2-85 kg	570	
	6.2-76 kg	600	
	7.7-90 kg	800	

Check list for clinical examination

History

Age, breed or supplier, sex, weight, animal's number, number in batch or litter, number affected, number died, diet + additives. Signs observed, treatment given. Sows - last litter/date served.

Examine in general

1. Housing of animals: type and arrangement of house
pen size
environmental temperature
ventilation
drainage
flooring
drinkers
feeding arrangements
and type of food
2. Attitude and behaviour of group
3. Is any feed left?
4. Appearance of dung
5. Respiratory rate

In detail

6. Skin colour and lesions/udder
7. Nervous signs such as convulsions or tremor
8. Feet/legs and gait
9. Mouth, nose and eyes
10. Rectum/perineum for diarrhoea
11. Respiratory rate/auscultate chest/heart (especially sows)
12. Vagina or prepuce for discharge
13. Rectal temperature
14. E.C.G. may reveal cardiac abnormalities.
15. Ultrasound for ovarian function and pregnancy

Sampling

Blood samples should be taken from the jugular vein, anterior vena cava or ear. Fine needles should be used for neonates. Milk can be obtained in quantity after oxytocin injection. Clean the udder before sampling.

Nasal secretion. Cotton-tipped fine nasal swabs can be used. The external nares should be cleansed if possible. Inoculation of plates on site improves recovery of respiratory pathogens.

Tonsillar swabs. A pig gag of metal shaped like a tuning fork with an appropriate-sized gap can be used to hold the mouth open and swabs can be taken from the tonsil. In neonates, a tube placed on the tonsil shields the swab used for sampling. Tonsillar biopy should only be performed under anaesthesia.

<u>Vaginal inspection</u> can be carried out using an endoscope and samples can be taken in the same way or using a speculum. If no speculum, use a guarded swab.

<u>Urine</u>. Urination frequently follows disturbance in resting sows. Samples for biochemistry and microbiology can be taken midstream. Dip slides can be used for bacteruria.

<u>Faeces</u>. Rectal faeces for parasitology, rectal faeces diluted in saline for E.M. examination for viruses, toxins, heat-resistant sporulating *C.perfringens* type A and phase contrast microscopy for spirochaetes, rectal swabs for culture and air-dried faeces smears for immunofluorescence or for cryptosporidium.

<u>Skin scrapings</u> and ear wax for mites, skin scrapings and plucked hair for fungi, swabs for bacteriology and vesicle fluid or swabs for virology.

<u>Submission of samples</u> (with full history).

<u>For virological examination,</u> swabs should be submitted in transport medium and chilled. Some can be frozen. Faeces should only be chilled.

<u>For bacteriological examination,</u> swabs should be submitted in transport medium without antibiotic and all samples chilled not frozen.

<u>For parasitological examination,</u> chilled never frozen.

<u>Blood samples</u> clotted for serum. Serum itself may be frozen, other blood samples must not be frozen. Unclotted blood for bacteriology or for biochemistry in the appropriate anticoagulant.

Samples should be sent first class post or rail, marked "Pathological Specimen" and packed according to the Postal Regulations or delivered chilled by hand. Consult the laboratory before samples are sent for specialist examinations.

Humane endpoints

U.K. farmers and veterinarians are always aware of the requirement of the consumer that animals produced for human food should not be kept alive if they have an injury which is not treatable and which is causing suffering. Both are aware of their legal and moral duty to prevent animal suffering. As a result of the clinical assessments described above, it may be necessary to decide whether each sick animal will -

a)   recover naturally
b)   can be treated and expected to recover fully or
c)   must be killed to prevent further suffering.

A decision must then be taken for all animals in categories b) and c) whether: they can be treated and fed to slaughter weight economically; kept until free from residues: and be suitable for human consumption of killed. If the animal is to be killed for human consumption, then its fitness to travel must be decided. If there is any doubt, the animal must be killed on farm and not transported regardless of whether the carcase can be salvaged.

To assist the decision process, some suggested humane endpoints are listed below and detailed ones are provided under the individual conditions in the main text. This list is provided also for the guidance of those concerned with welfare and for named veterinary surgeons under the Animals (Scientific Procedures) Act 1986.

General guide to conditions for which euthanasia is advised:

Sows:

Prolapsed uterus, rectum or vagina which cannot be repaired or is already damaged.
Wounds from fighting or accidents of such severity that healing is in doubt.
Severe and extensive burns.
Multiple open sores or wounds.
Cardiac failure from old age or endocarditis
Lameness from a broken leg, paralysis of hindlimbs, acute or chronic lameness such as from epiphyseolysis/osteochondrosis dissecans or arthritis.
Paralysis
Emaciation with condition score 1.
Dystocia which cannot be treated or where piglets remain in the uterus and cause untreatable clinical illness.

Growing and finishing pigs:

Wounds as above including open wounds from tail-biting.
Lameness as above including severe claw damage.
Rectal prolapse as above.
Strangulated hernias.
Paralysis
Emaciation.
Severe or terminal septicaemia, pneumonia or enteritis.

Piglets:

Those with congenital deformities incompatible with life such as epitheliogenesis imperfecta, kyphosis and atresia ani.
Emaciation.
Multiple arthritis and lameness.
Weakness at birth.
Umbilical abscessation (severe).
Wounds and overlaying.
Paralysis
Severe and terminal septicaemia, pneumonia or enteritis.

Euthanasia

Rapid and humane slaughter is routine in all pig units and the pig veterinarian frequently kills pigs for welfare reasons and for post-mortem examination. This section provides a brief guide to methods of humane destruction. Humane endpoints are given for each condition in which death or chronic disability might occur. The methods actually used will depend upon the person carrying out the procedure, the availability of barbiturates or firearms and whether the carcase will be used for pathological examination, human or animal consumption. Euthanasia should be rapid and painless regardless of the method used. As all methods can fail on occasions, always be prepared to repeat the procedure. Remember that injured pigs may be violent.

Location: Euthanasia must be carried out as soon as practicable after a decision has been taken about the animal. Pigs should only be moved to a convenient site if it is humane to do so. The requirement to kill *in situ* will restrict the methods used as free bullets should not be used in confined spaces or on concrete floors in case you or an assistant are injured. Any firearm may startle pigs and where possible euthanasia should take place out of sight and hearing of other pigs. Animals which are to be shot and those to be bled may bleed copiously and should be taken to an area which can be disinfected or cleaned if necessary.

Methods of humane destruction.

a)   Trauma

Only suitable for small piglets of less than 3 weeks of age and weighing up to 5kg. The pig should be held firmly by one person and killed by a second using a heavy blunt instrument directed downwards over the brain (between eyes and ears in the midline). If the animal does not appear to be dead, repeat the blow. The brain cannot be examined post mortem, so use another method if this is necessary. Swinging the pig by the hindlimbs and smashing the head against a wall or rail is not controllable or aesthetic.

b)   Barbiturate

Suitable for pigs of all ages but depends upon the availability of barbiturate solution of appropriate strength (20% sodium pentabarbitone weight/volume, w/v) and skill in administration. As a controlled drug (Schedule 3, U.K.) and prescription-only medicine (POM), users must be qualified to hold and administer the product. Pigs killed by this method are unfit for human or animal consumption and should not be left accessible to wildlife. It is the method of choice for most pathological examinations.

Young pigs 0-6 weeks of age (to 10kg).

Intravenous injection into the anterior vena cava is the preferred method. When 1-5ml is given rapidly, death is instantaneous. Restraint involves holding the pig on its back in a bleeding cradle if available with the forelimbs held vertical by an assistant. The operator should hold the chin down with one hand and locate the thoracic inlet with the other. The needle (at least 3cm) should be inserted at 45° to the vertical in a caudal direction (towards the heart) and when inserted to 2-3cm, the plunger should be withdrawn to ensure that the needle is in the vein. The barbiturate should be injected smoothly. Pigs should die instantly, but injection into the trachea or lung may result in coughing and into the pericardial sac in cardiac tamponade. If injected elsewhere outside the vein, the animal will gradually lose consciousness but will usually pass through a stage of anaesthetic excitement with paddling which may make subsequent injection difficult. As barbiturate suppresses respiratory movements in the pig, the heartbeat should be absent before the pig is left. Pigs killed in this way may be bled out to facilitate post-mortem examination. This process should not be carried out too soon after injection.

Intravenous injection by way of the ear vein is possible but is sometimes difficult because of the small diameter of the veins. See below for method. Intracardiac injection may also be used, injecting 2-3cm cranial to the apex beat and 2cm dorsal to it on the left side. Blood should be withdrawn before barbiturate is administered.

Older pigs

The ear vein is the route of choice. The pig should be restrained by the snout by a snare, the ear to be used should be cleaned and the ear veins assessed. The most prominent vein (usually that on the lateral side) should be selected. A needle of appropriate size should be used. It may be helpful to raise the vein by manual pressure or using a rubber band held by artery forceps, but any pressure should be released as soon as the needle is seen to be in the vein as pig ear veins are very fragile and tear easily. Infection should be slow and smooth for the same reason. Successful injection can be monitored by examination of the vein. The blue-purple colour is replaced by a clear colour in white pigs. Any problem results in interruption of the injection and the process should be stopped immediately. Haematomas occur rapidly and the injection site can no longer be used. For best results, begin at the periphery of the ear. Not only is it easiest, but it is possible to use the same vein further down if a blockage occurs. Very large pigs may collapse but the needle should be held in place as it may be necessary to administer a further injection. Death may occur rapidly, but, in larger pigs, it may require 20-50ml of solution to kill the animal. Apnoea usually follows barbiturate injection in pigs and it is particularly important to confirm death in large animals before leaving them or to bleed them out once anaesthetised. Bleeding should be carried out after complete anaesthesia has developed by cutting into the thoracic inlet with the edge of a sharp knife along the jugular channel lateral to the trachea. One or more reflex gasps may follow this procedure.

It is also possible to use the jugular route, but the potential for movement at this site is considerable and, although suitable for bleeding, injection may be more difficult. For the approach, see jugular bleeding.

c)   Shooting

Pigs other than piglets can be killed by shooting and the method must be used for farm slaughter for human consumption. Humane killers using a captive bolt; free bullets from rifle or pistol and shotguns may all be used. All these weapons are controlled in the U.K. under the Firearms Regulations and police permits are required for their purchase, carriage and use. Training in their safe handling, use and cleaning should be sought before use on live animals. All pigs which are shot may thrash around and this may be distressing, disruptive and dangerous. After humane killers and free bullets have been used, the animal should be pithed using a stiff wire or, if for human consumption, a stiff nylon/plastic pithing cane. This can be done in the period of quiet after the shot and before the onset of reflex movements. The cane is inserted into the hole and fed into the spinal cord through the foramen magnum. As this method destroys the spinal cord and much of the brain, the method is unsuitable if the carcase is required for neuropathological examination.

Humane killers

These operate by means of a bolt which penetrates the skull and brain, withdrawing automatically after firing. Before use, the cartridge size should be confirmed as adequate for the size of pig (0.22, 3 grain green cartridge, U.K.) and a second cartridge should be ready for use if failure occurs. A pithing cane and knife should be readily available. Pigs of up to 24 weeks of age may be killed directly, but older animals may be merely stunned. All should be pithed after shooting and may be bled out as described above. Animals to be stunned/killed are restrained by means of an easily released snout snare. The muzzle should be placed on the head in the midline 2cm above a line between the eyes and angled slightly upwards to hit the brain. Restraint by holding the ears is unwise because of the risk of accidental damage by the bolt following movement and use on piglets is dangerous.

Free bullets

Free bullet humane killers, 0.22 rifles (pigs less than 24 weeks only) and some handguns may be used. In all cases, use a soft-nosed lead bullet and carry out the operation outdoors as the bullet may pass through the pig and ricochet on walls or floor. Assistants or observers should stand behind the operator, and numbers should be restricted because of the risk. The muzzle of humane killers may be applied to the pig's head, but the other kinds of weapon should be held at least 2-5cm from it in the position described for humane killers above. Free bullets should not be used if there is an alternative and handguns and rifles should be used only in an emergency. This method is not suitable for pot bellied pigs.

Shotguns

Shotguns used to kill pigs are usually 12 bore. Restraint is by snare. The muzzle should be held 5-25cm away from the head and the gun aimed at the point described above, but are usually aimed at a point behind and below the ear pointing inwards towards the brain. A neat round hole results with some smoke staining and little blood. The brain and skull bones are smashed but shot remains under the skin at exit and the method is less dangerous than free bullets. The same precautions should be observed. Pithing is difficult with this method and may not be necessary. Post-mortem examination of the pharynx, brain and posterior nares may be impossible.

d) Commercial slaughter

This is by electric stunning or killing, humane killer or by carbon dioxide inhalation. Stunned pigs are then shackled and bled out.

Check list for post mortem examination

General

History as above, condition of carcase, weight for age, chilled, fresh, frozen. Length of time since death. Method of killing.

External features

Appearance of skin, presence of ectoparasites. Snout normal or twisted, discharge, eyes, normal or discharge, ears congested, bitten/mange, oral cavity, feet and coronary band, udder, rectum and vulva. For stillborn piglets note membranes on skin, gelatinous hoof tips and soft moist cord. Note post-mortem change indicating death *in utero*

Post mortem examination

Abdominal cavity. Umbilicus, peritoneal cavity, fluid or adhesions present, liver, gall bladder, spleen, kidney, adrenals, ureters, uterus, ovaries and bladder. Check mammary glands, testes and preputial diverticulum. Examine foetuses for placental necrosis, crown rump length, transudates, gross abnormalities, weigh thyroid and X-ray for growth arrests.

Alimentary tract. Pharynx: open and examine, oesophagus: open and note restrictions/mucosal ulceration, stomach: open and record feed present, appearance of pars oesophagea and mucosa, examine greater curvature for oedema, small intestine: record appearance of serosa, contents and mucosa, check villus height at several sites at least 10 cm from duodenum if enteritis present, Ileum, caecum, colon: - note serosa, contents and mucosa. Examine mesenteric nodes. Pancreas. Rectum: examine mucosa.

Thoracic cavity. Pleura and pleural cavities, the lungs, thymus, pericardium, pericardial cavity, heart - open to check valves and ventricular muscle. Examine bronchi, trachea and larynx including epiglottis. Bronchial lymph nodes.

Head. Tonsils, retropharyngeal lymph nodes, teeth, saw snout at premolar 2 for nasal cavity, septum and turbinates, remove brain in cases of meningitis and spinal cord in cases of paralysis. Take CSF before removing head. Note any cerebellar coning and obtain whole brain: cerebellar weight ratio in piglets

Carcase muscle, joints and lymph nodes not so far checked should be examined and any relevant nerves or ganglia dissected out and fixed.

Laboratory examinations are described under the individual conditions.

References

Wells, G.A.H. (1977). Proc.Pig Vet.Soc. **2**, 19-25
A Colour Atlas of Diseases and Disorders of the Pig. Smith, Taylor, Penny. (1989). Wolfe.
Pathology of the pig, a diagnostic guide (1996) Sims, L.D., Glastonbury, J.R.W. (Eds) Pig Research and Development Corporation and Agriculture Victoria, 456pp, ISBN 0 7306 65372

Carcase disposal

Clinical wastes such as carcases from post-mortem examinations should be diposed of safely and effectively. Carcases must be examined on washable and waterproof surfaces and drainage from those surfaces must not contaminate surface waters. Disinfection of the site with an appropriate disinfectant is essential. Sharps from euthanasia and the post mortem must be discarded into sharp safes and returned to the practice for disposal or placed in farm sharp safes for disposal.

Carcases may be collected by traditional knackers, the Fallen Stock scheme (UK) or incinerated. Storage until collection is best carried out in a separate building or depot (which may be refrigerated) sited on the periphery of the farm so that the knacker does not enter. It should have appropriate drainage and be capable of disinfection. Burial (not UK) should be carried out where carcases will not contaminate water supplies or surface water and should be deep enough not to cause nuisance to neighbours. Incineration should only be carried out in licensed incinerators capable of incinerating the quantity of material generated by the farm. Composting is not possible UK, but composting bins should be sited to avoid offence or contamination of water courses. When high mortality occurs, special plans may have to be made to dispose of carcases safely as ordinary farm mechanisms may be unable to cope. Planning is particularly necessary on sites with little land.

Safety on the farm

Pig farms contain a number of hazards to human health and all U.K. farmers should have carried out hazard analysis to reduce the risk to the workforce or visitors. The veterinarian is, however, in charge of hazards during procedures he/she initiates. The following hazards specific to pig farms should be considered :

Trauma: Pigs may be aggressive and injuries can kill. Restrain or tranquilise mature animals and ensure that an escape route is available. Avoid pig bites and needle stick injuries or cuts from knives or scalpels.

Electrocution: Power should be turned off prior to investigating electrocuted pigs. Avoid old electrical equipment.

Gassing: May occur in poorly ventilated houses.

Drowning: May occur in standing water or slurry lagoons.

Fire: This is a hazard in straw-filled units. If it occurs, evacuate buildings first, consider rescue of other humans next and of the pigs last. Do not endanger human life.

Allergy: Farm dusts are allergenic. Straw, hay, feed and pig urine may all provoke sensitisation. Wear masks or respirators to avoid sensitisation and carry antidotes if sensitised.

Infection: Some pig pathogens are zoonotic and infection should be avoided. Masks and gloves are essential at post mortem and disinfectants should always be available. Zoonotic conditions are listed in the text. Remember that farm rodents etc., also pose a hazard.

Medicines: Some affect human health and should be used carefully. They should be stored carefully, labelled correctly, used only after instruction and their use recorded. Used containers or unused drugs should be discarded as pharmaceutical waste. Prostaglandins are hazardous to female staff. Spills should be treated according to data sheet suggestions. Medical advice should be sought after ingestion of medicines and self-injection.

Public health

a)   On farm
The veterinarian visiting farms may advise on management practices which can affect the quality and safety of meat and affect risks from manures and effluent. He/she can provide early warning of diseases which may be zoonotic such as salmonellosis and monitor the use and withdrawal of medicines.

b)   At the abattoir
Ante-mortem and post-mortem inspection are vital elements in safeguarding the quality of meat and meat products. The health of the workers in the industry may also benefit from advice about zoonoses.

c)   In onward processing
A knowledge of the production systems used can be invaluable in tracing and eliminating public health hazards from food.

Xenotransplantation

Genetically modified pigs intended for xenotransplantation are strictly controlled. The herds from which they are obtained are derived by hysterectomy, maintained under stringent biosecurity and kept in conditions specified by a welfare code of practice (issued by the Home Office, UK). The presence of infections is closely monitored and those which must be absent are specified. Animals intended for organ donation may themselves be hysterectomy derived and maintained in isolators or under conditions which ensure high biosecurity until they reach the size required. Sibs are used for monitoring and a detailed code of practice will govern sampling, record keeping and screening of both pigs and staff. Harvested organs are treated as those of human origin and monitoring of recipients and their contacts will be obligatory. The xenotransplantation programme has been a significant source of information about the physiology, immunology, infection management and monitoring in the pig.

VIRAL DISEASES

A large number of viruses cause clinical disease in pigs and infections with many others have been recorded. Events within the last 10 years have highlighted the importance of awareness of virus disease. The industry has been profoundly affected in many countries by the appearance of Porcine Reproductive and Respiratory Syndrome (PRRS) and diagnosis in both the field and the laboratory has been complicated by its presence. The dramatic effects of swine fever on the Dutch pig industry and the identification of circovirus as a cause of Post-Weaning Multisystemic Wasting Disease (PMWS) have highlighted the importance of being able to recognise viral disease and to take measures appropriate to the disease concerned. Infections with Hepatitis E and retrovirus have also become more easy to recognise recently and are of unknown public health significance.

Viral diseases may be recognised as such by the identification of clinical signs, post-mortem findings or epidemiological picture with those of familiar or recorded diseases. These are described below and listed under the appropriate age group in the section on Differential Diagnosis. Appropriate laboratory tests can then be used to confirm their identity and control measures such as vaccination can be initiated. The infections which have been described in pigs are listed as an aid in the recognition of unknown syndromes. Others may also occur.

Virus diseases frequently spread from affected animals to susceptible animals after a recognisable incubation period. They are therefore recognisable as infectious. They may be identified as virus infections by:

a) the presence of clinical signs suggestive of viral disease such as vesicles or their identification as a known syndrome.
b) the failure of any antimicrobial to affect the course of the disease i.e., not a bacterial condition.
c) the presence of specific pathological findings including the presence of syncytia and inclusion bodies.
d) viral particles may be identified in lesions or extracts of lesions by electron microscopy, immunoperoxidase, in situ hybridisation, PCR or by immunofluorescence using recovered sera.
e) virus may be isolated in cell cultures such as established cell lines, primary cultures such as pig kidney cells or alveolar macrophages.
f) the demonstration of rising titres of antibody to specific virus infections in serological tests by a range of tests including ELISAs.
g) experimental animal transmission with bacteria/parasite-free inocula.

Parvovirus

Definition

Porcine parvovirus (PPV) infection causes infertility, mummified foetuses, stillbirths and small litters in sows. It may be associated with poor growth in the postnatal period. Parvovirus particles have been demonstrated in, and isolated from diarrhoeic faeces and skin lesions. The virus has been associated with PCV2 in PMWS.

Incidence

Porcine parvoviruses occur worldwide. Reports of individual surveys indicate that from 76% (Finland), 82% (U.S.), 93% (UK) and 95% (Switzerland) of herds may be infected. One survey of 499 herds in the UK indicated that 7% were negative for antibody to parvovirus and 30% contained both seronegative and seropositive animals. 18% of all sows, 44% of all gilts and 47% of all boars surveyed were seronegative. These figures are similar to those found in other countries and in subsequent surveys in the UK A US survey of unvaccinated herds suggested that at least 11% of all litters contain parvovirus-infected foetuses. In contrast, a Spanish survey in 2005 failed to demonstrate virus in aborted foetuses. An antigenically distinct enteric parvovirus has been shown by serological surveys to be widespread in Japan, the only country to be examined, but enteric parvovirus has also been detected in UK and US studies.

Aetiology

Porcine parvovirus is a small (20nm) non-enveloped single stranded DNA virus which appears to be stable over a wide range of pH (3-10 for 1 hour at 37°C) and can resist heating at 56°C for 2 days but is killed after exposure to 80°C for 5 minutes. The virus is not affected by ether or a number of proteolytic enzymes. The virus haemagglutinates guinea pig, human and chicken red cells. One antigenic type of the virus exists although isolates with different pathogenicity have been reported. The antigenicity appears to reside in the three capsid proteins, VPI (81kDa) VP2 (66kDa) and VP3 (62kDa). The virus replicates in cells about to divide and may be grown *in vitro* in primary pig kidney cell monolayers or continuous cell lines. Cytopathic effects (C.P.E) such as intranuclear inclusions and cell rounding may be transient on primary isolation and infected cells may have to be identified using immunofluorescence, immunoperoxidase, DNA probes, PCR, haemadsorption, haemagglutination reactions or ELISA.

The enteric parvovirus reported from the faeces of pigs with diarrhoea has 4 viral proteins and resembles bovine parvovirus, growing best in porcine thyroid and swine embryo kidney cells taking 9 days to produce C.P.E.

Pathogenesis

Porcine parvovirus enters by the oronasal or venereal routes. A viraemia ensues, followed after 10 days by a transient, barely detectable, leucopaenia. Viraemia results in passage of the virus into the reproductive tract taking 10-14 days from infection to cross the placenta. In boars it may be found on spermatozoa from days 5-9 post-infection and in seminal vesicles and testicular tissue from days 8-21.

The virus adheres to the zona pellucida of eggs and infects and kills embryos and foetuses until they reach immunocompetence at 67 days' gestation. The virus does not affect the products of conception in animals infected 1-4 weeks prior to service but crosses the placenta in those infected at service and for at least 90 days thereafter. Embryos and foetuses dying before 33-35 days may be resorbed completely while those dying later may become mummified, stillborn or, occasionally, aborted. Infection may spread from piglet to piglet along the uterus. In dams infected later in gestation, piglets which do not die from infection may develop high levels of neutralising antibody or become immunotolerant and remain infected for up to 8 months after birth. Recovered infected piglets may be stunted. Infection of the immuno-incompetent foetus appears to cause endothelial damage, perivascular haemorrhage in the brain and kidney and placental damage. In immuno-competent foetuses, meningoencephalitis with perivascular cuffing appears to develop but more extensive lesions have been described following infection with the Kresse (skin) strain. Maternal endometrial vessels may become surrounded by mononuclear cells. Serum antibody appears at 7-10 days after infection and rises rapidly. Virus is shed in low concentrations in urine, faeces, tonsillar debris and nasal secretions from 2 weeks after infection and pigs remain infectious for approximately 2 weeks. Recovered pigs are solidly immune and passive immunity is passed in colostrum to piglets and can be detected for 4-6 months after birth. The use of PCR and DNA probes may extend the period for which infection is detectable.

Studies of combined infections in experimental and natural cases of PMWS suggest that infection with PPV is most intense 20-24 days post infection.

Clinical signs

Returns to oestrus, failure to farrow, the production of small litters, mummified pigs, stillbirth and, rarely, abortion are the main clinical syndromes associated with parvovirus infections in pigs and are particularly prominent in newly introduced and first litter gilts in which a mean loss of 1.1 pigs per litter results from parvovirus infection. Farrowing rate to first service may be as low as 36% (first litter); small litters (especially those containing 5 or less) and the presence of mummified and stillborn pigs may all occur. Pseudocyesis and irregular returns to oestrus may also be seen. Clinical signs may occur in a whole susceptible herd if disease is introduced. Infection in boars is asymptomatic and appears to have no effect on semen quality or fertility. The virus has been recovered from a vesicular skin condition and from diarrhoeic faeces after weaning. Reports of the experimental production of pneumonia, leucopaenia, diarrhoea and encephalitis in piglets exist. The association of the virus with PMWS is described with that disease.

Pathology

Gross lesions are restricted to the uterus of the sow. Embryos may be shrunken and may die to appear as small areas of necrotic material on the uterine wall. Foetuses may be reduced in size, congested and oedematous prior to death. Dead foetuses become mummified. Mummified foetuses may increase in size along the uterus until stillborn animals are found. The virus has recently been identified in non-suppurative myocarditis in sucking pigs and in renal lesions in Canada. For microscopic lesions see Pathogenesis.

Epidemiology

Infection occurs most commonly in young sows and gilts or in susceptible animals introduced into an infected herd. Boars may transmit the virus in their semen (especially in seminal plasma) for up to 2 weeks after infection and both semen and embryos are potential sources of infection in clean herds as are congenitally-infected pigs. The disease is most common in herds where sows are stalled or tethered, especially where gilts have no contact with older animals. The brief period of virus shedding after infection and the small amount of virus shed in urine, faeces and nasal secretions prevents the rapid and thorough spread of infection from pig to pig. There is persistent environmental contamination for up to 4 months with virus from faeces, secretions and the products of parturition. The products of parturition may be the major source of infection in housed animals and lack of hygiene is important in spread. Piglets of immune sows which do not have active immunity at birth are protected from natural infection by colostral antibody and may become susceptible, seronegative gilts or sows. In some herds, immune sows may form a majority and infection may die out. Introduction of infection by pigs, germ plasm or fomites to such susceptible herds can lead to outbreaks of returns to service, small litters and increases in stillbirths and mummified piglets. Feral and wild pigs can maintain the infection. Virus can infect rats which in turn can shed infective virus for 2-3 weeks but subsequent transmission of infection to pigs is difficult.

Diagnosis

The occurrence of returns to service, small litters, mummified and stillborn pigs in gilts rather than sows with little or no abortion and no history of maternal illness suggests parvovirus infection. The diagnosis may be confirmed by the demonstration of virus in mummified foetuses of less than 70 days' gestation age, by isolation or more commonly, by the demonstration of parvovirus antigen in frozen or histological sections of lung and liver by specific immunofluorescence, immunoperoxidase, DNA probes or PCR. Extracts of foetuses may be tested for viral antigen by latex particle agglutination and by ELISA. Neutralising antibody may be detected in the sera of infected sows, of newborn piglets and in foetal fluids including exudates and transudates in stillborn piglets from infected litters. A haemagglutination inhibition test using guinea pig red cells has been used. Sera for this test should be absorbed with kaolin and the erythrocytes used in the test. Antibody levels may reach 1:10,000 or more. Titres greater than 1:256 indicate infection. ELISA tests are now widely used for the detection of serum antibody and antibody in foetuses. A rise in serum antibody level indicates infection in the absence of vaccination. Vaccinates may not produce antibody to nonstructural protein 1 (NS1) and wild type infections may now be distinguishable by this feature.

Control

Vaccination of susceptible stock is the best way to prevent losses from parvovirus infection and vaccinated stock do not experience the changes in productivity experienced by unvaccinated herds. Killed adjuvanted vaccines inactivated with acetylethyleneimine, formalin or ß-propiolactone prevent the disease if given i/m at least two weeks prior to service. Live viruses attenuated by passage and growth at low temperatures have been used as vaccines. A typical vaccine is inactivated and oil-adjuvanted and is administered as two doses, 3-4 weeks apart with boosters every two years and produces long-term immunity and overcomes waning passive immunity if given intramuscularly (i/m) at 5 months of age. Only killed vaccines are currently in use in the UK. Vaccination appears to protect even if low levels of serum antibody are present. Second or subsequent vaccinations should be given at least 2 weeks before service. Boars should also be vaccinated at 6 months of age, 6 months later and then annually. Maternal antibody may not disappear until 6-7 months of age and the ability of any vaccine used to overcome this will affect the vaccine schedule for gilts. Subunit vaccines based on capsid proteins VP1 and VP2 are under investigation. In countries where vaccines are not available 'feed back' may be practised. The foetal membranes and other products of parturition and faeces from weaned pigs are ground and administered to susceptible gilts 3 weeks before service. Variable amounts of virus are present in this material. Mummified foetuses represent the best source, followed by stillborn piglets (which may contain antibody) and the products of abortion. The procedure must be licensed under the Waste Foods Order in the UK and is not advisable anywhere vaccine is available.

In herds with solid immunity it may not be cost-effective to vaccinate, but it should be undertaken if the whole herd, a significant portion of the younger stock or introduced gilts are seronegative. If a decision is taken to test for antibody, at least 20 samples are needed from sows of different parities to give a profile of herd immunity. Herd immunity should be checked at intervals. Where a seronegative unvaccinated herd exists, and vaccination is not to be carried out, incoming stock should be vaccinated and disinfection practised. Where seronegative and seropositive stock exist, the control of rats and hygiene may reduce the spread amongst pregnant sows. The virus can be destroyed within 5 minutes using sodium hydroxide and sodium hypochlorite. Glutaraldehyde 2% and Formaldehyde 8% are also effective but take

longer. Steam cleaning may be used. Commercial disinfectants such as Virkon may also be effective.
Screening of boar semen for viral antigen by PCR has been advocated and oocyte decontamination using hyaluronidase can

References

Bachman, P.A., Sheffy, B.E. and Vaughan, J.T. (1975). Experimental *in utero* infections of foetal pigs with a porcine parvovirus. Infection and Immunity **12**, 455-460.
Bureau, M., Dea, S., Sirad, M.A. (2005). Evaluation of virus decontamination techniques for porcine embryos produced in vitro. Theriogenology **63** 2343-2355.
Jenkins, C.E. (1992). An enzyme-linked immuno-sorbent assay for detection of porcine parvovirus in fetal tissues. J.Virological Methods **39**, 179-184.
Kennedy, S., Moffett, D., McNeelly, F., Meehan, B., Ellis, J., Krakowka, S., Allan, G. (2000). Reproduction of lesions of PMWS by infection of conventional pigs with PCV2 alone or in combination with porcine parvovirus. J. Comp. Path. **122** 9-24
Kresse, J.I., Taylor, W.D., Stewart, W.N. and Eernisse, K.A. (1985). Parvovirus infection in pigs with necrotic and vesicle-like lesions.Vet.Microbiol. **10**, 525-531.
Madsen, E.S., Madsen, K.G., Nielsen, J., Jensen, M.H., Lei, J.C., Have, P. (1997). Detection of antibodies against porcine parvovirus nonstructural protein NS1 may distinguish between vaccinated and naturally-infected pigs. Vet Micro **54**, 1-16
Mengeling, W.L., Brown T.T., Paul, P.S. and Gutenkunst, D.E. (1979). Efficacy of an inactivated virus vaccine for the prevention of porcine parvovirus induced-reproductive failure. Am.J.Vet.Res. **40**, 204-207
Mengeling, W.L., Paul, P.S. (1986). The relative importance of swine and contaminated premises as reservoirs of porcine parvovirus infection. J.Am.Vet.Med.Ass. **188**, 1293-1295.
Molitor, T.W., Oraveerakul, K., Zharg, Q.Q., Choi, C.S. and Ludemann, L.R. (1991). Polymerase chain reaction for the detection of porcine parvovirus. J.Virological Methods **32**, 201-211
Nash, W.A. (1990). Porcine parvovirus survey. Veterinary Record **126**, 175-176.
Wrathall, A.E. (1988). Field trials of an inactivated oil-emulsion porcine parvovirus vaccine in British pig herds. Veterinary Record **122**, 411-418.
Yasuhara, H.,Yamanaka, M., Izumuda, A., Hirahara, T., Nakai, M., Inaba, Y (1995). Experimental infection of pigs with a parvovirus isolated from the diarrhoeic faeces of a pig. J. Vet. Med Sci **57**, 629-634

Enterovirus and Teschovirus Infections

Infection with enteroviruses may be asymptomatic, is associated with polio-encephalomyelitis (Teschoviruses) and less frequently with abortion, stillbirth and infertility. They are also associated with myocarditis and have caused pneumonitis and transient diarrhoea in experimental animals.

Incidence

Porcine enteroviruses occur worldwide and the infection rate in pig populations is high. Individual serotypes of Teschovirus may be restricted in their distribution.

Properties of porcine enteroviruses

Porcine enteroviruses and teschoviruses are spherical RNA viruses 25-31nm in diameter and are resistant to chloroform and ether. They are relatively heat stable and survive heating at 56°C for 3 hours relatively well, persist in infected tissue culture fluids for weeks or months at room temperature and have been shown to survive for up to 168 days at 15°C. They are stable between pH 2.0 and 9.0 and are relatively resistant to some disinfectants, e.g. lysol and cetrimide, but can be inactivated by formaldehyde, sodium hypochlorite, 70% ethanol and modern iodophors.

Porcine enteroviruses and teschoviruses grow readily in cultures of pig kidney cells and produce C.P.E. of three types. Isolates were classified initially according to the type of C.P.E. produced and on antigenic grounds. Strains of serogroups 1-7 and 11 e.g. Teschen produce Type 1 C.P.E. in which focal areas of rounded cells occur and are now classified as teschoviruses following sequencing and those of serogroup 8, e.g. V13 produce Type II C.P.E. in which cells become granular with cytoplasmic protrusions (now porcine enterovirus A , PEV A).The remaining groups are now classified as PEV B. Original isolates from infertility cases were identified by letters as follows: SMEDI (Swine mummification embryonic death and infertility) A-E etc. SMEDI A belongs to serogroup 8, B to 3, C to 1, D to 8 and E to 6.

Porcine enteroviruses multiply in the intestines of pigs but do not readily infect laboratory animals.

References

Doherty, M., Todd, D., McFerran, N., Hoey, E.M. (1999). Sequence analysis of a porcine enterovirus serotype 1 isolate: relationships with other picornaviruses. Journal of General Virology **80** 1929-1941

Knowles, N.J. (1983). Isolation and identification of porcine enteroviruses in Great Britain 1979-1980. Br.Vet.J. **139**, 19-22.

Knowles, N.J., Buckley, L.S. and Pereira, H.G. (1979). Classification of porcine enterovirus by antigenic analysis and cytopathic effects on tissue culture. Arch.Virol. **62**, 201-208.

Zell, R., Krumbholz, A., Henke, A., Birch-Hirschfeld, E., Stelzner, A., Doherty, M., Hoey, F., Prager, D., Wurm, R. (2000). Detection of porcine enteroviruses by nRT-PCR: differentiation of CPE groups I-III with specific primer sets. J.Virological Methods **88**, 205-218

Polioencephalomyelitis
(Teschen disease, Talfan disease, Benign Enzootic Paresis)

Definition

Infection with Teschovirus (Serogroup 1 porcine enteroviruses) can be asymptomatic or cause polioencephalomyelitis with varying degrees of fever, convulsions, tremors or paresis.

Incidence

Teschen is not seen in the UK but may still occur in Central and Eastern Europe. Talfan (a milder syndrome) is reported from time to time in the U.K. and less pathogenic Teschovirus infections may occur in countries such as the US and Germany.

Caused by Teschen virus (formerly Group 1 C.P.E.,Serogroup 1of the enteroviruses) and related Teschoviruses

Pathogenesis

The pathogenesis of the condition is similar to that of polio in man. Infection leads to multiplication in the ileum and large intestine and the associated lymph nodes, and, in non-immune animals, this is followed by viraemia associated with the pyrexia of 40-41°C, 104-106°F, and by localisation of the virus in the brain and spinal cord., where, within 7-10 days of infection, it affects the neurones of the grey matter to give rise to the clinical signs.

Virus is shed from multiplication sites in the reticuloendothelial tissue of the lamina propria of the intestine, especially in the ileum and the large intestine, for several weeks and may be isolated from the faeces. Recovery is associated with the development of systemic antibodies and with local IgA immunity in the gut. Passive immunity from the dam protects sucking pigs from infection until after weaning and infection is common as this immunity wanes at 3-8 weeks of age.

Clinical signs

Two clinical syndromes are recognised, the severe form (Teschen disease) which occurs in Central Europe and the mild form: Talfan disease, (G.B.); benign enzootic paresis (Denmark); or polio-encephalomyelitis (Canada, U.S., Australia).
Severe form: Affected animals develop fever of 40-41°C, 104-106°F, and show slight incoordination of the limbs, lassitude and anorexia. This stage is followed by irritability and then by stiffness, tremors, convulsions and paralysis often ending in death in 3-4 days. Mildly-affected animals may recover. This form affects non-immune pigs of all ages in herds where the disease is enzootic.
Mild form: This form affects young, unweaned and weaned pigs. 50-100% of a litter may be affected. Elevated temperature, diminished control of the hind legs and ataxia are succeeded by paresis or recovery. Mortality is unusual. Animals are frequently seen in the "dog-sitting" position.

Humane endpoint: animals with total paresis, or any degree of paresis which prevents eating and/or drinking, prevents use of all 4 limbs or leads to pressure sores or erosions. As neurones have been destroyed recovery is unlikely.

Pathological findings

Gross lesions other than muscle wasting in chronic cases are not apparent. Encephalomyelitis is found on microscopic examination and is more severe in the grey matter than in the white. Neuronal degeneration, perivascular cuffing, neuronophagia and meningitis may all be seen. The ventral columns of the spinal cord, the brain stem and the cerebellar cortex are chiefly affected. In mild forms, the lesions are milder and less extensive and have been restricted to the spinal cord in recent cases in the UK.

Epidemiology

Severe disease is only found in Central Europe. Mild forms are most common elsewhere. Inapparent infection is widespread and, in Britain, the clinical signs are rarely seen and are sporadic when they occur in a herd. Recovering pigs may pass infective faeces for several weeks. Manure and natural waters may remain contaminated for weeks. There is no documented risk to man.

Diagnosis

A presumptive diagnosis may be made on the basis of the clinical signs, epizootiology and the pathological findings. Confirmation may be obtained by examining for a rise in complement fixing, ELISA or virus neutralising antibody levels but isolation of the virus from the brain and spinal cord is necessary for a conclusive diagnosis. Chronically-affected pigs may not yield virus from the CNS. Recently the nRT-PCR and the related light-cycler PCR have been developed for use.

Control

Vaccination using live attenuated vaccine is practised in Central and Eastern Europe, but the milder forms of the disease are usually not treated or controlled in Britain. If the severe form should appear here, a slaughter policy might be used to control it coupled with isolation. The disease is notifiable under the Teschen Disease Order (1994) in domestic and EU legislation.

Reference

Pogramchny, R.M., Janke, B., Yoon, K.J. (2003). A prolonged outbreak of polioencephalomyelitis due to infection with a Group 1 porcine enterovirus. Journal of Veterinary Diaggnostic Investigation **15**, 191-194

Reproductive Failure, Stillbirths and Infertility (SMEDI)

Definition

Infection with enteroviruses may cause mummification (M) embryonic death (ED) and infertility (I).

Incidence

Infection is widespread In Britain but the reproductive effects are difficult to distinguish from parvovirus infections without laboratory tests.

Aetiology

The enteroviruses concerned have been called SMEDI viruses. Examples include V13 and F34, serotypes 3 and 8.

Pathogenesis

Infection of the foetuses takes place after viraemia in the sow or via infected spermatic or ovarian fluids. Infection of the litter is rarely complete and may never occur in immune animals, although maternal immunity cannot protect against intra-uterine infection.

The results of infection vary according to the period of gestation in which infection occurs. The most common sequelae of infection are death and resorption of the embryo if infection occurs before 35 days' gestation, resulting in delayed returns to service or death, mummification, abortion or malformation of the foetus and stillbirth if infection occurs after 35 days' gestation.

Clinical signs

Delayed returns to service, abortions and the production of litters containing variable numbers of mummified, dead or stillborn piglets or litters containing few piglets may follow the introduction of fresh breeding stock to a farm. Affected sows normally farrow satisfactorily on subsequent occasions. Reproductive failures due to enterovirus are rarely associated with clinical signs in the dam.

Epidemiology

Reproductive failure usually results from the introduction of a fresh strain of enterovirus to a non-immune herd and affects sows of all ages once only.

Diagnosis

Several other micro-organisms cause infertility of this type, especially porcine parvovirus and sometimes Aujeszky's disease virus, in countries where it still occurs. Leptospiral infection should be ruled out, also erysipelas and other systemic infections. If possible, virus should be isolated from the lungs of foetuses or stillborn piglets for confirmation. Frozen or chilled foetuses should be submitted for diagnosis. Paired serum samples may be of use in confirmation of the agent involved. Serum samples or samples of transudates from thoracic or abdominal cavities of piglets may also be used for antibody determination. A titre of 1:32 or more may indicate active infection.

Control

Isolation is probably the only method of prevention. When an outbreak occurs in a herd, the full economic effects can be mitigated and the immunity of the general population raised by dosing sows and gilts with ground faeces, foetal membranes and mummified foetuses at least 3 weeks prior to service. There are risks to health in this practice, but if used with care, it may maintain immunity to these viruses at a high level. In the UK the Waste Foods Order must be observed.

Reference

Huang, J., Gentry, R.F., Zarkower, A. (1980). Experimental infection of pregnant sows with porcine enteroviruses. Am.J.Vet.Res. **41**, 469-473.

Encephalomyocarditis

Definition

A condition of viral aetiology in which pigs of varying ages are found dead. Mortality varies between 10 and 100% and rates are highest in young pigs. Depression and staggering may occasionally be seen before death. The same virus is also associated with stillbirths and the birth of mummified foetuses of uneven size.

Incidence

Reported from the U.S., where 89% Iowa herds, 13.8% breeding stock and 8.5% finishing pigs had antibody in 1992, Central America and Australasia but the rodent viruses are found worldwide. Antibody to the virus has been found in pigs in the UK but the clinical syndrome has not been identified and the virus has not been isolated. Clinical disease has been identified in most European countries. Belgium had most outbreaks 1990-2001 (320), Italy (110 and 69% sera were positive in one survey), Greece (15) and Cyprus (6).

Aetiology

The condition is caused by encephalomyocarditis (E.M.C.) virus, a picornavirus of rodents assigned to the cardiovirus group. This virus is ether-resistant and resistant to a wide range of pH. Most isolates are inactivated at 60°C for 30 minutes. The virus haemagglutinates guinea pig red cells. There are four major viral proteins.

Pathogenesis

Infection is oral and follows exposure to infected rodents such as rats or consumption of their entrails. Virus multiplies in the pig intestine, becomes systemic and multiplies in heart muscle. Transplacental infection also occurs as soon as 2 weeks post-infection. Foetuses of all ages can be affected.

Clinical signs

Sudden death, particularly in piglets. Pigs with sub-lethal infections may show signs of fever to 41°C (105°F), cyanosis of extremities, depression, staggering or dyspnoea. Serum creatine kinase-MB and lactate dehydrogenase isoenzyme levels may be elevated. Sows and gilts may be fevered and abort at 107-111 days' gestation. Failure to farrow and the birth of litters containing stillborn piglets and mummies of different sizes may occur over a period of 2-3 months.

Animals with cardiac failure should be killed humanely. Heart damage is unlikely to resolve.

Post mortem findings

Carcases may be congested. Excess clear fluid is present in the thoracic, pericardial and peritoneal cavities and pulmonary oedema and hepatic enlargement are common. The heart is soft and pale with white areas 2-15 mm in diameter suggestive of necrosis, commonly on the right ventricular epicardium and extending for varying distances into the myocardium. Necrosis of the myocardium with lymphocytic and macrophage infiltration is seen in acute cases. Fibrosis of these lesions occurs in recovered animals. Mild meningo-encephalitis may be present. Affected foetuses may be mummified or have non-suppurative encephalitis including perivascular cuffing and focal myocarditis in addition to gross lesions of myocardial haemorrhage and excess pericardial fluid.

Epidemiology

Found in a wide variety of species but the main reservoir of infection is rats. Feed is contaminated by rats or their faeces. Pig-to-pig transmission has been confirmed. Virus is shed for 1-3 days after infection in young pigs, and as few as 4 particles may be sufficient to infect a pig by the oronasal route. Antibodies have been found in man, but have not been associated with heart disease. The virus is one of those which may be introduced to man by xenotransplantation, in monkey trials with infected pig pancreatic islet cells.

Diagnosis

The clinical picture and post-mortem findings are suggestive of encephalomyocarditis but other causes of sudden death such as Vitamin E deficiency may need to be considered. Encephalomyocarditis reproductive disease must be distinguished from parvovirus and other infectious forms of reproductive failure.

Virus demonstration by isolation, by PCR, RT-PCR and/or detection of serum neutralising or haemagglutination inhibition antibodies is necessary for confirmation

28

of a diagnosis. Virus may be demonstrated in myocardial cells, Purkinje fibres, endothelial cells and macrophages. Foetal transudates may contain antibody and can confirm intra-uterine infection.

Control

Prevention of exposure from rodents or pigs from infected farms. Disinfection with chlorine (0.5 ppm) disinfectants. An inactivated oil adjuvanted vaccine has been described and appears to prevent reproductive failures in experimental studies. The virus can be washed from infected blastocysts after hyaluronidase treatments.

References

Acland, H.M., Littlejohn, I.R. (1975). Encephalomyocarditis virus infection of pigs. I. An outbreak in New South Wales. Aust. Vet. J. **51**, 409-415.

Billins, C., Koutinas, A., Paschaleri-Papadopoulos, E., Papadopoulos, O. (1997). Serum creatine kinase-MB and lactate dehydrogenase-I isoenzyme activities in piglets with encephalomyocarditis virus. Vet Rec **140**, 628-629

Castryck, F., Miry, C., Koenen, F., Ducatelle, R. (1996). Clinical and pathological aspects of encephalomyocarditis virus infections in pigs in Belgium. Proc. IPVS **14**, 132.

Coulson, A. and Carlson, J. (1992). Encephalomyocarditis in Europe and America. Proc. IPVS **12**, 103.

Joo, H.S., Kim, H.S. and Leman, A.D. (1988). Detection of antibody to encephalomyocarditis virus in mummified or stillborn pigs. Arch. Virol. **100**, 131-134.

Joo, H.S., Kim, H.S. and Leman, A.D. (1988). Detection of antibody to encephalomyocarditis virus in mummified or stillborn pigs. Arch.Virol. **100**, 131-134.

Koenen, F., Vanderhallen, H. Castryck, F., Miry, C., Fockedey, M. (1996). Epidemiologic, pathogenetic and molecular analysis of the first encephalomyocarditis outbreak in Belgium. Proc. IPVS **14**, 96

Littlejohn, I.R. (1984). Encephalomyocarditis virus from stillborn pigs. Aust.Vet.J. **61**, 93.

Maurice, H., Nielen, M., Brocchi, E., Nowotny, N., Kassimi, L.B., Billins, C., Loukaides, P., O'Hara, R.S., Koenen, F. (2005). The occurrence of encephalomyocarditis virus (EMCV) in European pigs from 1990-2001. Epidemiology and Infection **133**, 547-557

Sangar, D.V., Rowlands, D.J., and Brown, F. (1977). Encephalomyocarditis antibodies in sera from apparently normal pigs. Vet Rec **100**, 240-241

Zimmerman, J.J., Owen, W.J., Hill, A.T., Beran, G.W. (1991). Seroprevalence of antibodies against encephalomyocarditis virus in swine of Iowa. J.Am.Vet.Med.Ass. **199**, 1737-1741.

Vomiting and Wasting Disease

Definition

A disease of neonatal piglets caused by Haemagglutinating Encephalomyelitis Virus (H.E.V.) and characterised by vomiting, constipation and anorexia leading to wasting and death as a result of encephalomyelitis and viral damage to gastrointestinal neurones.

Incidence

The disease was first recorded in Canada, but occurs in the U.K. and most of Europe, the U.S., Japan, Korea and Australasia. Clinical signs of infection are uncommon but antibodies to the virus occur widely in the pig population (up to 95% of sows in Britain although a survey in Japan suggested a lower figure there).

Aetiology

The disease is caused by infection of young piglets with H.E.V., a coronavirus. This RNA virus is ether and chloroform and heat sensitive, stable from pH 3-10 and agglutinates and becomes adsorbed to chick, rat and hamster erythrocytes, unlike T.G.E. virus. The mean size of H.E.V. is 120 nm with projections of 19 nm. There may be some antigenic similarity between the 2 viruses, but they are distinct in serum neutralisation tests and genomically. The virus grows in pig kidney cells to form syncytia within 12-16 hours. CPE is complete in 48 hours. There is only one serotype and a 2003 isolate from Canada was identical to virus isolated in 1962.

Pathogenesis

After oronasal infection, clinical signs develop within 3-5 days. Primary viral multiplication takes place in epithelial cells of the tonsil, lung, nasal mucosa and lungs. Virus spreads along nerves to the trigeminal, inferior vagal, superior cervical, solar and dorsal root ganglia and to the intestinal nervous plexuses. The trigeminal and vagal sensory nuclei in the brain stem become infected followed by other nuclei, the cerebrum, cerebellum and the spinal cord. Viral replication in the gastric nervous plexus causes damage and leads to delayed gastric emptying and eventual starvation. Passive colostral immunity protects against infection.

Clinical signs

Piglets aged between 5 days and 3 weeks are affected. The first signs to be noted are vomiting, huddling of the piglets which may be associated with a rise in temperature, depression, anorexia and constipation. Some affected animals may show signs of encephalomyelitis, e.g. hind leg weakness or difficulties in swallowing. Affected piglets die within 36-48 hours or become progressively emaciated. The contrast between affected and unaffected piglets in the same litter is striking. Clinical signs in piglets may be preceded by transient fever (to 40.6°C, 105°F) in the sows. Most infections occur in older pigs after maternal antibody has disappeared and are inapparent. Young pigs with progressive wasting or nervous signs should be killed by 7 days after development of clinical signs.

Post mortem lesions

No specific lesions are seen. The intestinal tract is normally empty with scanty faeces and there is pronounced wasting. In 25% of cases a nonsuppurative encephalomyelitis is found in which perivascular cuffing with mononuclear cells, glial node formation, neuronal degeneration and meningitis are seen in the grey matter of the mesencephalon, pons, medulla oblongata and in the upper spinal cord.

Epidemiology

A few litters may be affected in a herd at any one time (between 16 and 95% of the piglets at risk) and most of the clinically affected piglets die. Infection (monitored by serological means) spreads throughout the herd in nasal secretions. Frequently the clinical disease appears only in the litters of bought-in breeding stock and not in the herd at large. Maternal immunity is transferred in the colostrum but has disappeared by 15 weeks of age. The virus also spreads amongst weaned fattening pigs and active immunity develops within 8-16 weeks. The virus is rapidly destroyed by UV light.

Diagnosis

The disease occurs in piglets less than 21 days of age and may be suspected when vomiting, depression and constipation is followed by wasting and hairiness compared with uninfected littermates. Diagnosis may be confirmed by virus isolation from the respiratory tract, hindbrain and spinal cord of early cases. The C.P.E. can be confirmed as specific by haemagglutination, haemadsorption, serum neutralisation or immunofluorescence. Demonstration of antibody in the sera of wasting piglets and in sera from the dams of affected litters 14 days after the clinical signs are first noted is also of use. RT-PCR and nested RT-PCR have been described. Enteroviruses and Aujeszky's Disease may also cause encephalitis but are more severe and usually also affect older pigs. T.G.E. causes profuse diarrhoea and no encephalitis.

Treatment and control

There is no treatment and control in non-infected herds depends upon the maintenance of a closed herd or the purchase of stock from herds known to be free from the disease. In infected herds the only preventative measure is to ensure access to colostrum. It is possible that immunity may be stimulated in non-pregnant gilts by feeding affected piglets or the faeces of weaned pigs to them. This would require permission from the State Veterinary Service in the U.K. Disinfection is possible using lipid solvents.

References

Andries, K. and Pensaert, M.B. (1980). Virus isolation and immunofluorescence in different organs of pigs infected with H.E.V. Am.J.Vet.Res. **41**, 215-218.

Andries K. and Pensaert, M.B. (1980). Immunofluorescence studies on the pathogenesis of H.E.V. after oronasal inoculation. Am.J.Vet.Res. **41**,1372-1278.

Cartwright, S.F. and Lucas, M. (1970). Vomiting and Wasting Disease in piglets. Veterinary Record **86**, 278-280.

Cartwright, S.F. Lucas. M., Cavill, J.P., Gush, A.F. and Blandford, T.B. (1969). Vomiting and Wasting Disease in piglets. Veterinary Record **84**, 175-176.

Narita, M., Kawamura, H., Haritani, M. and Kobayashi, M. (1989). Demonstration of viral antigen and immunoglobulin (IgM and IgG) in brain tissue of pigs experimentally infected with H.E.V. J.Comp.Path. **100**, 119-128.

Transmissible Gastroenteritis (T.G.E.)

Definition

T.G.E. is a highly infectious viral disease of pigs, the chief clinical signs of which are diarrhoea, dehydration, occasional vomiting and a high mortality rate in young pigs. Disease in chronically-infected herds is less obvious.

Incidence

T.G.E. is currently (2006) rare in Britain but its effect on individual farms can be devastating. Up to 750 outbreaks per annum have been recorded, but none occurred between 1983 and 1996. The infection remains in some herds with more than 300 sows. U.K. survey data showed 0.6% sows seropositive in 1990, but 21.9% of 64 finishing herds surveyed in 1997 were positive. It is absent from Scotland and was first seen in Ireland in 1984 and then eradicated. Infection is present in many countries where the occurrence of disease is reduced by widespread infection by the porcine respiratory coronavirus (PRCV). In the mid-West United States antibody was present in 26% herds in 1989-90 and the disease is present in many Asian countries including China, India, Japan, Korea, Taiwan and Vietnam. It is absent from Australia and southern Africa.

Aetiology

The causal agent is an ether sensitive, spherical RNA corona virus approximately 135 nm in diameter composed of a filamentous nucleocapsid enclosed within an envelope with spikes or peplomeres 12-25 nm in length. The molecular biology of the virus and its growth in cells has been studied extensively. The RNA has been sequenced and the structure and functions of several genes are known. The major structural proteins are the M or membrane glycoprotein of 29-31 kDa, the S or spike peplomer glycoprotein of 195-220 kDa associated with attachment, membrane fusion and neutralisation. Monoclonal antibodies have revealed a number of antigenic sites on these proteins. The virus is not inactivated at pH 3.0, is partially sensitive to sodium desoxycholate but is fully resistant to trypsin. It is very thermolabile and treatment at 50°C for 45 minutes is sufficient to inactivate virus of pig intestinal origin. The half-life at 37°C is less than 2 hours. Some strains are very sensitive to light, but the virus is extremely stable when frozen. The virus is difficult to isolate as C.P.E. is very slight in the first 4-5 passages. However, more extensive C.P.E., syncytia and round refractile cells are produced in later passages if large amounts of virus are used to initiate infection. Pig kidney or testis cells are used. Serological tests have shown that only 1 serotype of T.G.E. virus exists but there are some relationships (shared gene sequences) with human and bovine coronaviruses and considerable homology with Porcine Respiratory Coronavirus. Serum neutralisation of tissue culture virus is used to assay antibodies and to compare viral isolates. ELISA tests using monoclonal antibodies have demonstrated minor antigenic differences between isolates and cDNA sequences of the viral RNA have also been used to study the relationships between isolates.

Pathogenesis

Infection takes place by ingestion or inhalation of infected droplets of faecal material. The virus multiplies in extraintestinal sites such as lungs and lymph nodes but principally in the cells of the alimentary tract, especially in those of the duodenum, jejunum and ileum. The cells chiefly affected are those at the tips of the villi, i.e. mature absorptive cells and their loss due to the effects of viral multiplication leads to their replacement by immature cells from the bases of the crypts. Loss of cells from the tips of the villi leads to lowering of the height of the epithelium, shortening of the villi and to an increase in the depth of the crypts. The ability of the small intestine to digest food (enzymes such as lactase are absent or in low concentration) and to absorb products of digestion is reduced by cell loss and damage. This results in hypoglycaemia and in osmotic diarrhoea which is exacerbated by a reduction in glucose-mediated sodium transport in the small intestine. Colonic absorption of water increases markedly but cannot prevent the diarrhoea and the subsequent death of piglets from dehydration. Superinfection with *E.coli* and *Clostridium perfringens* types A and C may occur and affect the clinical signs and pathology.

IgG serum antibodies develop in recovered pigs as do IgA, IgG and IgM antibodies in the lung but local IgA immunity in the small intestine is most important in protection against the disease. Specific IgA antibody in the colostrum and milk of immune sows protects piglets against infection for 36 hours after its withdrawal.

Maternal antibody levels rise before and after parturition and maternal antibody can be detected in the sera of piglets for 6-12 weeks after birth. Serum antibody from active infection develops within 7-8 days of infection and may persist for at least 6 months in finishers and 16 months to 2 years in sows. Cold stress has been shown to reduce the rate of antibody formation. Cell mediated immunity develops rapidly and may be important in recovery and immunity. It can last for over 100 days. Recovery from the disease is not always associated with elimination of the virus from the body. Virus can still be demonstrated in the lung 104 days after infection and in the gut for at least 104 days. Virus shedding in the faeces may not, however be easily detectable more than 14 days after infection but may continue for longer.

Clinical signs

The clinical signs of the disease are most characteristic in a non-immune herd. An explosive outbreak of diarrhoea occurs which involves pigs of all ages within a few days. The diarrhoea is profuse, watery and yellowish green in colour, sometimes with a foetid odour and containing curds of undigested milk. Vomiting may occur in piglets under 3 weeks of age and piglets under 1 week of age may show pink flushing of the skin. There is no febrile reaction and no nervous signs occur. Affected pigs become dehydrated - resulting in death in piglets within 24-48 hours and in agalactia in sows. The disease has a short incubation period of 1-2 days and occurs within 3-4 days of birth in susceptible piglets. The pattern of mortality in piglets is characteristic in a non-immune herd where water is not available to the piglets.

Age   0 - 7 days   100% mortality
       8 - 14 days   50% mortality
       15 - 21 days   25% mortality

Mortality is rare in piglets aged 3 weeks or more. Affected adults usually recover within 7-10 days. Some abortions and a reduced conception rate in sows bred after the deaths of their litters have been recorded. Where the disease is enzootic, its effects are most obvious in pigs aged between 10 days and 6 weeks. Diarrhoea and growth depression (F.C.R. may be reduced by 0.2) are the main clinical signs noted. In finishing pigs which seroconvert, growth depression may be the only clinical finding. Where wet feed is given with no supplementary water, weaned pigs may die from salt poisoning and these clinical signs may be superimposed on those of T.G.E.

Recent studies in enzootic infections in large herds suggest that disease occurs one week post-weaning and may persist for several weeks. Recrudescence of severe disease may occur in piglets aged 6 days or more and give rise to mortality. Such outbreaks rarely last more than 6-10 days. The litters of recently-purchased gilts may be most severely affected in such a herd.

Piglets which are comatose and cannot be treated should be killed humanely.

Pathological findings

Dead piglets are dehydrated but in good condition. The stomach is often distended with curdled milk and the small intestine is distended with foamy yellow fluid and is thin-walled. In some cases yellowish deposits or urate crystals may be seen in streaks in the kidney medulla. Areas of gastritis may also be present. The mesenteric lymph nodes may be enlarged. Villous atrophy may be seen in areas of the small intestine distal to the first 10 cm of the duodenum. Intestinal mucosa is best mounted in saline and viewed X 10 under a dissecting microscope.

Histological changes in the small intestine are those of villous atrophy with alteration of the crypt:villus ratio. Alteration of the cell types in the mucosal epithelium may occur. All lesions may be less obvious in recovering animals and those nursed by partially immune sows. Lesions of secondary infection may be superimposed on the basic lesions of villous atrophy.

Epidemiology

T.G.E. outbreaks commonly occur in winter and, in Britain, originated from foci in East Anglia or Yorkshire, spreading slowly to other parts of the country. Severe, widespread epizootics of T.G.E. have not occurred for many years. The last epizootic (winter 1969 - summer 1977) was unusual as a few outbreaks occurred in summer. This pattern was repeated in the 1980-88 period and infection has persisted in some finishing herds. A typical outbreak took place in 1999. The susceptibility of the virus to heat and light inactivation has been thought to account for the seasonal incidence of outbreaks. The severe widespread outbreaks reported in the Mid-West of the U.S. in winter may reflect this. Outbreaks usually last for 3-4 weeks. The virus is present in large amounts in the faeces of affected animals and may be excreted in the faeces of recovered pigs for up to 10 weeks. Carrier pigs may be important in the spread of the disease. Spread of the disease on a farm is by:

(a)   the ingestion of infected faeces by pigs in contact with affected animals.
(b)   inhalation or ingestion of droplets of faeces
(c)   movement of carrier or affected pigs
(d)   indirect transmission of faeces on implements, etc and when staff fail to wash and change between infected and naïve pigs..
(e)   direct transmission in the sows' milk

Spread of the disease between farms is usually by:

(a)   the introduction of affected or carrier pigs (usually weaners)
(b)   indirect carriage of infective faeces on boots, in contaminated lorries, etc.
(c)   wind transmission for distances of up to 1 mile/1.6km (possibly 3 miles in the US). (Slurry may be important here)
(d)   passive transmission of virus in the gut of starlings or by dogs. The virus can survive in dogs and remain infective for pigs for up to 14 days
(e)   persistence of virus in carcases. Fresh meat from infected pigs can transmit infection as can carcases frozen at -25°C for 30 days.

The reduction in clinical TGE in countries with widespread occurrence of porcine respiratory coronavirus has been shown experimentally to result from partial protection following active infection with PRCV or passive immunity from an immune sow. Recently, the concurrent circulation of PRCV and TGE in a US herd has been shown to result in mild disease although the virus was typical.

Diagnosis

T.G.E. is usually suspected on the basis of the epizootiology of the outbreak and clinical signs of diarrhoea throughout the herd, deaths in the young piglets and the pathological findings. T.G.E. may be distinguished from E.coli diarrhoeas by the extensive morbidity and mortality, the absence of enteropathogenic E.coli and the degree of inflammation and lack of villous atrophy in the small intestine in that disease. Rotavirus diarrhoea only affects piglets and weaned pigs but Epidemic Diarrhoea can affect all ages, usually without the mortality seen in piglets with T.G.E.

Recently dual infections with both viruses have been demonstrated and these can be distinguished only by laboratory means. In coccidiosis, clostridial and cryptosporidial infections there is marked necrosis of the intestine.

Diagnosis may be confirmed by:

(a)   by serum neutralisation tests, ELISA, or the bentonite agglutination test to detect serum antibodies in recovered pigs. In countries such as the U.K. in which the porcine respiratory coronavirus occurs, only tests such as the blocking ELISA using monoclonals specific for T.G.E. can now be used

(b)   by the demonstration of virus in frozen sections of the small intestine of freshly-killed piglets by the use of a specific fluorescent antiserum or specific monoclonal antibody. A positive diagnosis is made by finding fluorescence in epithelial cells at the tips or sides of the villi. Fluorescence is patchy in actively-infected pigs. Immunoperoxidase may also be used on fixed tissue as may in situ hybridisation using cDNA sequences of the S and M protein genes and reverse transcriptase-PCR (RT-PCR). DNA probes have been shown to be extremely sensitive in dot hybridisation in faeces and cell culture.

(c)   by virus isolation from mesenteric lymph node, tonsil and small intestine which may be frozen prior to examination. As C.P.E. is poor in initial cultures, virus may be identified by immunofluorescence or DNA probes.

(d)   by demonstration of virus in faeces by RT-PCR using a number of different primers and formulations (eg lightcycler PCR, nested RT-PCR)

Samples for laboratory examinations should include at least 1 moribund or live affected piglet for immunofluorescence, immunoperoxidase, in situ hybridisation, virus isolation and for examination of the villi. Faeces submitted for RT-PCR can be stored for up to 10 days at +4°C, but for shorter periods at higher temperatures.

Treatment and control

T.G.E. may cause massive and spectacular losses amongst young piglets, but acute outbreaks are relatively uncommon and are now localised in the U.K. Chronic infection in fattening houses may cause economic loss by affecting growth rate. The disease can be treated symptomatically with glucose:glycine electrolyte replacer solutions, given in cube drinkers. Early weaning, especially onto glucose - containing artificial feeds, the maintenance of high environmental temperatures and hygiene may all help reduce mortality. Cross suckling of litters onto immune sows may also help if they can be identified reliably e.g. by recording episodes of clinical disease. Water should be freely available to weaned pigs not treated as already described. Antimicrobials may control infections by *E.coli* and *Clostridium perfringens* in piglets and swine dysentery in weaned pigs. Experimental studies of support suggest that clonidine may be of value and combinations of specific monoclonal antibodies and hyperimmune sera or egg yolks given orally have been shown to reduce mortality. Human and porcine interferons have been given orally and also reduce mortality.

Control must be based on prevention by:-

(a)   Isolation. Unnecessary visitors or contaminated lorries should not be admitted to susceptible herds and all visitors entering a herd should do so via a disinfectant dip and change outer clothing. Stock should not be purchased during epizootics of T.G.E. Stock from infected farms may be non-infectious 40 days after the last clinical signs (but remember that carriage may persist 104 days).

(b)   An all-in, all-out policy should be operated in finishing and farrowing houses in herds where the disease is enzootic. Disinfection and control of rodents and birds may break the cycle of infection.

(c)   When outbreaks occur, sows due to farrow within 14 days should be maintained in isolation. The infected buildings may be re-occupied after 3 months or thorough disinfection.

(d)   Deliberate infection of sows. Sows which are more than 14 days from farrowing can be infected with intestinal contents from dead pigs and may develop immunity in time to protect their litters. This would require to be licensed but use of faeces does not.

(e)   Vaccination. The crude infectious materials mentioned above may be replaced by a number of vaccines. Virus killed by acetylethylenimine, detergent, and formalin has been administered by the intranasal and/or intramuscular routes. Live virus vaccines consisting of varying strains of attenuated virus have been developed. These have been administered by the oral, intranasal, intramuscular and intramammary routes. The oral or nasal route produces the best colostral and lactogenic immunity but virulent virus may infect susceptible pigs on the farm of use or on adjacent farms. Less virulent virus may not produce adequate immunity or even become established.
Strains which infect only a local area of gut and give good protective immunity have been described. The 200 kDa proteins from the spikes on the viral envelope have been engineered into vaccinia, porcine adenovirus, yeasts, plants such as maize and tobacco, *Salmonella typhimurium* and *E. coli* vectors and produce immunity and some degree of protection but have not been tested in the field and are not on available for use (2006). PRCV is not completely protective.

Vaccines are not available in the UK. In the US live attenuated virus vaccines are available. Vaccination should take place at least two weeks before farrowing to prevent mortality in the litter and more in the case of live virus vaccines. No vaccine has yet been shown to be more than 50% effective. T.G.E. eradication from a chronically infected herd has been described by whole herd vaccination in the US and by depopulation and serology in Ireland.

For differentiation of PRCV from TGE see PRCV section below.

References

Argenzio, R.A., Moon, H.W., Kemeny, L.J. and Whipp, S.C. (1984). Gastroenterology **86**, 1501-1509.
Brown, I.H., Paton, D.J. (1991). Serological studies of T.G.E. in Great Britain using a competitive ELISA. Vet.Rec. **128**, 500-503.
Drolet, R., Morin, M. and Fontaine, M. (1984). Hypoglycaemia: a factor associated with low survival rate of neonatal pigs infected with transmissible gastroenteritis virus. Canadian Journal of Comparative Medicine **48**, 282-285.
Fitzgerald, G.R., Welter, C.J. (1990). The effect of an oral T.G.E. vaccine on eliminating virus from a herd of swine. Agri.Practice. **11**, 25-29.

Gunn, H.M. (1996). Elimination of TGE virus from a pig farm by culling and serological surveillance. Vet. Rec. **138**, 196-198.

Kim, L., Hayes, J., Lewis, P., Parwani, A.V., Chang, K.O., Saif, L.j. (2000). Molecular characterisation and pathogenesis of TGE Coronavirus (TGEV) and porcine respiratory coronavirus (PRCV) field isolates co-circulating in a swine herd. Archives of Virology **145**, 1133-1147.

Pritchard, G.C. (1982). Observations on clinical aspects of transmissible gastroenteritis of pigs in Norfolk and Suffolk. Vet.Rec. **110**, 465-469.

Pritchard, G.C. (1987). TGE in endemically infected breeding herds of pigs in East Anglia. 1981-1985. Vet.Rec. **120**, 226-230.

Pritchard, G.C., Paton, D.J., Wibberley, G., Ibata, G. (1999). Transmissible Gastroenteritis and Porcine Epidemic Diarrhoea in Britain. Vet.Rec. **144**, 616-618.

Siegel, J.P., Hungerford, L.C., Hall, W.F. (1991). Risk factors with TGE in swine. J.Am.Vet.Med.Ass. **199**, 1579-1583.

Smerdou, C., Urniza, A., Curtis R. III, Enjuanes, L. (1996). Characterisation of Transmissible Gastroenteritis coronavirus S protein expression product in avirulent *Salmonella typhimurium* Δcya Δcrp, persistence, stability and immune response in swine. Vet. Micro **48**,87-100

Wesley, R.D., Woods, R.D. (1996). Induction of protective immunity against Transmissible Gastroenteritis virus after exposure of neonatal pigs to Porcine Respiratory Coronavirus. Am. J. Vet. Res. **57**, 157-162

Porcine Epidemic Diarrhoea

Definition

Porcine Epidemic Diarrhoea is a highly contagious disease characterised by vomiting, diarrhoea and inappetence in pigs of all ages. Mortality in young piglets is less common than in TGE.

Incidence

First described in Britain in 1972, it has now been identified in most European countries, China, Korea, Japan, India, Indonesia and Taiwan but antibody was absent from sera from small numbers of pigs from Sweden, Australia, Northern Ireland and the US. Similar diseases not confirmed as epidemic diarrhoea have been identified in Canada. In Austria and Switzerland serological surveys suggest that the incidence is low in contrast to Belgium.

Aetiology

The causal agent is a coronavirus distinct from TGE, PRCV and H.E.V. The virus is 95-150 nm (mean 130 nm) in negative stain and 60 nm in section. The peplomeres are 18-23 nm in length. There are three major protein antigens, the S or spike glycosylated protein of 85-130 kDa, the M protein of 27 kDa and an N protein of 58 kDa with some relationship to Feline Infectious Peritonitis virus. All isolates appear to belong to a single serotype. It can be cultivated in Vero cells with added trypsin and produces syncytia on subculture and has been sequenced. The virus is destroyed at >60°C within 30 minutes, but is stable at 50°C. At 37°C it is stable between pH 6.5 and 7.5 but at 4°C only between pH 5.0-pH 9.0.

Pathogenesis

The virus does not replicate in the respiratory tract but otherwise pathogenesis resembles that of TGE. It attaches to a 150 kb receptor on epithelial cells. Those at the tips and sides of the villi are infected and can shed virus without being destroyed, but, by the onset of diarrhoea, epithelial cell shedding has already begun. Six hours later it occurs in the ileum. Levels of alkaline and acid phosphatase, succinic dehydrogenase and monoamine oxidase fall. In older pigs lactase levels have also been shown to fall. Villous fusion and atrophy are widespread within 24 hours of the onset of clinical signs. In partially-immune piglets, a very localised area of the small intestine may show villous atrophy. Serum antibody levels become detectable 2-4 weeks after infection and rise to levels of up to 1:10,000 declining rapidly to lower levels of 1:20-1:640. Passive antibody has disappeared from the sera of piglets within 5-13 weeks and active immunity then develops. The presence of serum antibody in a nursing sow does not rule out epidemic diarrhoea in her litter. Antibody levels on infected farms peak at 4 months and decline from then onward.

Clinical signs

The disease occurs as an explosive outbreak of diarrhoea in non-immune weaned pigs (Type I) or in pigs of all ages (Type II). After an incubation period of 1-3 days, piglets develop a TGE-like watery diarrhoea and may vomit but although morbidity in non-immune pigs approaches 100%, mortality can be low. The disease spreads rapidly in the unit. Twenty to thirty per cent of the older pigs may be affected with vomiting and diarrhoea. One hundred per cent inappetence may occur, especially in breeding stock. In Type I, sucking and young weaned pigs under 32 kg liveweight are rarely affected. Affected weaned pigs are dull and unwilling to rise. Pyrexia is rare. The diarrhoea is greenish-brown in colour and very fluid, often coating the pigs completely. Signs of dehydration are common. Vomiting is prominent in some outbreaks and less obvious in others. The acute stage of vomiting and diarrhoea lasts approximately 3 days but recovery takes a further 7-8 days. Mortality is rare in the absence of intercurrent disease and where water is freely available. Affected feeding pigs take about 14 days longer to reach 90 Kg due to the effects of inappetence and loss of condition. Clinically-recovered pigs show no after effect. Agalactia may occur in sows and result in some indirect mortality in unaffected litters.

Severely dehydrated, wasted piglets not responding to supportive therapy should be humanely destroyed.

Pathological findings

Few weaned pigs have been examined as mortality is low. The stomach is usually empty or filled with bile-stained fluid, and both large and small intestines are pale and thin-walled, often with fluid contents. Villous atrophy is present. Some villous atrophy may be seen in the small intestines of baby pigs affected by this condition and they may have a gastritis

Epidemiology

Separated from TGE on epidemiological grounds in the 1969-1977 TGE outbreak in 1971, the disease continued until spring 1972 and then died down in the summer to reappear in winter 1972-73. Pig contact is important and spread has occurred through markets and by pig transport lorries. Type II disease was first described in 1977. Epidemic diarrhoea is usually introduced by carrier pigs and introduction may be followed by an explosive outbreak. Severe outbreaks involving sows and piglets are now unusual and clinical disease may be confined to individual litters or occur in recently purchased grower pigs.

Diagnosis

Type I disease may be suspected by its history and clinical signs of an acute, rapidly spreading scour with vomiting and inappetence not affecting sucking pigs. The only similar condition is TGE. which can be eliminated by laboratory tests.

Type II disease may be suspected by the pattern of mortality in a non-immune herd. In a partially immune herd, only a few piglets may develop the disease and differentiation from _E.coli_ (absence of agent, villous atrophy) clostridia, cryptosporidia and coccidia (no blood or necrosis of the small intestinal epithelium) and rotavirus and TGE (laboratory methods including immunofluorescence, RT-PCR and ELISA must be carried out).

Confirmation can be obtained by immunoelectron microscopy of the intestinal contents or faeces of affected pigs when coronavirus particles may be seen. The virus may be demonstrated using RT-PCR or nested RT-PCR. Specific fluorescent antibody or immunoperoxidase demonstrates the virus in intestinal epithelium and an ELISA test is available for the detection of specific antibody in the sera or milk of recovered pigs. Only rising titres in paired serum samples are diagnostic. A number of ELISAs have been evaluated. The most efficient appears to be one using whole, tissue culture virus as antigen although the S protein can also be used. It has become clear that dual infections of TGE and PED can occur in the same pig.

Treatment and Control

Provide adequate water and provide milk substitute for any piglets of affected sows which may lose their milk and adequate water for all affected stock at all times. Piglets may be treated using glucose: glycine electrolyte solutions . There is no specific treatment, although pig interferon has been used to reduce weight loss and mixed monoclonal antibodies and egg yolk antibody have also been found to protect. The effects of an outbreak of the disease may be controlled by isolating all sows within 14 days of farrowing, and by infecting all those due to farrow in more than 14 days. Weaners may also be infected in order to reduce the duration of the outbreak. Where swine dysentery or other intercurrent disease is present, recovery from epidemic diarrhoea is hastened by the treatment appropriate to the intercurrent disease. Experimental vaccines attenuated by passage (83 times) have been described and protect 94.6% pigs after 21 days, but are not available commercially and genetically-engineered plant protein vaccines have been produced..

References

Bollwahn, W. (1983). Epizootic viral diarrhoea of pigs. Pig News and Information 4, 141-144.

Chasey, D. and Cartwright, S.F. (1978) Virus-like particles associated with porcine epidemic diarrhoea. Res. Vet.Sci. 25, 255-256.

De Bouck, P., Pensaert, M. and Coussement, W. (1981). The pathogenesis of an enteric infection in pigs experimentally induced by the coronavirus-like agent CV777. Vet.Microbiol. 6, 157-165.

Ducatelle, R., Coussement, W., De Bouck, P. and Hoorens, J. (1982). Pathology of experimental CV777 coronavirus enteritis in piglets. I. Histological and histochemical study. Vet.Path. 19, 46-56.

Ducatelle, R., Coussement, W., Charlier, G., De Bouck, P. and Hoorens, J. (1982). Pathology of experimental CV777 coronavirus enteritis in piglets. II Electron microscopic study. Vet.Path. 19, 57-66.

Egberink, H.F., Ederveen, J., Callebaut, P. and Horzinek, M.C. (1988). Characterisation of the structural proteins of PED virus strain CV777. Am.J.Vet.Res. 49, 1320-1324.

Hofmann, M. and Wyler, R. (1988). Propagation of the virus of porcine epidemic diarrhoea in cell culture. J.Clin.Micro. 26, 2235-2239.

Hofmann, M. and Wyler, R. (1989). Quantitation biological and physicochemical properties of cell culture adapted P.E.D. coronavirus.Vet.Microbiol. 20, 131-142.

Hofmann, M. and Wyler, R. (1990). ELISA for the detection of porcine epidemic diarrhoea virus antibodies in swine sera. Vet.Microbiol. 21, 263-273.

Ishikawa, K., Sekiguchi, H., Ogino, T., Suzuki, S. (1997). Direct and rapid detection of porcine epidemic diarrhoea virus by RT-PCR. J. Virol. Methods **69**, 191-195.

Wood, E.N. (1977). An apparently new syndrome of porcine epidemic diarrhoea. Vet.Rec. **100**, 243-244.

Porcine Respiratory Coronavirus Infection

Definition

Infection with porcine respiratory coronavirus (PRCV) causes rapid seroconversion of a herd to some tests for T.G.E. virus and can cause fatal bronchopneumonia with fever coughing and anorexia in experimental pigs. In the field infection can cause a similar syndrome or be subclinical.

Incidence

First reported from Belgium in 1986 it has been found in the UK, France, Germany, Denmark, Canada and The Netherlands and many Asian countries. Related viruses have been identified in the U.S. In the UK antibody became widespread in 1986 but antibody-free herds still exist.

Aetiology

A coronavirus resembling TGE virus and causing spreading cytopathic effects and syncytia in pig kidney cell cultures has been isolated from the lungs of infected pigs. Antibody to it neutralises T.G.E. virus and the syncytia fluoresce with sera specific to TGE. Epitopes common to both viruses have been demonstrated on all virus proteins examined but monoclonal antibodies which react with TGE virus and not with PRCV have been found. The genomic differences between TGE and PRCV are slight and the major antigenic difference appears to be a truncated S protein.

Pathogenesis

Infection is by aerosol and the virus multiplies chiefly in the lungs. Virus has been demonstrated in nasal mucosal epithelial cells, those of the trachea, bronchi, bronchioles and alveoli. Alveolar macrophages are also affected. A viraemia follows respiratory tract multiplication and some viral antigen may be found in the small intestinal submucosa but not in the epithelium. Varying degrees of interstitial pneumonia result from infection. IFNα is produced. The virus is shed as an aerosol and in nasal secretions for 1-6 days after infection. It does not appear to cross the placenta but has been found in the semen for up to 6 days post infection in boars. Antibody to the virus becomes detectable in sera within a week. Experimental dual infections of PRCV with swine influenza and Aujeszky's Disease viruses result in an initial decrease in colonisation by the other virus and more severe lesions in the lung

Clinical signs

No clinical signs have been observed prior to seroconversion at 3-5 months in some herds in which maternal antibody is present but coughing and anorexia have been reported in others. Anorexia, reluctance to move, laboured respiration and fever (40°C, 104°F) have been reported 1-5 days following the experimental infection of antibody-free conventional pigs. No clinical signs were noted in gnotobiotes in some studies. Experimental infection with PRCV alone or together with influenza virus has little effect on growth rate.

Pathological findings

No lesions have been reported in some cases and in others severe catarrhal bronchopneumonia has been seen. Lesions are restricted to the lung and bronchi. The lesions include mild interstitial pneumonia, hyperplasia of the bronchiolar epithelium and epithelial cell loss. Syncytia occur in the alveoli and airways. Virus may be demonstrated in the bronchiolar and bronchial epithelial cells, in alveolar macrophages and septal monocytes.

Epidemiology

Aerosol infection appears to occur within a herd and seroconversion spreads rapidly to pigs of all ages. Maternal immunity appears to persist for up to 3-4 months when active seroconversion occurs. Spread between herds appears to have been by movement of infected carrier pigs. Experimental infections do not protect against TGE infections, but field infections with TGE are milder where PRCV occurs

Diagnosis

The clinical signs are not sufficiently consistent to reach a diagnosis on clinical grounds alone. The spread of mild respiratory disease throughout a herd previously free from TGE, coupled with seroconversion to TGE virus in the absence of enteric signs may allow diagnosis. Blocking ELISA tests for serum antibody have been described using monoclonal antibodies specific for TGE. The virus can be demonstrated in tissue using immunoperoxidase, biotin labelled monoclonal antibody and in situ hybridisation. PCR primers, RT-PCR and DNA probes have been developed.

Treatment and Control

The only indication for control at present is the problem of certification of herds for freedom from TGE. This has been approached in the UK by founding and maintaining antibody-free herds by rigorous testing and isolation. Disinfect as for TGE. A recombinant adenovirus vaccine expressing the glycoprotein has been shown experimentally to produce some protection.

References

Ahn, K., Chae, C., Kweon, C.H. (1997). Immunohistochemical identification of PRCV antigen in the lung of conventional pigs. Vet. Path. **34**, 167-169.
Callebaut, P., Enjaunes, L., Pensaert, M. (1996). An adenovirus recombinant expressing the glycoprotein of porcine respiratory coronavirus is immunogenic in swine. J.Gen.Virol. **77**, 309-313.
Cox, E., Hooyberghs, J. and Pensaert, M.B. (1990). Sites of replication of a P.R.C.V. related to T.G.E. virus. Res.Vet.Sci. **48**, 165-169.
Garwes, D.J., Stewart, F., Cartwright, S.F. and Brown, I. (1988). Differentiation of porcine coronavirus from TGE virus. Vet.Rec. **122**, 86-87.
Pensaert, M., Callebaut, P. and Vergote, J. (1986). Isolation of a porcine respiratory non-enteric coronavirus related to TGE and VWD of pigs. Veterinary Quarterly **88**, 257-261.
Reeth, K. van, Nauwynck, H., Pensaert, M., (2000). A potential role of tumour necrosis factor α in synergy between porcine respiratory coronavirus and bacterial lipopolysaccharide in the induction of respiratory disease in pigs. Journal of Medical Microbiology **49**, 613-620
van Nieuwstadt, A.P. and Pol, J.M.A. (1989). Isolation of a TGE-related respiratory coronavirus causing fatal pneumonia in pigs Vet.Rec. **124**, 43-44.

Rotavirus

Definition

Rotavirus infections are associated with profuse diarrhoea in young piglets and result in varying degrees of mortality. Less severe diarrhoea may occur in weaned animals

Incidence

Infections with porcine rotavirus appear to occur in all pig rearing areas. In both Britain and the U.S. 100% slaughter pigs have antibody to at least one rotavirus group in the UK. Groups A, B, C and E are most common.

Aetiology

Rotaviruses contain double stranded RNA arranged in 11 segments and particles are ultrastructurally indistinguishable from calf and human isolates which have been shown to cause disease in gnotobiotic pigs. Particles measure 75nm with the outer capsid (a double-shelled smooth outer layer) and 58nm without it. The two major surface proteins are VP4 non-glycosylated 90 kDa protease sensitive 'P' protein which can haemagglutinate and VP7, a glycosylated 37 kDa protein ('G' protein). There is also a common core antigen.

Rotaviruses are divided into groups based on antigenicity and polyacrilamide gel electrophoresis banding of the DNA Groups A, B, C and E have been recorded in pigs. Classification is now expressed as Group (A) strain (OSU) subgroup (II) G protein type (3, 4, 5, 11) and P type (6, 7). The genes for these two proteins have been synthesised and cDNA probes can be used for typing as can monoclonal antibodies.

Rotavirus may resist $60^{o}C$ for 30 minutes in faeces and survive for 7-9 months at $18\text{-}20^{o}C$ and 32 months at $10^{o}C$, is stable between pH 3 and 9 but can be inactivated by 3.7% formaldehyde, 70% ethanol, 2% glutaraldehyde, 1% hypochlorite and 0.01% iodine, and heat at $63^{o}C$ for 30 minutes. It may remain infective for three days in 1% formaldehyde. Rotaviruses may be cultured in calf and kidney cells but require exposure to trypsin and agitation for continued subculture. Cytopathic effects and plaque formation can be produced on monkey cell line MA104 with pancreatin and dextran. Viral antigen can be present in the cytoplasm of cells without CPE. It must be detected by IF, immunoperoxidase, RT-PCR or DNA probes.

Pathogenesis

Oral infection with as few as 90 particles results in replication of the virus in the cells of the epithelium of the middle small intestine from upper jejunum to lower ileum. Virus particles attach to a monosialoglycoside receptor and enter cells by pinocytosis between the microvilli of enterocytes and are then seen in the endoplasmic reticulum. Infected cells do not become vacuolated as in T.G.E. but swell, lose their microvilli and are shed. Replication is most intense 24-96 hours after infection but later becomes restricted to villus tips. Mature absorptive cells are shed and villous atrophy, crypt hyperplasia and villous fusion occur. Lactase levels fall but lactose digestion may not be affected. Recovery may be complete within 7 days of infection. Virus particles are shed in large numbers ($10^{7}\text{-}10^{8}$ml) in the faeces. Other infectious agents are often present and rotaviruses of more than one group or serotype may occur in the same animal. Colostral and milk antibody is important in

42

the development of clinical disease and protects for 3-5 weeks. Passive antibodies have normally disappeared by 7 weeks of age. Active IgA and IgM antibodies first appear 7-13 days after infection and serum antibody, principally IgG, 17-24 days after infection. Antibody in sows passes into colostrum (IgG and IgM) but IgA is the principal antibody class in milk. Sow serum IgG rises with each parity, IgA remains constant and IgM declines progressively.

Clinical signs

The incubation period is 18-24 hours after which depression, anorexia and reluctance to move are noted. Vomiting may be seen. A few hours later, profuse diarrhoea develops and in milk-fed pigs this is yellow with floccules floating in a whey-like fluid, while in others it may be yellow or dark grey. There is a rapid loss of condition. Anorexia continues for 24-72 hours after which appetite returns. Clinical signs regress 4-6 days after infection but loose yellow faeces may persist for 7-14 days. Thirty-three per cent of affected young pigs may die in field outbreaks but mortality can be up to 100% in experimental animals. Weaned pigs may also be affected, but in them no diarrhoea or only transient diarrhoea (mean duration 3 days) results when rotavirus is demonstrated in the faeces. Rotavirus diarrhoea may recur as immunity to one type does not prevent infection with others.

The effects on growth rate range from nothing to at least 5 days to 25kg. Piglets suffering from dehydration and hypoglycaemia such that they cannot rise, should be killed.

Pathology

Dead pigs may appear dehydrated, the stomach is filled with milk and the small intestine is distended with creamy fluid contents. There is desquamation of the epithelial cells of the villi lining the distal three quarters of the small intestine resulting in stunting of the villi and flattening of the remaining epithelial cells with loss of the brush border and the presence of cuboidal cells and multinucleate syncytia. Crypt depth is increased and villous fusion occurs. Infection with other agents such as *E.coli*, clostridia, adenovirus and T.G.E. may also occur, complicating the picture described.

Epidemiology

Infection is transmitted in herds directly from sow to litter as 30% sows pass virus in their faeces during farrowing. Within litters, infection begins in one or two pigs and then spreads to the others over a period of 10-14 days, beginning at 19 days and being complete at about 40 days of age. Infection may also be contracted from the environment as rotavirus is stable in faeces for up to 9 months and persists in water.

Group A infections tend to occur early in life, followed by B and C based on the detection of active immunity. Exceptions are known and Group C infections have been recorded in neonates and Group A infections in pigs of 2-20 weeks in extensive husbandry systems. Piglets of 0-7 days of age may be less susceptible to Group A infections. All infections in a herd may belong to a single electrophoretic type for up to 2 years and then change. Infection may be transferred from group to group in carrier pigs, by man, implements or rodents. Rotaviruses from other species such as calves and man may cause disease in pigs. There is a close resemblance between some pig Group C rotaviruses and human strains but it is not clear whether human infection with porcine strains can occur.

Diagnosis

The clinical signs may suggest rotavirus and are distinct from those of T.G.E. and epidemic diarrhoea in non-immune herds. The ubiquity of rotavirus infection should lead to its consideration as a component of most diarrhoeas of sucking and recently-weaned piglets. Pathological findings may suggest a viral condition and the use of a hand lens or dissecting microscope will reveal the presence of villous atrophy which is often more restricted than in T.G.E. or epidemic diarrhoea. There is no necrosis on the epithelium in uncomplicated rotavirus infections, unlike in cryptosporidial, clostridial or coccidial infections. The presence of rotavirus can be confirmed by the electron microscopical examination of faeces or colon contents for the characteristic particles or by polyacrilamide gel electrophoresis to detect the characteristic double-stranded RNA. These two methods detect all groups of rotavirus. cDNA probes usually based on the VP7 gene have been developed for virus in tissue, and PCR and RT-PCR methods have also been described, detecting as little as 5ng of virus. ELISA tests have been described for the detection of faecal antigen and commercial reversed passive latex agglutination tests (RPLA) and immunochromatic tests can be used on faecal filtrates on farm. All serological tests may give false negatives if prepared against individual serotypes of Group A only. Immunofluorescence may be used to detect antigen in frozen sections of intestinal material. Unfortunately, up to 25% of outbreaks of diarrhoea in pigs are said to contain rotavirus particles and mixed infections are common so that it is up to the clinician to decide the relevance of their presence. Serum antibody can be detected by indirect fluorescent antibody and by ELISA tests but serum titres are low. Up to 80% of adults may possess titres of up to 1:80 in serum and 1:640 in colostrum but IgA is more important after 7 days post-partum. Passive antibody levels persist for 2-3 weeks (IgA and M) and 7 weeks (IgG) and active antibody levels increase from 5-8 weeks. IgA antibody is present in the faeces.

Treatment

Withholding milk from affected piglets may enhance recovery. but may have an adverse effect on energy balance. Bacterial and protozoal complications should be controlled. Fluid replacement using glucose:glycine electrolyte solutions may be of value. Recent studies suggest that glutamine stimulates sodium uptake in damaged intestine. Water should always be available. Growth depression in weaned pigs is reduced if high protein rations are given but milk protein is better than vegetable protein. Prevention may be achieved by stimulating maternal immunity by feed-back of faeces from affected piglets at least 14 days prior to farrowing or by vaccinating. No vaccines are currently available in the U.K. Live vaccines given intramuscularly or orally have been described and may contain serotypes A1 and A2, human rotavirus, or constructs containing viral proteins VP3 and 7 from serotypes 4 and 5 for protection against both serotypes. Significant improvement in performance may result from vaccination of the sow 4 and 2 weeks prior to farrowing followed by oral or i/m vaccination of piglets at 2 or 4 weeks. Viral excretion may not be prevented by dead vaccines and transient diarrhoea may occur. Protection against other rotavirus serotypes or groups may be poor. Cow colostrum containing antibodies to bovine rotavirus will protect if fed to piglets. Disinfection can be carried out using hypochlorite on clean surfaces and proprietary disinfectants such as 'Virkon', Antec, a mixture of surfactant, organic acid, oxidising agents and buffers. Phenolic disinfectants are less effective.

44

References

Bridger, J.C., Brown, J.F. (1988). Porcine rotaviruses and their role in disease. Pig News and Information **9**, 23-26. Review:

Bridger, J.C., Brown, J.F. (1985). Prevalence of antibody to typical and atypical rotaviruses in pigs. Vet.Rec. **116**, 50.

Bywater, R.J. and Woode, G.N. (1980). Oral fluid replacement by a glucose:clycine electrolyte formulation in *E.coli* and rotavirus diarrhoea in pigs. Vet. Rec. **106**, 75-78.

Chasey, D., Bridger, J.C., McCrae, M.A. (1986). A new type of atypical rotavirus in pigs. Arch.Virol. **89**, 235-243.

Chasey, D. and Davies, P. (1984). Atypical rotaviruses in pigs and cattle. Vet.Rec. **114**, 16-17.

Corthier, G., Vannier, P. (1983). Production of coproantibodies and immune complexes in piglets infected with rotavirus. J.Inf.Dis. **147**, 293-296

Fu, Z.F., Hampson, D.J., Wilks, C.R. (1990). Transfer of maternal antibody against group A rotavirus from sows to piglets and serological responses following natural infection. Res.Vet.Sci. **48**, 365-373.

Gelberg, H.B., Patterson, J.S., Woode, G.N. (1991). A longitudinal study of rotavirus antibody in a closed specific pathogen-free herd. Vet.Microbiology **28**, 231-242.

Gelberg, H.B., Woode, G.N., Kniffen, T.S., Hardy, M., Hall, W.F. (1991). The shedding of Group A rotavirus in a newly-established closed SPF swine herd. Vet.Microbiology **28**, 213-229.

Hoshino, Y., Saif, L.J., Sereno, M.M., Chanock, R.M., Kapikian, A.S. (1988). Infection immunity of piglets to either VP3 or VP7 outer capsid protein confers resistance to challenge with a virulent rotavirus bearing the corresponding antigen. J.Virol. **62**, 744-748.

McAdaragh, J.P., Bergeland, M.E., Meyer, R.C., Johnshoy, M.W., Stotz, I.J., Benfield, D.A. and Hammer, R. (1980). Pathogenesis of rotaviral enteritis: A microscopic study. Am. J. Vet. Res. **41**, 1572-1581.

Rosen, B.I., Saif, L.J., Jackwood, D.J. and Gorziglia, M. (1990). Hybridisation probes for the detection and differentiation of 2 serotypes of porcine rotavirus. Vet.Microbiology **24**, 327-329.

Saif, L.J., Terret, L.A., Miller, K.L., Cross, R.F. (1988). Serial propagation of porcine group C rotavirus (pararotavirus) in a continuous cell line and characterisation of the passaged virus. J.Clin.Microbiol. **26**, 1277-1282.

Welter, M.W. and Welter, M.J. (1990). Evaluation of killed and modified live porcine rotavirus vaccines in caesarian-derived colostrum-deprived pigs. Vet.Microbiology, **22**, 179-186.

Woode, G.N., Bridger, J., Hale, G.A., Jones, J.M. and Jackson, G. (1976). The isolation of reovirus-like agents (rotavirus) from acute gastroenteritis of piglets. J.Med.Microbiol. **9**, 203-209.

Verdier Klingenberg, K.de, Estudiari, J. (1996). Evaluation of a one-step test for rapid, in practice detection of rotavirus in farm animals. Vet. Rec. **138**, 393-395.

Caliciviruses in diarrhoea

Caliciviruses are RNA-containing viruses 37 nm in diameter with a petal-like arrangement of capsomeres and have been identified in cases of post-weaning diarrhoea in pigs in Britain, the US and Japan. Porcine isolates have a major structural and immunogenic protein of 58 kDa and have been shown to be antigenically distinct from the calicivirus of vesicular exanthema. Porcine calicivirus has been grown in pig kidney cells with and without the presence of gnotobiotic intestinal content and eventually causes rounding and detachment of cells. Infection of gnotobiotic piglets caused diarrhoea lasting 3-7 days. Virus was present in the epithelial cells of sides and base of villi in the duodenum and jejunum and caused significant villous atrophy. It could be demonstrated in intestinal contents.

Calici-like viruses must be considered potential contributors to diarrhoea in piglets.

References

Bridger, J.C. (1980). Detection by electron microscopy of caliciviruses, astroviruses and rotavirus-like particles in the faeces of piglets with diarrhoea. Vet. Rec. **107**, 532-533.

Flynn, W.T., Saif, L.J. (1988). Serial propagation of porcine enteric calici-like virus in primary porcine kidney cell cultures. J.Clin.Microbiol. **26**, 206-212.
Flynn, W.T., Saif, L.J. and Moorhead, P.D. (1988). Pathogenesis of porcine enteric calici-like virus in four day old gnotobiotic pigs. Am.J.Vet.Res. **49**, 819-825.
Parwani, A., Saif, L.J., Kang, S.Y. (1990). Biochemical characterisation of porcine enteric calicivirus: analysis of structural and non-structural viral proteins. Arch.Virol. **112**, 41-53.

Astroviruses in diarrhoea

Astroviruses are 29 nm in diameter and have a star-shaped pattern on their surfaces. They have been seen in the faeces of pigs with post-weaning diarrhoea with other viruses in the UK and South Africa, and isolated from outbreaks of diarrhoea in Japan. The virus can replicate in primary calf kidney cells and has been grown in porcine embryonic kidney cells with added trypsin where CPE consisting of enlargement of cells and granularity of the cytoplasm occurs.

It is an RNA virus producing 13 kDa, 30 kDa, 31 kDa, 36 kDa and 39 kDa polypeptides. It is stable to lipid solvents and for 30 minutes at $50^{O}C$ but is killed by acid at pH 3.0. The virus is antigenically distinct from calf astrovirus. Infected 4 day old hysterectomy-derived colostrum-deprived piglets developed mild diarrhoea. Seroconversion occurs and antibody was widespread in Japan in 50% of pigs tested, 0-83% in individual herds.

References

Bridger, J.C. (1980). Detection by electron microscopy of caliciviruses, astroviruses and rotavirus-like particles in the faeces of piglets with diarrhoea. Vet.Rec. **107**, 532-533.
Shimizu, M., Shirai, J., Narita, M., Yamane, T. (1990). Cytopathic astrovirus isolated from porcine acute gastroenteritis in an established cell line derived from porcine embryonic kidney.). J.Clin.Microbiol. **28**, 201-206.

Toroviruses in Diarrhoea

Kidney-shaped torovirus-like particles I00 x 38nm and spherical particles 80 x 67nm were found in a 3 week-old piglet with diarrhoea. They have also been identified from Italy in 4 week-old weaned pigs with greenish yellow diarrhoea, 30% morbidity, 8-10% mortality also infected with *E. coli* and in 60-90% 8-10 week old pigs in the presence of *Trichomonas* and *Balantidium* sp.

Reference

Lavanza, A., Candotti, P., Perini, S., Vezzali, L. (1996). Electron microscopical identification of torovirus-like particles in post-weaned piglets with enteritis. Proc IPVS **14**, 131
Scott, A.C., Chaplin, M., Stack, M.J. and Lund, L. (1987). Porcine torovirus. Vet. Rec. **120**, 583.

Picobirnavirus in Diarrhoea

Electron microscopy of faeces from pigs with and without diarrhoea has identified featureless virus particles 35nm in diameter, sometimes with a hexagonal profile and associated with bisegmented double stranded DNA in PAGE profiles in both the U.K. and Venezuela.

Their significance is currently unknown but 11% of samples from 15-35 day old pigs were positive on one farm.

References

Chasey, D. (1990). Porcine picobirnavirus in U.K.? Vet.Rec. **126**, 465.
Ludert, J.E., Hidalgo, M., Gil, F., Lipandi, F. (1991). Identification in porcine faeces of a novel virus with a bisegmented double stranded RNA genome. Arch.Virol. **117**, 97-107.

Orbiviruses in Diarrhoea

Orbivirus-like particles and RNA have been demonstrated in pig faeces. Their significance is not clear.

Bredaviruses in Diarrhoea

Particles resembling Breda virus have been demonstrated in diarrhoeic piglet faeces and have been associated with a sudden increase immortality in 6-8 week old piglets, reduction in appetite, weakness, tremor, recumbency and death.

Reference

Penrith, M.L., Gerdes, G.H. (1992). Breda virus-like particles in pigs in South Africa. J.South African Vet.Ass. **63**, 102.

Adenovirus Infection

Definition

Mild diarrhoea in pigs from 5 days to 24 weeks of age. Also involved in pneumonia and encephalitis.

Incidence

Adenovirus diarrhoea has been identified in the U.K., United States, Canada, Belgium, Germany, Hungary, Japan, South Africa. Antibody to the virus has been identified in 70-80% slaughter pigs in the U.K. and the incidence of antibody increases with the age of the pigs. Similar findings are reported from Japan.

Aetiology

Adenoviruses are DNA viruses 75nm in diameter with 252 capsomeres arranged in cubic symmetry. Peripheral fibres exist. The virus can be cultivated in epithelial cell cultures eventually producing rounded cell cytopathic effects and intranuclear inclusions. They are resistant to ether, bile, detergents and acid and can persist for periods of up to 1 year at 4°C. They are susceptible to disinfectants. Seven serological types have been identified in pigs, of which 1-4 are most common. The genomes of 1-5 have been mapped and genes such as the penton base gene and fibre genes have been sequenced. Porcine and human adenoviruses have been studied widely as vectors for vaccines against diseases such as Foot and Mouth Disease and Classical Swine Fever (Hog Cholera).

Pathogenesis

Type 4 adenovirus has been shown to produce lesions repeatedly in experimental primary SPF piglets. Infection of week old piglets results in interstitial and proliferative pneumonia with thickened alveolar septa containing some intranuclear inclusions in septal cells. In the presence of *Mycoplasma hyopneumoniae* more severe lesions were produced. Encephalitis is also produced. Intestinal strains colonise the tonsil and in the intestine they infect epithelial cells of the villi of the lower jejunum and ileum. Intranuclear Cowdry Type A inclusions (eosinophilic or amphophilic) develop in the epithelial goblet cells and are surrounded by a clear halo. Affected nuclei swell and often lie above the line of normal nuclei. Affected cells lose microvilli and their loss may be accelerated to cause villous shortening. Diarrhoea develops and affected cells are found progressively nearer the villus tips. Dehydration may result. Serum antibody can be demonstrated in recovered pigs.

Clinical signs

Infection can occur in pigs aged 5 days - 24 weeks but is commonest in piglets of less than 3 weeks of age. The incubation period is 3-5 days and diarrhoea lasts 3-6 days and is yellow, intermittent and of variable consistency. Diarrhoea has been associated with infection in 53% cases. Dehydration may occur in piglets but mortality is rare. Virus has been isolated from nasal discharge, abortions, from stillborn piglets following transplacental infection, from piglets with cutaneous and visceral haemorrhages and from normal animals.

Severely dehydrated piglets unable to rise should be killed.

Pathology

Thinning of the intestinal wall with shortening of jejunal and ileal villi is described. Intranuclear inclusions are most commonly present in the epithelial cells of the short villi over Peyer's patches and in M cells but may occur more widely in the base and sides of the villi.

There may be an interstitial pneumonia or kidney tubule lesions.

Epidemiology

Rarely diagnosed at present but in one study 24% of piglets to 8 weeks, 60% of finishing pigs and 90-93% sows had antibody to adenovirus group antigen. Infection is clearly widespread. Infection persists in herds for long periods.

Diagnosis

Based on histological finding of adenovirus intranuclear inclusions in histological sections or or the detection of viral particles in gut contents. A rise in serum precipitating antibody levels to adenovirus group antigen might also confirm. Cultivation in porcine thyroid cells has been described for Type 4 but blind passage in tissue culture is required isolation.

Treatment and control

Symptomatic treatment with fluid replacers and, possibly, feedback to sows.

References

Coussement, W., Ducatelle, R., Charlier, G. and Hoorens, J. (1981). Adenovirus enteritis in pigs. Am.J.Vet.Res. **42**, 1905-1911.
Ducatelle, R., Coussement, W and Hoorens, J. (1982). Sequential pathological study of porcine adenovirus enteritis. Vet.Path. **19**, 179-189.
Sanford, S.E., Hoover, D.M. (1983). Enteric adenovirus infection in piglets. Can. J.Comp.Med. **47**, 396-400.
Tang, K.N., Baldwin, C.A., Mansell, J.L., Styer, E.L. (1995). Disseminated adenovirus infection associated with cutaneous and visceral haemorrhages in a nursing piglet. Vet. Path. **32**, 433-437.

Swine Influenza

Definition

A respiratory tract infection with Influenza A viruses resulting in coughing, dyspnoea and prostration which spreads rapidly through a herd and resolves within a week. Influenza may contribute to respiratory disease in weaned pigs in herds where infection is enzootic.

Incidence

Infection with classical swine influenza virus (HIN1) is a significant cause of respiratory disease in pigs in North America and since 1976 in most of Europe and Eastern Asia. Clinical disease was absent from Britain until 1986 when it occurred widely in England. Neither clinical disease nor serum antibody has yet been reported from Australia. While H1N1 remains the commonest strain (100% farms North Germany, H3N2 is widespread (88% herds North Germany) and H1N2 has been identified in the UK and in many countries of the world where it is less prevalent than either of the other main serotypes

Aetiology

Caused by Influenza A virus, an orthomyxovirus 80-120nm in diameter. These (and B and C viruses) have an RNA and protein core and surface spikes bearing haemagglutinating (H) and neuraminidase (N) antigens. They can be grown in embryonated eggs or on a number of porcine cell lines. The genes governing H and N antigens have been sequenced and the information has been used to identify the causal agents further. Classical swine influenza is associated with influenza virus A HIN1 in the U.S. but elsewhere in the world other strains are present in addition. H1N1 A/swine/Eng/195852/ 92 was identified in UK in 1992 and is related to the avian swine group of viruses circulating in Europe. In many European countries, including Britain, Japan and other South East Asian countries H3N2 also causes disease. Many H3N2 isolates from Europe are closely related antigenically to A/7/Port Chalmers/1/73, a human strain that appears to have persisted in pigs, but is now changing. In the US these strains have arisen recently (1998) and appear to contain US avian sequences. In addition recombinants may occur and HIN2 has been reported from Japan and the UK, H3N2 has been reported in Italy, Japan, Hungary, Czechoslovakia and France and H1N7 (a horse/human recombinant) and H2N1 have been recorded in UK. H3N3 has been reported from Quebec and the Andaman Islands and H9N2 from China where H5Ni may also occur. Influenza viruses are sensitive to heat, drying, detergents and disinfectants. They are sensitive at high dilutions to modern disinfectants which contain oxidising agents and surfactants such as Virkon (Antec).

Influenza C infection has been reported in Japan and China and antibody was recently found in 26% of pigs in South Germany.

Pathogenesis

In classic swine influenza, the virus enters the respiratory tract and multiplies rapidly from 2 hours in cells of the bronchial epithelium until at 24 hours post-infection most cells are infected and infected exudate is present in the bronchioles. Infection has largely disappeared by day 9. Infection of the alveolar septae and ducts occurs at the same time. The microscopic lesions develop as congestion followed by focal necrosis of bronchial epithelium. Small bronchi become blocked by neutrophil-rich exudate within 24 hours, alveolar necrosis and hyperplasia of the bronchial epithelium develop with increased levels of the cytokines IFNα, TNPα and IL1 to give rise to the clinical signs. Affected animals rapidly recover. The alveolar septae become thickened and cellular infiltrations of the alveolar septae and bronchial mucosa build up as recovery occurs. Serum IgM, IgG, and secretory IgA antibodies are produced. Viraemia can occur and transplacental infection has been recorded following infection up to 40 days before parturition and may result in failure of the lungs to develop. Antibody and antigen can be detected in foetuses. The severity of swine influenza infection may be much increased by the concurrent migration of Ascaris larvae through the lung and by infection with Aujeszky's disease virus, A.pleuropneumoniae, H.parasuis or P.multocida and , sometimes, with PRRS. Porcine respiratory coronavirus did not appear to exacerbate infection experimentally. In some cases "influenza-like" illness is not accompanied by the isolation of the swine influenza virus and other agents may also be responsible for the syndrome.

Clinical signs

In typical outbreaks in non-immune herds, the incubation period is 1-2 days and there is rapid, virtually 100% involvement of all susceptible animals. Affected animals are apathetic, develop prostration, erythema of the skin, anorexia and fever (to 41.8°C, 107°F). Coughing occurs commonly and may be sufficiently severe for pigs to appear to vomit mucus exudate. Sneezing and dyspnoea are accompanied by reddened eyes and conjunctival discharge. Loss of condition rapidly becomes apparent. Recovery usually occurs suddenly at 5-7 days after the onset and mortality is low (usually less than 1%). Some pigs may remain depressed and growing pigs may reach slaughter up to 14 days later than expected. Piglets born to sows affected in pregnancy may develop disease at 2-5 days of age and adults kept in cold conditions may develop the clinical signs to a greater extent. In some herds infection or infection with some serotypes may be completely subclinical and only be detected by seroconversion. Outbreaks may end abruptly or continue in finishing pigs with new cases for periods up to 7 months. In atypical outbreaks only a few animals develop acute signs, others are scarcely affected and the disease spreads slowly. Influenza may be followed 3 days to 3 weeks later by abortions in sows in the second half of pregnancy. Conception to service during the outbreak may be reduced by up to 50% and litter sizes may be reduced.

Animals which remain prostrate or fevered for more than 7 days should be re-assessed and treated rather than killed.

Pathology

Animals with uncomplicated disease rarely die but sharply demarcated purple-red pneumonic lesions are present in the apical and cardiac lobes of the lung and may occur in the other lobes. Mucus and exudate are present in the bronchi and the mucosae are congested. Old lesions are depressed, greyish pink and firm on section. Microscopic lesions include thickened alveolar septae and bronchial epithelial changes. Bronchi are filled with neutrophils and later mononuclear cells. Finally, interstitial pneumonia and hyperplasia of the bronchial epithelium also occur. In some cases only congestion may be seen.

The necrotising pneumonia reported from the U.K. and Canada both appear to be associated with infection with H1N1 variants. The U.K. H1N1 variant causes more pulmonary consolidation and congestion and the lesions are more severe with proliferative alveolitis, extensive necrosis of bronchioles and bronchi and peribronchial and peribronchiolar infiltration. The airways are filled with eosinophilic material. Virus antigen may be demonstrated by immunofluorescence, immunoperoxidase or labelled DNA probes in bronchial epithelium, bronchial exudate and the alveolar septae.

Epidemiology

Virus spreads from pig to pig by snout to snout contact, by aerosol or droplet infection and does not persist for long in the environment. Disease may remain in large units for long periods, occurring particularly in newly-introduced susceptible breeding stock or feeder pigs. Maternal immunity may be demonstrable for up to 4 months. It may not prevent infection and virus shedding but may interfere with the production of active immunity. The disease is usually introduced to piggeries in carrier pigs. The virus survives best in the cold and disease is more common in cool conditions and in winter. Wind transmission to pigs kept partly outdoors may have occurred in France and some British outbreaks. Carrier pigs appear to have introduced the classical disease to Denmark, Japan, Italy and, possibly, the U.K. It appears that H1N1 occurs as a U.S. type (A/New Jersey/8/76/H1N1) and a European type in Europe. Oligonucleotide analysis has confirmed that some Swedish, Danish and Italian types, as well as those elsewhere in the world, are of U.S. origin.

The virus can persist on chilled meat for 8 days and in meat frozen at $-20^{o}C$ for 15 days, but there is no documented account of infected meat as a source of infection for herds.

Influenza may be carried by birds. Turkeys have been shown to be capable of carrying and transmitting the disease to pigs and vice versa. Influenza C in Japan and Germany occurs in dogs and influenzas in ducks are closely linked to pig disease in China and can carry H5N1 in many parts of the world..

Man may introduce clinical infections with H3N2 which result in disease in pigs. Cases of influenza of porcine origin have been demonstrated in piggery workers in Europe and the U.S. In one U.S. case, a human fatality was caused by H1N1 shown to be of pig origin by RNA fingerprinting. Others attending the same pig fair were infected and the disease spread to hospital staff.

Diagnosis

Clinical signs of a rapidly-spreading respiratory disease affecting all pigs in a herd which does not respond to antimicrobial treatment is suggestive of influenza. The chronic disease is less easily identifiable on clinical grounds. Infection may be confirmed by a rise in serum antibody in paired serum samples taken 3-4 weeks apart. Antibodies to the virus can be detected using the haemagglutination inhibition (HI) test, single radial immunodiffusion or virus neutralisation tests. A four-fold rise in HI titre is considered diagnostic. HINI and H3N2 antigens should both be used. ELISAs for all the common serotypes have been developed and tested and may be used to detect antibody if available. A blocking ELISA using a nucleoprotein monoclonal antibody has been described but still requires HI and N inhibition tests for typing. Specific antibody to H1 antigen may be detected as early as 3 days post infection in serum and IgA antibody may be present in nasal secretions after 4 days. Virus isolation from nasal or tonsillar swabs and lung samples is possible if samples are taken within 2-5 days of the onset of clinical signs and submitted in virological transport medium. Egg inoculation is the method of choice, but MDCK cells support growth after trypsinisation. Fluorescent antibody to H1N1 and H3N2 can be used on lungs and nasal cells to demonstrate virus and immunoperoxidase may be used on fixed sections. RT-PCR has been used to demonstrate the specific H and N genes and the matrix gene (for all serotypes) in multiplex tests and real-time RT-PCR has also been described. Pathology is often complicated by the presence of other diseases. Influenza must be distinguished from PRRS, porcine respiratory coronavirus infection and from Aujeszky's Disease in countries where these occur and in chronic disease or restricted outbreaks from pneumonic pasteurellosis, pleuropneumonia and chlamydial infection. It may be present together with other agents.

Treatment and Control

Vaccination with 2 doses of an oil adjuvanted vaccine 3 weeks apart has been used widely in Europe (not yet U.K.) to protect against both clinical disease and loss of production. Common vaccine strains such as A/Swine Ned/25/80 against European H1N1 viruses, A/Port Chalmers/1/73 against most H3N2 strains and A/Philippines/2/82 for protection against "Bangkok" H3N2 strains are frequently evaluated to confirm that they are still protective. Alum or Quil A adjuvanted subunit, DNA, recombinant vaccinia, adenovirus and live virus vaccines have been described. Intranasal vaccination appears to provide complete protection. Control within herds consists of symptomatic treatment and antimicrobial treatment of secondary bacterial infection. Disinfectants can be used to prevent introduction on fomites. Sero-negative herds should only introduce pigs from similar herds. Total eradication from enzootically-infected herds must be by depopulation and restocking.

References

Abusugura, I.A., Linne,T., Klingeborn, B. (1989). Analysis of some swine influenza H1N1 viruses by oligonucleotide fingerprinting. J.Vet.Med. B. **36**, 63-68.

Brown, I.H., Done, S., Hannam, D., Higgins, R.J., Machie, S.C., Courtenay, A. (1992). An outbreak of influenza in pigs. Vet.Rec. **130**, 166.

Brown, I.H., Harris, P.A., McCauley, J.W., Alexander, D.J. (1998). Multiple genetic reassortment of avian and human influenza viruses in European pigs resulting in the emergence of H1N2 virus of novel genotype. J.Gen. Virol. **79**, 2947 - 2955.

Brown, I.H., Ludwig, S, Olsen, C.W., Hannoun, C., Scholtissek, C., Hinshaw, V.S., Harris, P.A., McCauley, J.W., Strong, I., Alexander, D.J. (1997). Antigenic and genetic analysis of H1N1 influenza A viruses from European pigs. J.Gen. Virol. **78**, 553-562.

Brown, I.H., Manvell, R.J., Alexander, D.J., Chakraverty, P., Hinshaw, V.S., Webster, R.G. (1993). Swine influenza outbreaks in England due to a new H1N1 virus. Vet.Rec. **131**, 461-462.

Chambers, T.M., Hinshaw, V.S., Kawaoka, Y., Easterday, B.C., Webster, R.G. (1991). Influenza viral infection of swine in the U.S. 1988-89. Arch.Virol. **116**, 261-265.

Choi, Y.K., Goyal, S.M., Kang, S.W., Farnham, M.W., Joo, H.S. (2002). Detection and subtyping of swine influenza H1N1, H1N2 and H3N2 viruses in clinical samples using two multiplex RT-PCR assays. J.Virol Methods **102**, 53-59

Grosse Beilage, E., Schenk, L., Suss, J., Schrader, C. (1996). The influence of maternal antibody on the frequency, severity and serology of the infection with influenza virus. Proc IPVS **14**, 130.

Kaufman, J., Hassan, M. and 13 others (1988). Human infection with swine influenza virus - Wisconsin. J.Am.Med.Ass. **260**, 3116.

Lee, B.W., Bey, R.F., Baarsch, M.J., Larson, M.E. (1995). Class specific antibody response to influenza H1N1 infection in swine. Vet. Micro. **43**, 241-250.

Madec, F., Kaiser, C., Gourreau, J.M., Martinat-Botte, F. (1989). Consequences pathologiques d'un épisode grippal severe (virus swine A/H1/N1) dans les conditions naturelles chez la truie non immune en debut de gestation. Comp. Imm. Micro. and Inf.Dis. **12**, 17-27.

Nerome, K., Sakamoto, S. et al. (1983). The possible origin of H1N1 virus in the swine population of Japan and antigenic analysis of the isolates. J.Gen.Virol. **64**, 2611-2620.

Onno, M., Jestin, A., Vannier, P. and Kaiser, C. (1990). Diagnosis of swine influenza with an immunofluorescent technique using monoclonal antibodies. Vet.Quarterly **12**, 251-254.

Pritchard, G.C., Dick, I.G.C., Roberts, D.H., Wibberley, G. (1987). Porcine influenza outbreak in East Anglia due to influenza A virus (H3N2). Vet.Rec. **121**, 548.

Reeth, K. van, Gucht, S. van, Pensaert, M. (2003). Investigation of the efficacy of European H1N1 and H3N2-based swine influenza vaccines against the novel H1N2 subtypes. Vet Rec. **153**, 9-13

Reeth, K. van, Nauwynck, H., Pensaert, M. (2001). Clinical effects of experimental dual infections with PRRSV followed by swine influenza virus in conventional and colostrum-deprived pigs. J.Vet.Med. Series B **48**, 283-292

Roberts, D.H., Cartwright, S.F., Wibberley, G. (1987). Outbreaks of classical swine influenza in pigs in England in 1986. Vet.Rec. **121**, 53-55.

Romijn, P.C., Swallow, C. and Edwards, S. (1989). Survival of influenza virus in pig tissue after slaughter. Vet.Rec. **124**, 224.

Wells, D.L. and 6 authors (1991). Swine influenza virus infections: transmission from ill pigs to humans at a Wisconsin Agricultural Fair and subsequent probable person-to-person transmission. J.Am.Med.Ass. **265**, 478-481.

Paramyxovirus infection

Paramyxoviruses have been recorded from pigs in many parts of the world. They include Sendai virus, Parainfluenza 3 and the virus of 'Blue Eye', a rubula virus (resembling human mumps) which can cause encephalomyelitis and opacity of the eye in young pigs and stillbirths and infertility in adults and viruses associated with fruit bats such as Nipah virus and Menangle virus. They generally cause respiratory and central nervous system disease such as interstitial pneumonia and bronchioloitis and encephalitis with lymphocytic perivasculitis and diffuse gliosis.

Reference

Janke, B.H., Paul, P.S., Landgraf, J.G., Halbur, P.G., Huinker, C.D. (2001). Paramyxovirus infection in pigs with interstitial pneumonia and encephalitis in the United States. J.Vet Diagn.Invest. **13**, 428-433.

Rubula virus infection and 'Blue Eye'

Encephalomyelitis and corneal opacity associated with anterior uveitis have been recorded in young pigs 2-21 days of age in Mexico. The causal rubulavirus (La Piedad Michoacan Paramyxovirus, LPMV) also produces stillbirths, mummified piglets, returns to oestrus and orchitis. It is a paramyxovirus of 135-360nm, is usually spherical and is related most closely to SV5 and human mumps virus.The Haemagglutinating and Matrix genes have been sequenced and code for proteins of 63.3 kDa, and 41.6 kDa respectively. Other proteins, 59 kDa, 52 kDa, a nucleoprotein of 52 kDa and a large protein of 200 kDa have all been identified. The virus grows in Pig Kidney cells (PK15). CPE can be seen at 48 hours with cell rounding, death and syncytia. The virus haemagglutinates chicken, pig and human erythrocytes. Infectivity is destroyed by ether, formalin, beta propiolactone and heat for 4 hours at 56°C. There is no cross neutralisation with other paramyxoviruses.

Infection is oronasal and spreads to brain, lung and reproductive tract in pregnant sows (where it crosses the placenta to infect the foetuses) and to the male reproductive tract in boars. Infection appears to spread by retrograde transmission along nerves, particularly from the nasal mucosa to the olfactory lobes of the brain where virus levels are highest at 5 days post infection in piglets. Viraemia occurs from day 4 post infection, initially on erythrocytes and later in leucocytes. Antibody can be demonstrated from 8 days and peaks at 16 days post infection. Cellular immunity has also been demonstrated.

Affected piglets are usually 2-15 days old. Fever occurs suddenly and is accompanied by arching of the back, ataxia and rigidity. Conjunctivitis and corneal opacity may occur. Older piglets may develop listlessness and pneumonia. Ataxic piglets should be killed. Boars develop mild fever (40.5-41°C, 105-106°F), anorexia and apathy 2-3 days after infection and may develop corneal opacity and testicular changes such as epididymitis, atrophy and scrotal oedema after 10 days. Reproductive effects in the sow include the production of small litters and increased numbers of mummified pigs.

Encephalomyelitis is the most obvious pathological feature with some interstitial pneumonia, and corneal oedema occurs in 'Blue Eye'. Epidydimitis and orchitis may be identified in boars. Focal congestion and haemorrhage in the placenta and endometrium may be seen in sows, together with mummified foetuses. Virus may be identified in affected tissues (including the foetuses) by immunostaining.

The disease appears to be confined to central Mexico. 'Blue Eye' alone has been reported from Northern Ireland and, possibly, Czechoslovakia, but its relationship if any with the syndrome described here is unknown. Disease is maintained in continuous flow operations but is self-limiting in closed herds. The virus may be present in semen for up to 45 days after infection.

Diagnosis is based upon the clinical signs and the histological findings backed up by serology using HI and a blocking ELISA to LPMV haemagglutinin: neuraminidase glycoprotein. The virus is most easily isolated from brain (particularly olfactory bulb) 4-9 days post infection or from tonsil 3-9 days post infection on PK15 cells.

Control is based on isolation although a killed vaccine has been produced.

References

Allan, G.M., McNeilly, F., Walker, I., Linne, T., Moreno Lopez, J., Hernandez, P., Kennedy, S., Carrol, B.P., Herron, B., Foster, J.C., Adair, B. (1996). A sequential study of experimental porcine paramyxovirus (LPMV) infection of pigs: immunostaining of cryostat sections and virus isolation. J.Vet. Diagnostic Invest. 8, 405-413.

Hernandez Jauregui, P., Ramirez Mendoza, H., Mercado Garcia, C., Moreno-Lopez, D., Kennedy, S. (2004). Experimental porcine rubulavirus (La Piedad Michoacán Virus) infection in pregnant gilts. J.Comp. Path 130, 1-6.

McNeilly, F., Walker, I., Allan, G.M., Foster, J.C., Linne, T.,Merza, M., Hernandez, P., Kennedy, S., Adair, B. (1997). A comparative study on the use of virus and antibody detection techniques for the diagnosis of La Piedad Michoacan Paramyxovirus (LPMV) infection in pigs. J.Vet. Diagnostic Invest. 9, 3-9.

Moreno-Lopez, J., Correa-Giron, P., Martinez, A. and Ericsson, A. (1986). Characterisation of a paramyxovirus isolated from the brain of a piglet in Mexico. Arch.Virol 91, 221-231.

Stephano, H.A., Gay, G.M., Ramirez, T.C. (1988). Encephalomyelitis, reproductive failure and corneal opacity in pigs associated with a new paramyxovirus infection ('Blue Eye'). Vet.Rec. 122, 6-10

Sundquist, A., Berg, M., Hernandez-Jauregui, P., Linne, T., MorenoLopez, J. (1990). The structural proteins of a porcine paramyxovirus (LPMV). J.Gen. Virol. 71, 609-613.

Vizuet, A.O., Martinez, G.R., Carreon, N.R., Lopez, M.J.R., Pradal Roa, P., Mendoza, G.R., Hernandez, M.L. (1996). Experimental inoculation in Mexican Hairless boars with the paramyxovirus of the Blue Eye disease. Proc IPVS 14, 127.

Menangle Virus

A single outbreak of this rubulavirus (Paramyxoviridae) occurred in Australia in a large piggery. The virus has been sequenced and came from a fruit bat (Pteropus poliocephalus). It depressed reproductive performance from a farrowing rate of 80-82% to 63-78% and numbers of live born piglets decreased to fewer than 6 in some litters. Mummified foetuses, stillborn piglets with arthrogryposis and craniofacial deformities were produced and there were a few abortions. Degeneration of the brain and spinal cord was present and eosinophilic inclusion bodies were visible in neurones of the cerebrum and spinal cord of affected piglets, sometimes with a non-suppurative meningitis, myocarditis and hepatitis. Two piggery workers developed disease and seroconverted, so infection is transmissible to humans. Diagnosis should be based on history of exposure to fruit bats and the clinical signs of depression of reproductive performance coupled with the birth of affected piglets. It can be confirmed by passage of the virus on BHK12 cells after which the prominent vacuolation of cells and the development of syncytia appear. Virus neutralisation and detection of serum antibody confirm.

Eradication was carried out by serological testing followed by segregation of the uninfected stock, cleaning and prevention of access by fruitbats.

Reference

Love, R.J., Philbey, A.W., Kirkland, P.D., Ross, A.D., Davis, R.J., Morrissey, C., Daniels, P.W. **(2001)**. Reproductive Disease and congenital malformations in pigs caused by Menagle Virus. Aust.Vet.J. **79**, 192-206.

Nipah Virus.

Infection with two strains of this Henipavirus (Paramyxoviridae) was recorded as a cause of fatal respiratory disease in pigs in Malaysia during1999 and was responsible for a number of deaths in humans. There have been subsequent reports of seropositive animals outside the original affected area. To protect human life, a slaughter campaign was carried out.

The virus is a negative-stranded RNA virus varying in size but about 500nm in diameter and bearing surface spikes 10 nm long. The nucleocapsid has a distinctive herringbone pattern. The virus grows readily in Vero and BHK-21 cells to produce large plaques containing syncytia.

Pigs can be infected by the oronasal route and virus can be demonstrated in respiratory tract secretions, confirming this route of transmission from pig to pig. Affected weaner and grower pigs develop fever (> 40°C) and develop a harsh barking cough (described as the most characteristic clinical sign) and mouth breathing, particularly when disturbed. Hind limb weakness is followed by recumbency and thrashing. Head pressing, tetanic spasms and fits have been described in adults which may die suddenly.

There are few gross lesions although there may be pulmonary consolidation with froth in the trachea. Histological findings include pneumonia with syncytial cells, macrophages and neutrophils. Viral antigen can be demonstrated with tagged monoclonal antibodies in most parts of the respiratory tract. There is a non-suppurative meningitis.

The virus originates in Pteropid fruit bats but can be maintained in other species. Pigs were the major host in Malaysia and the disease was spread by pig movement, but dogs and cats can be infected. Humans in contact with pigs in Malaysia and

Singapore were affected and some died. Others seroconverted. The virus has been classified as Category 4, is Notifiable in the EU and is an OIE List A Disease.

Diagnosis was based on history of exposure, on the distinctive barking cough and neurological signs and confirmed by demonstration of the virus in tissues using tagged monoclonal antibody. Serology can be carried out using a solid phase blocking ELISA confirmed by serum neutralisation. Fixed plaque assays have been used to reduce risk.

Control was carried out by isolation followed by slaughter of pigs and species such as cats and dogs on infected farms. Goggles were found to be effective in protecting eradication teams.

Reference

Middleton, D.J., Westbury, H.A., Morrissy, C.J., Heide, B.M.van der, Russell, G.M., Braun, M.A., Hyatt, A.D. (2002). Experimental Nipah Virus Infection in pigs and cats. J. Comp. Path. **126**, 124-136.

Respiratory Syncytial Virus (Pneumovirus)

Antibody to this virus has been found using indirect immunofluorescence and human RSV in the early 1980s in the sera of Scottish slaughter pigs at levels which indicate that active infection had occurred. Similar findings were subsequently made in Northern Ireland in 1998 using bovine antigen. No clinical or pathological changes have yet been correlated with these. Virus established in the bronchi when hysterectomy-derived colostrum-deprived piglets were inoculated with human RSV, but lesions were confined to syncytia in the bronchiolar epithelium.

Reference

Allan, G.M., McNeilly, F., Walker, I.W., Young, J.A., Fee, S., Douglas, A.J., Adair, B.M. (1998). Serological evidence for pneumovirus infections in pigs. Vet. Rec. **142**, 8-12.

Pig Inclusion Body Rhinitis, Porcine Cytomegalovirus Infection (PCMV)

Definition

Infection with the porcine cytomegalovirus has been associated with rhinitis (Pig Inclusion Body Rhinitis, IBR, PIBR) and with lethal, generalised infection in very young pigs. It may cause disease in older animals in non-immune herds, crossing the placenta to cause an increase in embryonic and foetal mortality. It is a potential cause of failure in xenotransplantation

Incidence

Found worldwide and present in at least 90% of herds in Britain. The disease is usually identified when it enters a non-immune herd and may not be recognised in a given country until a clinical outbreak is investigated. Recently shown to be present in 41% herds in Iowa, US and 50% in Germany.

Aetiology

Porcine cytomegalovirus or porcine inclusion body rhinitis virus is a typical enveloped cytomegalovirus approximately 150 nm in diameter which can only be cultured with difficulty and which is most easily isolated by the culture of alveolar macrophages from 3-5 week old pigs. . It can be cultivated *in vitro* in these or porcine testis or fallopian tube cell lines. In alveolar macrophage cultures C.P.E. does not occur although infected cells enlarge and form basophilic intranuclear inclusions which may be demonstrated by immunofluorescence or Giemsa stains.

The virus is inactivated by chloroform and ether but other physicochemical properties have not been reported. All UK isolates appear to belong to one antigenic type, although serological differences have been found amongst recent isolates from Japan and sequence differences between isolates have now been identified.

Pathogenesis

Primary replication appears to be in the nasal mucous glands in non-immune piglets infected by the oronasal route, in neutrophils in the viraemic stage 14-16 days p.i. and finally in epithelial sites such as nasal mucosa, seminiferous and kidney tubules at 3 weeks of age. Virus may cross the placenta and infect the foetus during the viraemic stage at 14-21 days after infection in non-immune sows. Viral isolation from the nose at 14-21 days post infection (dpi) is followed at 30-35 dpi by isolation from the cervix. Virus takes 14-20 days to multiply in the foetus and cervical virus may be of foetal origin. Multiplication occurs in foetal leptomeninges, hepatic sinusoidal cells, peritoneal macrophages and periosteal cells. Embryonic death occurs in early gestation. Foetuses exposed late in gestation are born seronegative. Boars can excrete virus in urine and nasal secretions. Serum antibody responses develop but low levels of antibody may not prevent infection of the products of conception.

Clinical signs

Few clinical signs other than anorexia and pyrexia occur in pigs of more than 3 weeks of age in herds where the infection is enzootic. Where individual sows or whole herds are non-immune, pigs may be infected *in utero* or within 2 weeks of birth and may develop rhinitis, sneezing and respiratory distress. Mortality in an affected litter may reach 25%. Piglets may be born dead, die without clinical signs or be pale anaemic and oedematous in the generalised form of the disease. A reduction in growth rate frequently occurs. Disease may occur in recently-weaned pigs and be associated with anorexia, respiratory distress, conjunctivitis and copious nasal exudate. Severe disease in adults has been recorded when infection enters non-immune herds. Anorexia, fever, coughing and serous, purulent and haemorrhagic nasal discharge have been recorded. Stillbirths and mummified foetuses may result and there may be an increase in returns to service and of small litters. Severely affected piglets should be assessed and killed as soon as they can no longer rise.

Pathology

Gross lesions are rarely visible in animals with localised upper respiratory tract infection but may appear as severe nasal congestion of the nasal septum with adherent tenacious mucus. Histological examination reveals cytomegaly with basophilic intranuclear inclusions in cells of the nasal mucus glands and other epithelial sites such as duodenum and renal tubules. Affected glands may be surrounded by macrophages and lymphocytes. Generalised lesions in young pigs and foetuses may be seen in the lung where pulmonary oedema occurs, and serous effusions and widespread haemorrhages may be seen, particularly in the kidneys. Inclusions may be seen in reticuloendothelial cells in lymphoid tissue, in the leptomeninges and hepatic sinusoidal cells, peritoneal macrophages, penosteal cells and, rarely in alveolar macrophages. Growth arrests may be present in the long bones. In field outbreaks, lesions may sometimes be complicated by other agents.

Epidemiology

Enzootic in many herds, virus can cross the placenta and therefore occur in hysterectomy-derived herds. There appear to be no vectors and infection appears to survive in carrier pigs, being spread to unaffected herds by the introduction of infected pigs. Infection can spread by direct contact with urine or respiratory secretions or by aerosol. Virus is shed in nasal secretions mostly between 3 and 8 weeks of age. Infection may occur even up to slaughter weight and may be reactivated by stress and mixing. There appears to be little persistence outside the host. Pig organs used for xenotransplantation may be affected by the activation of latent virus.

Diagnosis

Serum antibody can be detected by indirect immuno-fluorescence or ELISA tests. The clinical signs must be distinguished from those of Bordetella infection and Progressive Atrophic Rhinitis in piglets. The presence of the inclusions in sections or smears from nasal mucosa confirms the presence of infection. In sows and neonates the lack of abortion and the relatively low mortality distinguishes the disease from Aujeszky's disease. Viral isolation can be carried out but with difficulty. PCR testing can demonstrate the virus in a wide range of tissues. Spleen is always infected and it is recommended that it is always tested in xenotransplantation.

Control and treatment

Secondary infection can be controlled e.g. using parenteral ceftiofur, and disease-free herds can be founded if hysterectomy-derived pigs are screened serologically for 70 days after birth. Where severe infection occurs, neonatal piglets should not be exposed to it. Gancyclovir and cidofovir are active against the virus and could be used in non-food animals.

References

Clark, D.A., Fryer, J.F.L., Tucker, A.W., McArdle, P.D., Hughes, A.E., Emery, V.C., Griffiths, P.D. (2003) Porcine cytomegalovirus in pigs being bred for xenograft organs: progress towards control. Xenotransplantation 10, 142-148

Edington, N., Plowright, W. and Watt, R.G. (1976). Generalised cytomegalic inclusion disease: distribution of cytomegalic cells and virus. J.Comp.Path. 86, 191-202.

Edington, N., Broad, S., Wrathall, A.E. and Done, J.T. (1988). Superinfection with PCMV initiating transplacental infection. Vet.Microbiol. 16, 189-193.

Edington, N., Wrathall, A.E. and Done, J.T. (1988). Porcine cytomegalovirus in early gestation. Vet.Microbiol. 17, 117-128.

Koon, K.J., Anderson, M.S., Zimmermann, J.J. (1998). Assessing the significance of porcine cytomegalovirus in respiratory disease of young swine. Proc. IPVS 15, 173.

Orr, J.P., Althouse, E., Dulac, G.C., Durham, P.J.K. (1988). Epizootic infection of a minimal disease swine herd with a herpesvirus. Can.Vet.J. 29, 40-53.

Solignac, T., Le Bris, E. (1996). Use of ceftiofur in two outbreaks of Inclusion Body Rhinitis (Porcine Cytomegalovirus) complicated by Pasteurella multocida in piglets. Proc IPVS 14, 666.

Reovirus

Reovirus has been isolated from a number of clinical syndromes including respiratory, enteric and nervous problems and from aborted foetuses in the U.K.

(Type 1). Type 2 has been recovered from the faeces of diarrhoeic and clinically-normal pigs in Japan. Type 3 has been recovered from respiratory disease and untyped virus from outbreaks of abortion and foetal and early neonatal death. Mild microscopic lesions including infiltration of the interalveolar septae by macrophages, lymphocytes and fibroblasts have been described following experimental infection. Infection with the 75nm icosahedral double-stranded RNA virus may be demonstrated by culture in primary pig kidney cell lines where they eventually form intracytoplasmic eosinophilic inclusions or by serological methods such as the haemagglutination inhibition test. Paired sera are necessary to confirm a diagnosis. Antibodies to Type 1 and Type 2 were found in 30-40% of pig sera in Britain in 1971. Fifty-seven per cent of herds were found to be infected. Type 1 virus was most common in S.W. England and W. Scotland and Type 2 in the E. Midlands and N. Scotland. Higher prevalences have been detected in Japan and Brazil where the development of antibody occurred between 2 and 3 months of age.

Reference

Fukutome, T., Sanekato, T., Akashi, H. (1996). Isolation of reovirus type 2 from diarrhoeal faeces of pigs. J.Vet. Med. Sci. **58**, 555-557.

Swine Pox

Definition

A mild infectious disease caused by the swine pox virus in which red, circular pox lesions appear on the skin of the belly, axillae, face and head in young pigs. Rare congenital infections are fatal within 24 hours of birth.

Incidence

Widespread but rarely reported. Clinical case reports often represent a formal declaration of its presence in an area. In a 1990 survey of 150 sera from 69 herds in the U.K., 19.3% sows in 28.9% herds were antibody-positive.

Aetiology

Caused by the swine pox virus, a large ether-sensitive (300-400 x 176-200nm) DNA virus of the swinepox group or in the past by Vaccinia virus. These viruses are extremely resistant to drying and may persist for years in exudates in which it can resist temperatures of 100°C for 10 minutes. Swine pox virus grows in pig kidney cell lines or on the chorioallantoic membranes of eggs to cause C.P.E. and intracytoplasmic inclusions. The genome of the virus has recently been sequenced and found to be of 146 kbp, code for around 150 genes and to be most closely related to capripox. The virus has been used as a vector for vaccines against swine fever and other diseases..

Pathogenesis

The virus enters locally via skin abrasions and multiplies there or attacks the skin after viraemia. The incubation period is 4-5 days from infection to the development of pustules and these last 10-14 days. All stages from vesicle, macule, pustule to ulcer may develop. Viraemia in sows results in the birth of congenitally-infected piglets. Serum neutralising antibody develops at 7 days, peaks at 20 days and has largely gone by 50 days post infection. Cellular immunity peaks at 11-21 days post infection.

Clinical signs

The incubation period is 3-6 days but may be up to 14 days and the lesions persist for 1-3 weeks. Slight pyrexia (to 40°CF, 104°F) may accompany the appearance of the lesions. Red 1 cm. papules appear on the ventral abdomen and rapidly form circular red brown scabs, which soon blacken. In young piglets the bursting of the vesicular stage on the face may lead to wetting, scab formation and conjunctivitis. Slight inappetence may accompany the development of the lesions. Affected pigs appear hairy and growth may be depressed. A large percentage of successive litters of sucking and recently-weaned pigs may be affected but the disease is rare in adults. Mortality is rare although transplacental infection in newborn pigs can cause deaths. Lesions may be seen on the edge of the tongue, lips and all over the body. Badly affected neonates may have to be killed, but all other age groups normally recover.

Pathology

The skin lesions are those of a typical pox virus. Nuclear vacuolation and cytoplasmic inclusions may be seen at the papular stage in the cells of the epidermis. A mild vesicular stage occurs but the pustular and crusting stages are most prominent. Secondary bacterial infections may occur.

Epidemiology and Occurrence

The disease is widespread but is rarely reported, occurring in successive litters of sucking pigs, often becoming less common in the winter. Because good immunity is produced, adults are rarely affected. The virus may persist in a farm for years between outbreaks in dust and dried secretions in unused pens and fittings. The progeny of newly purchased pigs are often affected as are weaned pigs from non-immune farms when mixed with carriers. Lice and flies may transmit the disease within a farm.

Diagnosis

The size and colour of the lesions is characteristic. Flank biting, "spirochaetal granuloma" and local infections with *Staphylococcus hyicus* may also resemble pig pox but the agents of these are usually demonstrable. Local lesions of PDNS do not usually form crusts. Electron microscopy or culture can confirm and differentiates from Orf.

Treatment and Control

Treatment or control are rarely attempted because of the mildness of the disease, but the use of insecticide to eliminate lice if present and the thorough cleaning and disinfection of pens in which outbreaks of the disease have occurred help to reduce the incidence. Vaccines have been produced experimentally but do not protect completely as fever may still occur on challenge.

References

Borst, G.H.A., Kimman, T.G., Gielkens, A.L.J., Kamp, J.S. van der (1990). Congenital swine pox. Vet.Rec. **127**, 61-63.

Gorg, S.K., Chandra, R., Roo, V.D.P. (1989). Swine Pox. Vet.Bull. **59**, 441-448.

Jubb, T.F., Ellis, T.M., Peet, R., Parkinson, J. (1992). Swine pox in Northern Western Australia. Aust.Vet.J. **69**, 99.

Paton, D.J., Brown, I.H., Fitton, J., Wrathall, A.E. (1990). Congenital pig pox: a case report. Vet.Rec. **127**, 104.

Williams, P.P., Hall, M.R., McFarland, M.D. (1989). Immunological responses of crossbred and inbred miniature pigs to swine pox virus. Vet.Immunol. Immunopath. **23**, 149-159.

The Porcine Reproductive and Respiratory Syndrome (PRRS)

(Porcine Epidemic Abortion and Respiratory Syndrome PEARS, Blue Ear)

Definition

A viral infection causing inappetance, laboured breathing, occasional fever, abortion and returns to service occurs in sows, accompanied by an increase in stillbirths and piglet mortality from birth to the early post-weaning stage. Respiratory distress, poor growth rates and increased mortality in weaned piglets are major features of the disease in chronically infected herds. Infection may be inapparent.

Incidence

The disease is widespread in most pig-rearing countries especially in North America, where it was first seen in the US in 1987 and in Europe where it was seen first in Germany in 1990, and in 1991 was recorded in The Netherlands, Spain, Belgium and UK (May 1991, Humberside). It was identified in France in 1992. It has been recorded in South America in Venezuela and is present in China, Korea, Taiwan, Thailand and Japan but is absent from Australia. In most of these infected countries, serological surveys suggest that over 50% of herds are infected. In all infected countries serologically negative herds exist.

Aetiology

PRRS is caused by an enveloped RNA virus 45-55 nm in diameter (62 nm negatively stained) with a 30-35 nm nucleocapsid. The genome is 15 kb and has been cloned and sequenced. PRRS virus is an arterivirus related to lactose dehydrogenase elevating virus of mice, equine arteritis virus and simian haemorrhagic virus. Sequence and antigenic analysis suggest that European (EU) isolates are closely related to the first isolate, the Lelystad virus (LV), with minor variations, but that US (VR 2332) and Canadian isolates are more distantly related to it (55-79%) and form a separate group (NA isolates). Several different genomic and antigenic variants have been described from North America and there are differences in pathogenicity amongst these isolates. The gene sequences and the proteins themselves are used in diagnosis. Six structural viral proteins have been identified, produced from open reading frames (ORF) 2-7. They are: a 15 kDa nucleocapsid (N) protein (ORF7); an 18 kDa membrane (M) protein (ORF6) and 4 glycosylated proteins (GPs), of which the major envelope (E) protein is of 25 kDa (ORF5, GP5), GP 4 (ORF4) is of 31-35 kDa, GP 3 (ORF3) is of 49-50 kDa and GP 2 (ORF2) is of 29-30 kDa. Serum neutralisation tests, PCR and monoclonal antibody panels can distinguish between US and European strains and also individual isolates.

The virus grows in the cytoplasm of cells, principally porcine alveolar macrophages but also in cell lines such as CL2621, MA 104 and MARC-145, budding into the smooth endoplasmic reticulum and accumulating within it. Infected cells such as macrophages may lyse within 12 hours but lysis and cytopathic effect do not occur in peripheral blood monocytes and some other permissive cells. Levels of >10^7 particles per ml can be produced by exocytosis. The virus has been shown to be stable at -70°C and -20°C, to persist for one month at +4°C, to be 93% inactivated and to be inactivated after 48 hours at 37°C and to persist less than 45 minutes at 56°C. Survival is reduced at pH 6.5 and by drying.

Pathogenesis

Infection is usually by the respiratory route or contact, although infection can follow insemination. Oral infection may require $10^{5.3}$ Tissue Culture Infectious Doses (TCID), nasal inoculation $10^{4.0}$ and parenteral infection only $10^{2.2}$. The virus multiplies in alveolar macrophages, peripheral monocytes, follicular dendritic cells, other elements of the reticuloendothelial system including microglia and testicular epithelial germ cells. Alveolar and other macrophages may be destroyed, have a shorter lifespan or be rendered less effective and the effects of cytokines (especially TNFα) give rise to vascular lesions including swelling of the endothelial cells of capillaries and veins allowing plasma proteins to leak into the tissue. Secondary damage may result in thrombosis or complete occlusion of vessels. Many features of the disease depend upon these properties of the virus. Viral antigen and nucleic acid may be found in a wide variety of other cell types (such as endothelial cells) but it may not multiply in them.

Following infection in gnotobiotic pigs, viraemia develops within 12-24 hours and virus can be demonstrated in both serum and monocytes, in tonsillar epithelium and macrophages, in bronchiolar epithelial cells, arteriolar endothelial cells and both alveolar and intravascular macrophages in the lung. There is a transient reduction in circulating white cells about four days post-infection and this affects neutrophils and lymphocytes. CD4, CD8 and B cells are all affected in lymph nodes within the first week of infection. Infection may result in interstitial pneumonitis, myocarditis, encephalitis, rhinitis, renal lesions, vasculitis and lymphoid necrosis within 14 days. Interstitial pneumonitis is accompanied by an absence of alveolar macrophages in weeks 2 and 3 post infection. The virus may penetrate the reproductive tract. In boars the virus occurs in macrophages within the bulbourethral glands, the testes, within testicular epithelial cells, spermatocytes, spermatids and infection results in giant cell formation and apoptosis. Virus and these cells are shed in the semen and infection can be transmitted to the sow in semen. Conception does not appear to be affected, but, following implantation, infection can lead to resorption and to mummification and stillbirths, particularly when transfer across the placenta occurs from 72 days and particularly between 85-91 days' gestation. Virus is present in lesions in both maternal and foetal placenta, and arteritis, myocarditis and encephalitis have been identified in foetuses although infection and antibody may be present in normal foetuses. Virus can be shed in mammary secretions. Infection in young piglets can lead to destruction of the alveolar macrophages rendering the lung susceptible to infection with bacteria such as *P.multocida*, *A.pleuropneumoniae*, *H.parasuis* and *Chlamydophila sp.*. An interstitial pneumonia develops associated with capillary damage.

Virus can be demonstrated by RT-PCR in serum for up to 210 days after birth in transplacentally-infected pigs, but viraemia more often lasts for 1-9 days in sows and up to 3-8, or even 12 weeks in young pigs and can continue in the presence of antibody. Throughout this period, virus is shed in nasal secretions and faeces. Virus persists in the tonsil for at least 105 days post infection.

IgM antibody can be demonstrated from 4 days and IgG antibody from 7-9 days onwards and may persist more than 20 weeks in some animals.

Clinical signs

These are at their most severe when infection enters a non-immune herd, but infection may be inapparent.

In sows, there is usually an inappetance lasting 24-36 hours - 4 days in individuals and 7-10 days in the herd. They may be listless, with laboured breathing but fever is not consistent, rarely exceeds 40°C and is transient, often lasting a single day. Abortion may occur at any stage of gestation, and is first apparent at 22 days, but most cases occur later. 2-3% of sows in a house may abort, many not even showing prior inappetance. There may be accompanying skin changes such as hyperaemia or congestion of the ears, nose and tail, but only 1-2% of animals develop these changes. Farrowing problems develop with a rise in stillbirths and increased mortality in piglets aged up to 1 week. This is partially due to premature farrowing (the herd gestation length may be reduced by two days). Lactation is affected in some sows and inappetance in lactation may lead to anoestrus. Returns to service may also occur although this may be partly attributed to boar fertility. A general rise in other diseases such as cystitis may be expected in stalled sows.

Boars may be listless and occasional animals develop blue ears. A drop in semen quality may occur but cannot be linked in every case to clinical signs.

In piglets, antenatal infection or effects on the sow may lead to antepartum deaths which result in large mummified piglets and an increase in stillbirths. Many of the piglets born are weak, may have splayleg and do not survive (up to 54% infected pilets may die). Affected piglets may have oedema of the eyelids which gives a spectacled appearance and there may be conjunctivitis. Bleeding from interference such as tail docking and tooth clipping is common and bruising may occur at iron injection and may be apparent as discolouration of the skin. Haemorrhage into the gut may lead to melaena and the appearance of a greyish diarrhoea. Laboured breathing may also be apparent. Occasional cases of meningitis have been reported.

In weaners and growers there is an increase in respiratory disease and skin changes may be seen in recovering pigs, 5-7 days after infection. An increase in any other disease endemic on the farm becomes apparent.

In the herd, the first 8 weeks of the disease are characterised by a rise in pre-weaning mortality (average 33%) and a dramatic rise in the number of stillbirths (average 18%). Later, mummified piglets appear and live births decrease (average reduction of 1.0 piglet/litter). Post-weaning mortality may increase (average 9%) and the number of treatments required increases markedly. In the second period of 6 weeks, there is an overall improvement but mummified piglets remain common and livebirths are still low. Returns to service increase (average 18%). Illness in piglets and weaned pigs remains common and numbers of treatments are still raised. In the third period, a drop in total births occurs as a result of continuing low numbers born and the increase in returns to service. A return to near normal levels of production can be expected 26 weeks after infection.

Annual levels of production may be affected as follows:

Returns to service	2.0% increase
Abortions	0.3% increase
Numbers born alive per littler	0.3% decrease
Stillbirths	2.7% increase
Piglet mortality	3.7% increase
Weaned pig mortality	1.1% increase

An overall loss of 2.54 pigs/sow/year may be expected and increases in the costs of feed medication may occur. Weight gain may be depressed during viraemia, and be made more severe by the presence of influenza infection.

Once infection becomes enzootic, clinical disease is restricted to non-immune animals exposed to the disease for the first time. These are usually non-immune gilts introduced to an infected herd, weaners and growers. The disease in weaners and growers appears as fever (to 41°C), weakness and occasional cyanosis and raised respiratory rates. Diseases present on the farm may develop 5-7 days after infection. In gnotobiotic pigs or on SPF farms there may be no clinical signs and weight gains may be unaffected.

Humane destruction may be indicated in sows with blue-ear in severe and prolonged distress, particularly if they begin to lose condition or develop subnormal temperatures. Piglets with respiratory distress, weakness or severe splayleg should be destroyed. Weaners rarely require euthanasia in uncomplicated disease, but severe and prolonged respiratory distress which does not respond to treatment would be an indication.

Pathology

Infected piglets may have no gross lesions. Stillborn piglets may have haemorrhagic areas 1-2 cm in length in the umbilical cord associated with necrotising arteritis. There may be extensive focal haemorrhage around bronchial buds and large bronchi, and myocarditis, arteritis and encephalitis may be present. In infections contracted after birth there may be skin haemorrhages and bruising with bleeding into tissues, particularly where interference has occurred. The most consistent change is pulmonary congestion or anterior lobe pneumonia appearing as tan discolouration of the cranial, middle and accessory lung lobes which are firm or rubbery, and excess pericardial or pleural fluid. Lymph nodes are enlarged. Interstitial pneumonia and type 2 pneumocyte proliferation are present with perivascular cuffing. Alveolar macrophages are absent. Tracheal and nasal lesions are rare and there is vacuolation and surface blebbing of the bronchiolar epithelium which may not be functional. Canadian cases have had a more severe proliferative necrotising pneumonia with lymphocytic rhinitis and perivascular cuffing. *Pneumocystis carinii* infection has been identified in some of these lesions. Necrotising pneumonia such as reported in Quebec is atypical and has not been reported in the UK. Lymph nodes are enlarged with necrotic lymphocytes, syncytia and spaces lined by giant cells. There may be myocarditis with myocardial foci of lymphocytes and the occasional brain lesions include lymphohistiocytic perivascular cuffing in both the grey and white matter. Renal lesions may be found in animals infected for more than 14 days. There is marked lymphohistiocytic interstitial nephritis with interstitial oedema especially in the medulla, focal mild non-suppurative periglomerular and peritubular infiltration in the renal cortices and vasculitis. The Porcine Dermatitis and Nephropathy Syndrome is commonly associated with PRRS.

All post-mortem findings may be complicated by the presence of disease normally present in the herd. Influenza, *M. hyopneumoniae*, porcine respiratory coronavirus, pleuropneumonia and *H.parasuis* infections are particularly important in the lungs and streptococcal meningitis and salmonellosis have also been recorded. Increases in enteric infections have also been reported.

Epidemiology

The disease spreads within a unit by direct contact between pigs and, to a lesser extent by aerosol although experiments suggest that the distances involved are normally short (+/- 1 metre) and that aerosol transmission is strain dependent.

Nasal secretions are the main source of infection but faeces may also be infective. Milk may contain virus for 1-2 days after infection. Serological studies have shown that infection may be confined to weaners and growers on a farm and that active infection may be absent from sows and sucking pigs. Infection tends to appear as maternal antibody levels fall (days 30-35 of age). Serology has also confirmed that spread amongst this age group is rapid and often complete within one or two weeks, and that antibody levels reach a peak at 6-12 weeks of age and are often declining by slaughter. Viraemia (and infectivity) may last for 8-12 weeks (and sometimes much less) in infected groups and pigs may be virus-free at slaughter. Congenitally-infected pigs may remain infected for up to 210 days, but more commonly, serum remains infective for 21 days, urine up to 14 days, tracheal secretions 35 days, saliva 42 days and oropharyngeal secretions for 84 days, although virus has been demonstrated in tonsillar scrapings up to 250 days after infection by RT-PCR. Sow to sow transmission has been demonstrated for up to 86 days. Semen has been shown to contain virus for up to 92 days.

Studies of the survival of the virus in the farm environment have used virus isolation, RT-PCR, nested RT-PCR and sentinel pigs. Outside the host the virus has been demonstrated to survive on fingernails (5 hours) human saliva and nasal washings (48 hours) does not survive for long on clothing, rubber boots, feed or bedding. It can only be demonstrated for a day in saliva, urine, faeces but survives longer in slurry (12 days, 4°C, more commonly 1-8 days), and water (up to 11 days). Insect vectors transmit the disease mechanically in their gut. Mosquitoes (*Aedes vexans*, North America) mechanically transmit virus by biting, and infection rapidly disappears from the surface of houseflies (*Musca domestica*) but can still be demonstrated in the gut (48h) An individual housefly can contain enough virus to initiate infection.

Spread within groups of gilts, sows or boars varies in its speed and completeness. Infected sows may In some cases the introduction of an infected animal may not result in the infection of a farm and some infected farms spontaneously become seronegative and virus-free. Infection can be transmitted at service and virus has been isolated from semen from 13 to 43 days in one study. Natural service and artificial insemination with infected semen have both been shown to result in infection of the sow. Infection at day 1 of gestation (service) may not always result in reproductive failure but infection at 30 days may lead to 20% litters being affected and the most severe effects are produced by infections at around 90 days gestation

The disease is most commonly spread between farms by the introduction of carrier pigs which may remain infected for at least 12 weeks. It may also move locally and clusters of related virus have been identified by sequencing viral isolates. Aerosol transmission has been suggested in spite of the difficulty in demonstrating spread by this means experimentally. Spread between farms appears to occur over at least 3 km and occasionally up to 20 km, usually in low ambient temperatures and high humidity on dull days. Studies of the persistence of virus on vehicles and boots in freezing conditions confirm these as a probable means of farm to farm transmission and infected flies have been found up to 1.7 km from infected sources. Semen produced by boars in the viraemic stage of infection is capable of introducing infection to non-immune herds. Birds such as mallard ducks and chickens have been shown to carry virus infective for pigs and shed it in their faeces. Their importance in spread between farms is unknown.

Serological surveys suggest that inapparent infections are common and, in a UK survey of 22 breeding herds and 10 feeding herds with no history of PRRS, 50% were found to be seropositive. The development of clinical signs may depend upon the virulence of the virus involved (North American virus may be more virulent), the number of pigs present on the unit, their density and the hygienic conditions.

Although PRRSV survives for up to 8 days in muscle, abattoir surveys have failed to recover it from meat and the virus appears not to pose a risk to human health.

Diagnosis

Clinical signs such as an increase in stillbirths to 20%, in abortions to 8% and in pre-weaning mortality to 26% should lead to suspicion of PRRS. Lesser levels of these parameters and the other clinical signs described above may also lead to suspicion. The development of respiratory disease which is difficult to control in weaners or growers may also be associated with PRRS infection. The presence of the disease may also be suspected at post-mortem examination. Anterior lobe lung lesions, lymphadenopathy and the presence of haemorrhages in the carcase may suggest the disease. Histological findings of the presence of an interstitial pneumonia and the absence of alveolar macrophages may also be noted. The presence of the virus in tissue may be confirmed by immunofluorescence or by immunoperoxidase using antibody to the p15 nucleocapsid protein (appears to react with all types) and by *in situ* hybridisation using DNA probes.

Virus isolation may be carried out on using porcine alveolar macrophages or one of the permissive cell lines such as CL2621. Cytopathogenic effects may be seen within 12 hours but not all isolates grow in both systems. Isolates should be further characterised as a number of other viruses may be isolated in this system. Lung tissue, porcine alveolar macrophages harvested directly by bronchoalveolar lavage and co-cultivated, tonsil (if biopsied, this requires analgesia), serum, buffy coat and lymph node may be used. Blood samples should not be taken in heparin which inhibits viral isolation and samples should be refrigerated or frozen for transport. Where vaccine virus is likely or novel variants are suspected, restriction fragment polymorphism and sequencing of ORF 5 and 6 may help to identify the type present.

Viral RNA may be demonstrated by RT-PCR and nested RT-PCR which may detect as few as 1-10 particles per ml. Lelystad and US primers may be required. Real time PCR (ReTi RT-PCR) has been used for quantitative estimates of viral load. Indirect ELISAs use monoclonal antibody for viral capture.

The detection of serum antibodies to the virus is the most commonly used way of confirming a diagnosis and may be used to construct serum profiles of infection in a herd and for disease monitoring. The most commonly used tests are:

ELISAs using cultured virus or recombinant proteins such as nucleocapsid (from ORF 7) (Lelystad and North American isolates may both be required as in HerdChek™PRRS , IDEXX)
Chromatic penside assay strips (Biosign™PRRSV) have also been described
Blocking ELISAs used to distinguish vaccine and wild-type antibodies
Immunoperoxidase monolayer assay (IPMA) is used less frequently than the ELISA but detects antibody from 7-14 days.
Indirect fluorescent antibody test (IFA) from 7-14 days peaking at 30-50 days.
Serum neutralising test (SNT) which is strain specific. It can therefore be less useful in confirmation but very useful in identifying antibody to individual strains of virus and is useful in chronic infection (up to 1 year).

Samples for serological testing can be taken from piglets at birth (precolostral antibody), 0-4 weeks of age (colostral antibody) and 10-12 weeks of age in enzootically-infected herds. Samples taken from slaughter pigs may be less satisfactory.

Other diseases which may need to be considered from a clinical point of view are Aujeszky's disease, African and Classical Swine Fever, Swine Influenza, Porcine Respiratory Coronavirus, Encephalomyocarditis, Porcine Parvovirus infection, Haemagglutinating Encephalomyelitis Virus infection, TGE, Porcine Epidemic

Diarrhoea, Talfan, *Chlamydophila psittaci*, erysipelas and leptospirosis. Serological testing will eliminate their involvement.

Treatment and control

There is no specific treatment but a series of measures have been recommended to reduce the economic and welfare impact of the disease:

1. Proved electrolytes for all weak/diarrhoeic pigs.
2. Delay iron injection to 3 days and tail docking to 3-5 days. Do not clip teeth.
3. Stop induced farrowings.
4. Give artificial colostrum to piglets at birth and 4 hours of age.
5. Treat sows with acetyl salicylic acid (aspirin) daily for 7 days prior to farrowing at 8g/sow/day by top dressing of feed for first 4-6 weeks of outbreak.
6. Do not serve sows until 21 days after farrowing regardless of the fate of the litter. Do not restore depleted litters to full size.
7. Sows weaned during the acute phase of the disease should be given high energy diets to reduce the effects of inappetance on reproductive performance.
8. Allow minimum of 21 days before re-service following abortion of litters of 70 days' gestation.
9. Re-serve immediately sows aborting earlier litters.
10. Check all sows for pregnancy weekly from 4-5 weeks' gestation onwards.
11. Supplement all services with A1 for 6 weeks from appearance of acute disease due to effects on semen quality.
12. Be prepared for the onset of disease in the feeding herd and treat as appropriate.
13. Maintain normal health procedures if possible.

Vaccination is possible in many countries using modified live virus vaccines. Vaccines generally contain either North American or European virus and the type of wild virus present should be established before use. Killed vaccines have been described. Protective programmes usually involve vaccination of gilts at arrival, or sows at service followed by a second vaccination 14 days later and a third at 70 days' gestation. Piglets may be vaccinated at 3 weeks of age or at 6 weeks. Vaccination does not prevent colonisation with wild-type virus and if given to pregnant sows for the first time late in gestation may result in clinical signs. Vaccination according to approved programmes reduces reproductive losses in breeding stock and production losses and disease in growing pigs. Vaccination may not prevent virus shedding in semen by boars. Vaccine virus has been shown to spread within a herd and should not be used in a previously uninfected herd or area. It may become virulent by recombination or reversion in some cases.

A number of systems for reducing and eliminating infection from herds have been devised. Serological profiles can be used to determine whether virus is actively circulating in a breeding herd, rearing accommodation or in growing and finishing accommodation. Active circulation of virus can be arrested by closing the sow herd to fresh breeding stock for some months or by a vaccination programme. If active circulation is not taking place in a breeding herd, the introduction of clean breeding stock can maintain freedom from infection and the removal of infected weaners from the site may allow infection to die out. More frequently, test and removal and partial depopulation policies are used to eliminate antibody positive animals and establish clean herds. Cleaning, removal of slurry, disinfection and three weeks' rest of the accommodation, followed by restocking, is essential for elimination of the infection. Ensuring that cleaned and disinfected equipment is dried is critical.

Continuous medication with antibacterials over the period of risk may reduce the economic effects. Regional schemes can be carried out by quarantine, partial or complete depopulation.

References

Albina, E., Baron, T. and Leforban, Y. (1992). Blue eared pig disease in Brittany. Vet.Rec. 130, 58-59.

Albina, E., Leforban, Y., Baron, T. and Duran, J.P. (1992). Blue eared pig disease in Brittany: a new test. . Vet.Rec. 130, 83-84.

Albina, E., Leforban, Y., Baron, T., Duran, J.P., Vannier, P. (1992). An ELISA for the detection of antibody to the PRRS virus. Annales de Recherche Veterinaires 23, 167-176.

Albina, E., Madec, F., Cariolet, R., Torrison, J. (1994). Immune response and persistence of the PRRS virus in infected pigs and farm units. Vet.Rec. 134, 567-573.

Amass, S.F., Stevenson, G.W., Anderson, C., Grote, L.A., Dowell, C., Vyverberg, B.D., Kanitz, C., Raglund, D. (2000). Investigation of people as mechanical vectors for PRRSV. Swine Health and Production 8, 161-166.

Anon (1992). Porcine reproductive and respiratory syndrome (PRRS or blue-eared pig disease). Vet.Rec. 130, 87-89.

Benfield, D.A. Nelson, E., Collins, J.E., Harris, L., Goyal, S.M., Robison, D., Christianson, W.T., Morrison, R.B., Gorcyca, D. and Chladek, D. (1992). Characterisation of swine infertility and respiratory syndrome (SIRS) virus (isolate ATCC VR2332). J.Vet.Diagn.Invest. 4, 127-133.

Beyer, J., Fichtner, D., Scirrmeier, H., Polster, U., Weiland, E., Wege, H. (2000). PRRSV (PRRSV): kinetics of infection in lymphatic organs and lung. J.Vet.Med. series B.47, 9-25.

Bureau, M., Dea, S., Sirard, M.A. (2005). Evaluation of virus decontamination techniques for porcine embryos produced in vitro. Theriogenology 63 2343-2355.

Christianson, W.T., Collins, J.E., Pijoan, C., Joo, H.S., Benfield, D.A., McCullough, S.J. (1991). Swine Infertility and Respiratory Syndrome. Pig Vet.J. 27, 9-12.

Christopher-Hennings, J., Holler, L.D., Benfield, D.A., Nelson, F.A. (2001). Detection and duration of PRRSV in semen, serum, peripheral blood mononuclear cells and tissues from Yorkshire, Hampshire and Landrace boars. J.Vet. Diagn Invest. 13, 133-142.

Cooper, V.L., Hesse, R.A., Doster, A.R. (1997). Renal lesions associated with experimental porcine reproductive and respiratory syndrome virus (PRRSV) infection. (1997) J. Vet. Diagn. Invest. 9, 198-201.

Dee, S.A., Joo, H.S. (1994). Prevention of the spread of PRCV in endemically infected herds by nursery depopulation. Vet.Rec. 135, 6-9.

Dee, S.A., Joo, H.S., Polson, D.D., Park, B.K., Pijoan, C., Molitor, T.W., Collins, J.E., King, V. (1997). Evaluation of the effects of nursery depopulation on the persistence of PRRSV and the productivity of 34 farms. Vet. Rec. 140, 247-248.

Dee, S.A., Martinez, B.C., Clanton, C. (2005). Survival and infectivity of PRRSV in swine lagoon effluent. Vet. Rec. 156, 56-57.

Dee, S.A., Molitor, T.W., Rossow, K.D. (2000). Epidemiological and diagnostic observations following the elimination of PRRSV from a breeding herd by a test and removal protocol Vet. Rec 146 211-213.

Done, S.H., Spencer, Y., Paton, D.J., Drew, T.W., Hannam, D., Higgins, R., Twiddy, N., Simmons, J.R., White, M.E.C. (1996). The pathology of natural infections with (porcine reproductive and respiratory virus (PRRSV) in the UK. Pig J. 36, 18-30.

Gordon, S.C. (1992). Effects of blue-eared pig disease on a breeding and fattening unit. Vet.Rec. 130, 513-514.

Horter, D.C., Pogranichniy, R.M., Chang, C.C., Evans, R.B., Yoon, K.J., Zimmerman, J.J. (2002). Characterisation of the carrier state in PRRSV infection. Vet. Micro. 86, 213-228.

Mengeling, W.L., Lager, K.M., Vorwald, A.C. (1994). Temporal characterisation of placental infection of porcine fetuses with PRRSV. Am. J. Vet. Res. 55, 1391-1398.

Morin, M. and Robinson, Y. (1991). Porcine reproductive and respiratory syndrome in Quebec. Vet.Rec. 129, 367-368.

Nielsen, J., Botner, A., Tingstedt, J.E., Aasted, B., Johnson, C.K., Riber, U., Lind, P. (2003). In utero infection with PRRSV modulates leucocyte subpopulations in peripheral blood and bronchoalveolar fluid of surviving piglets. Vet Immunol and Immunopath. 93, 135-151.

Paton, D.J., Brown, I.H., Scott, A.C., Done, S.H., Edwards, S. (1992). Isolation of a Lelystad virus-like agent from British pigs and scanning electron microscopy of infected macrophages. Vet.Microbiol. 33, 195-201.

Petry, D.B., Holl, J.W., Weber, J.S., Doster, A.R., Osorio, F.A., Johnson, R.K. (2005). Biological responses to PRSSV in pigs of two genetic populations. J.Anim. Sci. 83 1494-1502.

Robertson, I.B. (1992). Transmission of blue-eared pig disease. Vet.Rec. 130, 478-479.

Rossow, K.D. (1998). Porcine reproductive and respiratory syndrome. Vet. Path. 35, 1-20.
Rossow, K.D., Bautista, E.M., Goyal, S.M., Molitor, T.W., Murtaugh, M.P., Morrison, R.B., Benfield, D.A., Collins, J.E. (1994). Experimental PRRS virus infection in 1, 4 and 10 week-old pigs. J.Vet.Diagn. Invest. 6, 3-12.
Rossow, K.D., Benfield, D.A., Goyal, S.M., Nelson, E.A., Christopher-Hennings, J., Collins, J.E. (1996). Chronological immunohistochemical detection and localisation of porcine reproductive and respiratory syndrome virus in gnotobiotic pigs. Vet. Path. 33, 551-556.
Rowland, R.R.R., Lawson, S., Rossow, K., Benfield, D.A. (2003). Lymphoid tissue tropism of PRRSV replication during persistent infection of pigs originally exposed in utero. Vet Microbiol. 96 219-235.
Stevenson, G.W., Alsine, W.G. van, Kanitz, C.L. (1994). Characterisation of infection with endemic PRRS virus in a swine herd. J.Am.Vet.Med.Assn. 204, 1938-1942.
Swenson, S.L. and 10 other authors (1994). Excretion of PRRSV in semen after experimentally-induced infection in boars. J.Am.Vet.Med.Assn. 204, 1943-1948.
Wensvoort, G., Terpstra, C., Pol, J.M.A. (1991). Mystery Swine Disease in the Netherlands: the isolation of Lelystad virus. Vet.Quarterly. 13, 121-130.
Wills, R.W., Zimmerman, J.J., Swenson, S.L., Yoon K. J., Hill, H.T., Bundy, D.S., McGinley, M.J. (1997). Transmission of porcine reproductive and respiratory syndrome virus by direct, close or indirect contact. Swine Health and Production 5, 213-218.
Wills, R.W., Zimmerman, J.J., Yoon, K.J., Swenson, S.L., Hoffman, L.J., McGinley, M.J., Hill, H.T., Platt, K.B. (1997). Porcine reproductive and respiratory syndrome virus: routes of excretion. Vet. Micro. 57, 69-81.
Woensel, P. van., Wouw, J. van der, Visser, N. (1994). Detection of PRRSV by the polymerase chain reaction. J.Virol.Methods 47, 273-278.
Yoon, I.J., Joo, H.S., Christianson, W.T., Kim, H., Collins, J.E., Morrison, R.B., Dial, G.D. (1992). An indirect fluorescent antibody test for the detection of antibody to SIRS virus in swine sera. J.Vet.Diagn.Invest. 4, 144-147.
Zimmerman, J.J., Yoon, K.J., Pirtle, E.C., Wills, R.W., Sanderson, T.J., McGinley, M.J. (1997). Studies of porcine reproductive and respiratory syndrome virus (PRRSV) infection in avian species. Vet. Micro. 55, 329-336.

Porcine Circovirus (Postweaning Multisystemic Wasting Syndrome)

Definition

Infection with porcine circovirus Type 2 (PCV2) is present in weaned and growing pigs with the Postweaning Multisystemic Wasting Syndrome (PMWS) which can cause unthriftiness, pallor, rough hair coat, dyspnoea, jaundice, lymphadenopathy, diarrhoea and high mortality in naïve pigs. It can contribute to the Porcine Dermatitis and Nephropathy Syndrome (PDNS) and may be found in reproductive problems. Type 1 virus (PCV1) causes few if any clinical signs.

Incidence.

PMWS was first associated with PCV2 in Canada in 1996, since when infection with the virus has been identified in most countries and is widespread, although the syndrome has not been confirmed in Australia. Infection with PCV1 is widespread and it is common in pig tissue cultures.

Aetiology

Porcine circoviruses are small circular single-stranded DNA viruses 15-24nm which can grow in a wide range of porcine cell lines. There are two types known at present, PCV1 is related to plant circoviruses, is widespread and not associated with disease, while PCV2 differs from it in terms of DNA sequence (80% homology) and antigenicity. The PCV2 genome consists of 1767-1768 nucleotides with two open reading frames (ORF1 and ORF2). ORF 1 codes for a replicating enzyme and ORF 2 codes for a major structural protein of 30 kDa which self-assembles to produce capsid and which gives rise to antibody in infected pigs. Its nucleotide sequence has been used to study differences between isolates and produce recombinant proteins for diagnostic purposes. Minor differences in the sequence of ORF2 have identified subgroups of PCV2 in China and Canada, UK, and Western Europe. Some wild boar strains from Europe are of the Chinese subtype. The virus is stable at 70°C for 15 minutes and resists pH3 and inactivation by chloroform and ethanol.

Pathogenesis

The syndrome has been reproduced experimentally in gnotobiotic, colostrum - deprived and conventional pigs from unaffected herds using PCV2 alone. Infection with porcine parvovirus, PRRSV or reduced immune function appear to exacerbate the clinical signs. Infection is oronasal, although transplacental infection occurs. Infection with circovirus results in virus multiplication in a number of tissues, but the exact identity of those cells which permit multiplication is not yet clear, as virus antigen and DNA accumulates in many cells. RT-PCR for mRNAs is being used to resolve this. In the foetus, myocytes, hepatocytes and macrophages may be affected, while in older pigs dendritic cells retain viable, non-replicating virus for long periods. The lymphoid system is affected by increased cytokine expression (especially IL10) and reductions in lymphocyte numbers occur but not by apoptosis. The changes in the lymphocyte populations include an early reduction in B lymphocytes and CD4 T cells and CD8 cells in peripheral blood fall. Histiocytes replace lymphocytes in the lymph nodes. Viraemia develops and both virus and viral protein can be demonstrated in tissues. Clinical signs of PMWS appear at 10-14 days post infection when particle loads in tissue reach $10^{7.0}$ per ml, but do not do so at viral loads below $10^{5.0}$ per ml. This association of disease with particle load may explain the occurrence of infection in the absence of disease. Virus is shed in nasal secretions and faeces within 2 days of infection. Antibody can be demonstrated after 14 days. Passive immunity protects against clinical disease but not against infection. High levels of antibody appear to predispose to PDNS. Foetal infection at 57 days causes lesions more repeatably than infection later in gestation.

Clinical signs

Both epidemic and endemic forms have been reported. In non-immune herds, an increase in preweaning mortality (13%) may occur to give low numbers weaned (6.3), but the effects are seen mainly in weaned pigs, where disease is most obvious between weeks 6-8 and mortality peaks at week 9. Mortality rates of 64.3% have been recorded in affected recently-weaned pigs, up to 92.3% in those weaned for 4 weeks and up to 64.3% in growers but it does not affect finishers or adults. In immune herds, the first clinical signs appear at 42+/- 13.5 days, in the flat deck or early grower stage and may give rise to 6.5+/- 5.1% mortality. Affected pigs may be the progeny of naïve sows or those which have not ingested colostrum. In all cases, affected pigs are dull, unthrifty, may be fevered (to 41.7° C), may lose condition and waste, have dyspnoea, pallor, rough hair coat, jaundice, lymphadenopathy (most noticeable in the inguinal lymph nodes) and diarrhoea and may die after 2-8 days. There is a marked lymphopaenia. The clinical signs may not be present in all members of an affected group. Approximately 40 % of severely affected animals will recover completely but both they and unaffected members of the group may have reduced growth rates. Abortions and the birth of mummified piglets, stillborn pigs and small litters have been described but are not the norm.
As mortality rates are high in this disease, animals should be destroyed humanely as soon as they become too weak to feed or stand and assessment should be carried out at least twice daily, as disease progresses rapidly in its later stages.

Pathology

Variable degrees of wasting are seen, the skin may be pale, there may be icterus and there may be wasting of carcase muscle. The lungs do not collapse, there may be lobular mottling and a tan colour, particularly in the caudal lobes. All body lymph nodes are enlarged, firm, homogeneous in texture and whitish on the cut surfaces. The liver may be atrophic, pale, with white foci and the kidneys may be normal, have white foci or be enlarged, pale and oedematous with oedema of the renal pelvis. The spleen is often enlarged. Ulcers may be present in the pars oesophagea of the stomach and the wall may be slightly oedematous. There may be oedema around the pancreas, the small intestine is thin-walled, the contents watery and the caecum distended. There may be reddening of the caecal wall.

Histopathological changes are most prominent and consistent in the lymphoid tissues. Follicular B cells are rapidly replaced by histiocytes and multinucleate giant cells which may obliterate sinusoids and T cell regions. Inclusion bodies which are intensely basophilic and form grape-like clusters in the cytoplasm are common, especially in tonsils and Peyer's patches of the ileum. Liver lesions begin as lymphoid infiltrations of the periportal areas, then single cell necrosis of hepatocytes occurs and eventually progresses to widespread loss of hepatocytes. Mixed lymphocytic and eosinophilic interstitial nephritis with arteritis, phlebitis and lymphangitis occur in the kidney. There is a Johnes Disease-like villous atrophy and granulomatous enteritis in the intestines and necrosis of crypts and subsequent sloughing can occur with subsequent infiltration by monocytes. Acinar cell atrophy and loss of zymogen granules may occur in the pancreas and there may be non-suppurative myocarditis or cerebral meningitis. A diffuse interstitial pneumonia is present, and an unusual slow, progressive destruction and sloughing of the bronchial and bronchiolar epithelium can lead to marked bronchial stenosis in the final stages of the disease. Secondary bacterial infection is common. PCV2 can be demonstrated in histiocytes, giant cells and lymphoid tissues, usually as cytoplasmic inclusions, but in the nucleus of acinar cells of the pancreas and the liver cells by immunoperoxidase using polyclonal sera, and by in situ hybridisation. Stillborn piglets have cardiac hypertrophy, a severe fibrotic or necrotic myocarditis and passive congestion of the carcase and especially, the liver.

Epidemiology

PCV2 infection has been demonstrated in archived material from 1978 (Japan) and the 1980s (Europe, Canada) and it occurs in countries where PMWS has not yet occurred (Sweden in the 1990s, Australia). The spread of PMWS has, however, resembled that of an infectious disease, spreading from foci of infection. This fact and the requirement for additional infections or the suppression of immunity in experiments may indicate the involvement of some underlying initiator. Infected animals shed virus in nasal secretions, saliva and faeces within 1 day of infection and continue to do so for some weeks. The virus can be shed in semen from day 5 post infection for at least 47 days and can be found on eggs and supporting tissues harvested for embryo transfer. Infection is oronasal in most cases, but transplacental infection can occur. Venereal transmission cannot be ruled out.

Serious outbreaks of clinical PMWS occur after first introduction in non-immune herds, but within chronically-infected herds, piglets appear to be protected by maternal antibody until 10 weeks of age after which active infection appears to occur and antibody levels rise from 12 weeks of age to reach >80% by 20 weeks of age. Factors which appear genuinely to exacerbate or prolong the occurrence of severe clinical disease include those that reduce maternal antibody levels in piglets (naïve sows or gilts, poor colostral uptake in piglets), the presence of active circulating parvovirus, PRRSV and possibly, other infections and poor hygiene which increases virus challenge to young pigs as their protection wanes. The severity and duration of disease is usually least in SPF herds. The evidence that vaccination or immunostimulation predispose to or exacerbate clinical disease is equivocal. Vaccination against *M.hyopneumoniae* can reduce disease severity.

Infection is introduced to a herd by carrier pigs, but fomites could introduce infection and the importance of contaminated or infected semen is not yet clear. PCV Type 1 infections are widely distributed, but some herds are free from PCV Type 2 infections.

The Porcine Dermatitis and Nephropathy often occurs on farms where PCV2 infection is present and appears to develop in older pigs with high levels of antibody to PCV2.

Diagnosis

PMWS is suspected on clinical grounds, confirmed at farm level by post mortem examination and then confirmed in the laboratory by histopathology and demonstration of virus in the lesions. The presence of antibody can inform the veterinarian of the dynamics of infection in the herd.

Clinical signs suggesting PMWS include stunting/wasting, pallor, dyspnoea, enlarged inguinal lymph nodes and diarrhoea, coupled with high mortality rates (5-15% or more) in weaned pigs aged 6-13 weeks (depending on the health status of the herd). On farm confirmation is by post mortem findings of enlarged whitish, firm carcase lymph nodes, failure of the lungs to collapse, and their tan colour, particularly in the caudal lobes. The liver may be atrophic, pale, with white foci and the kidneys may be normal, have white foci or be enlarged, pale and oedematous with oedema of the renal pelvis. The post mortem findings do not occur in every pig, so 5-10 affected pigs may be required to reach a diagnosis on pathological grounds.

In the laboratory, diagnosis is confirmed by the presence of histiocytes and giant cells in lymphoid tissues, especially in tonsil and ileal Peyer's patches, the typical bronchiolar lesions and the presence of inclusion bodies. The presence of antigen of PCV type 2 in cells by immunoperoxidase using monoclonal antibodies particularly to peptides from ORF2 is supportive and viral DNA can be demonstrated in lesions by in situ hybridisation using a variety of probes. PCR of tissues confirms the presence of PCV2 in the animal but cannot be used alone to confirm diagnosis. Antibody may be demonstrated using an indirect immunofluorescence test using infected PK cells in multiwell plates, the IPMA assay or ELISAs using whole virus or capsid proteins from tissue culture or recombinant sources. The presence of antibody in foetal fluids is diagnostic.

Treatment and control

There is no treatment. Secondary infections should be controlled and individual animals can be removed from the herd and nursed as they may grow normally if they recover. This is not possible on any large scale and high mortality often persists under farm conditions until predisposing factors are addressed.

Where PMWS is absent, strict isolation should be practised. Semen or ova can be imported with appropriate safeguards such as hyaluronidase treatment of ova, but replacement breeding stock should be home-bred.

Short term measures which may reduce the severity of an outbreak include ensuring that all piglets receive colostrum, that all in, all out husbandry is practised and coupled with thorough cleaning and disinfection with an effective disinfectant such as Virkon S (Dupont). Strict hygiene between pens and houses is essential and other diseases present should be controlled by therapy or vaccination as appropriate. Mixing and movement should be reduced to a minimum. Delaying weaning and routine vaccinations have been reported to help in control. Feed quality to sucking and recently-weaned piglets may be improved. Feeding spray dried plasma has been found to be beneficial in countries where it is in use.

Longer term measures involve closing the herd to incoming susceptible gilts and ensuring that all gilts and sows are immune. This can be ensured by vaccination of sows and gilts using a killed vaccine where this is licensed. Colostral uptake must be ensured.

Herds free from PCV2 and PMWS can be derived by segregated early weaning, snatching or hysterectomy derivation, rearing in isolation in small groups and testing for freedom. These techniques are of potential use in xenotransplantation.

Isolation appears to have maintained some herds free from the disease.

References.

Allan, G.M. (1996). Porcine circoviruses: epidemiology and pathogenesis. (Pig J. **37**, 14-19.

Allan, G.M., McNeilly, F., Cassidy, J.P., Reilly, G.A.G., Adair, B., Ellis, W.A., McNulty, M.S. (1995). Pathogenesis of porcine circovirus: experimental infections of colostrum-deprived piglets and examination of pig foetal material. Vet. Micro. **44**, 49-64.

Allan, G.M., Meehan, B., Todd, D., Kennedy, S., McNeilly, F., Ellis, J., Clark, E.G., Harding, J., Espuna, E., Bother, A., Charreyre, C. (1998). Novel circoviruses from pigs with wasting disease syndromes. Vet. Rec. **142**, 467-468.

Clark, E.G., Harding, J.C.S. (1998). The pathology of post weaning multisystemic wasting syndrome. Proc IPVS **15**, (2) 212.

Harding, J.C.S., Clark, E.G., Strokappe, J.H., Willson, P.I., Ellis, J.A. (1998). Post weaning multisystemic wasting syndrome (PMWS): epidemiology and clinical presentation. Swine Health and Production **6**, 249-254

Kennedy, S., Allan, G.M., McNeilly, F., Adair, B., Hughes, A., Spillane, P. (1998). Porcine circovirus infection in Northern Ireland Vet. Rec. **142**, 495-496.

Le Cann, P., Albina, E., Madec, P., Canolet, R., Jestin, A. (1997). Piglet wasting disease. Vet Rec. **141**, 660.

Nayar, G.P.S., Hamel, A., Lin, L. (1997). Detection and characterisation of porcine circovirus associated with post weaning multisystemic wasting syndrome in pigs. Can. Vet. J. **38**, 385-386.

Opriessnig, T., Yu, S., Thacker, E.L., Halbur, P.G. (2004). Derivation of swine porcine circovirus type 2-negative pigs from positive breeding herds. J.Swine health and Production **12**, 186-191

Rosell, C., Segales, J., Plana-Duran, J., Balasch, M., Rodriguez-Arrioja, G.M., Kennedy, S., Allan, G.M., Meehan, B., Todd, D., Kennedy, S., McNeilly, F., Latimer, K.S., Domingo, M. (1999). Pathological, immunohistochemical, and in situ hybridisation studies of natural cases of post weaning multisystemic syndrome (PMWS) in pigs. J. Comp. Path. **120**, 59-78.

Royer, R.L., Nawagitgul, P., Halbur, P.G., Paul, P.S. (2001). Susceptibility of porcine circovirus type 2 to commercial and laboratory disinfectants. J. Swine Health and Production **9**, 281-284.

Sanchez, R.E. Jr., Nauwynck, H.J., McNeilly, F., Allan, G.M., Pensaert, M.B. (2001). Porcine circovirus 2 infection in swine foetuses inoculated at different stages of gestation. Vet. Micro. **83**, 169-176.

Aujeszky's Disease (Pseudorabies)

Definition

Aujeszky's disease is a herpes virus infection of pigs characterised by nervous and respiratory signs associated with a rise of temperature and often leading to death in young pigs. Infection in adults may be inapparent or associated with stillbirths or abortion.

Incidence

Once widespread in the United States and Europe, eradication campaigns have dramatically reduced ithe number of countries affected. It is present in South America and South East Asia and in some European countries. Aujeszky's disease occurred sporadically in Britain; 3 outbreaks occurred in 1970, rose to 12-20 p.a. and in 1982 43 outbreaks were recorded. 470 infected herds were found in 1983-84 when eradication began in Great Britain and by 1988 only 6 infected herds were recorded, some as serological reactors. Five were recorded in 1989 and eradication was then complete. The disease is still present in Ireland.

The disease has been eradicated from Denmark, Germany, Sweden, is absent from Switzerland, Australia and Canada and other parts of the world. Eradication campaigns in major pig-keeping countries such as the United States and The Netherlands have been successful. The use of effective vaccines makes the clinical disease uncommon in countries where it is present, but between 40% and 90% of farms may be infected in countries where eradication has not been attempted.

Aetiology

The causal agent of Aujeszky's disease is an alphaherpes virus, Suid herpesvirus I (SHVI), the complete enveloped particle of which has a diameter of 150-180nm. It may be cultivated in tissue cultures of porcine origin or in embryonated hens' eggs. Cowdry Type A intranuclear inclusion bodies are produced in tissue culture and *in vivo* and the C.P.E. produced in tissue culture is characterised by the formation of syncytia. The virus consists of a DNA core 75nm in diameter, a nucleocapsid of 105-110nm consisting of 162 capsomeres and an envelope bearing glycoproteins. The genes and proteins of Aujeszky's Disease Virus have recently been renamed. Earlier names are given in brackets. The glycoproteins include gG(gX), gD(gVI,gp50), gI(gp63), gE(gI), gB(gII), and gC(gIII). Other important viral proteins include the thymidine kinase (TK) and nucleocapsid proteins. The genes for these proteins have been identified, sequenced, cloned from two parts of the genome, the short (US) part e.g. gE,US8 and the long (UL) part e.g. TK,UL13 and used to produce recombinant proteins, primers for the polymerase chain reaction (PCR) and probes. Cell penetration appears to be associated with gE(gI), gB(gII) and gD(gp50), cell fusion with gE(gI) and gD(gp50) and central nervous system spread with gE(gI). Monoclonal antibodies have been used to study epitopes on the proteins and for diagnostic tests. Restriction endonuclease fragment analysis has been used on the whole genome to sub-divide Aujeszky's Disease Virus into RF types. Molecular biology has been vital in the development of new vaccines, diagnostic tests, control measures and epidemiology and additional information appears below.

Only one major antigenic type of the virus is recognised, but strains of virus producing predominantly nervous lesions and others producing predominantly pneumonic lesions have been described. Other biological differences include a few entirely genital strains and some isolates which do not produce syncytia in tissue culture. The virus is ether sensitive and is readily inactivated by heat (30 minutes exposure to 57°C). It is stable between pH 6 and 11 at 23°C when suspended in tissue culture fluid. Low concentrations of disinfectant e.g. 2% lysol and 5.25% sodium hypochlorite will inactivate it as will formaldehyde and detergents. Disinfectants combining surfactants and other agents are particularly useful.

Pathogenesis

Infection with Aujeszky's disease virus occurs via the epithelium of the upper respiratory tract and multiplication of the virus in this site is followed by invasion of the central nervous system and by passage of the virus along the course of the olfactory, trigeminal and glossopharyngeal nerves to the medulla and pons. Venereal infection can localise in the sacral ganglia. A non-suppurative meningo-encephalitis and myelitis is produced. Strains of the virus found in Northern Ireland and Central Europe also produce pneumonia. Local multiplication in the upper respiratory tract also occurs. Viraemia may accompany the invasion of the C.N.S. or lungs and give rise to lesions elsewhere in the body, but viraemia is not essential to the production of the clinical signs of the disease. Virus is shed in nasal and respiratory tract secretions. 10^{10} tissue culture infectious doses may be present per ml of nasal secretion. Infected alveolar macrophages are less effective as phagocytes and lymphocyte lysis and focal necrosis in lymph nodes depress the immune response. Invasion of the uterus, maternal and foetal placentas and foetuses occurs and can cause abortion, foetal death, mummification and foetal resorption if it occurs in the first half of gestation, and mummification in some cases in the last third. The virus can be adsorbed onto the zona pellucida of embryos and can infect recipient sows in embryo transfer. Infection of the genital tract may occur in boars and virus may be shed in the semen for up to 10 days. Virus shedding from animals infected by any route may occur between 2 days post-infection and continue until 10-14 days post-infection in most cases and exceptionally until 19-20 days. Latent infections commonly develop. Virus can be demonstrated by co-cultivation, PCR and labelled DNA probe in trigeminal ganglia and other areas of the brain for up to 7 months after infection and, following immunosuppression using corticosteroids for up to 18-19 months. Immunosuppression, whether artificial or natural by means of stress can be followed by a period of virus shedding for 4-11 days after the event. Latent virus may be present in nervous tissue only as viral DNA sequences. Up to 30 copies of viral genome may be present in infected cells. Restriction endonuclease techniques and in situ hybridisation confirm its identity and that of re-isolated virus with initial infecting virus. Recovered animals develop both humoral and cellular immunity. The humoral response can be demonstrated by day 8 post exposure at titres of 1:2-1:4 and rises to 1:128 or 1:512 at which level it remains for some weeks. IgM, IgG1 and IgG2 antibodies are most important in quantity and for protection but an IgA response has been demonstrated in the nasal mucosa. Cellular immunity develops by day 7-14 post infection and persists for up to 170 days post infection. Colostral antibody levels may be double or treble those in maternal serum and piglet serum levels are the same as those in colostrum by 1 day post partum. Maternal antibody cannot be demonstrated by 14 weeks post partum. The presence of neutralising antibody may not prevent colonisation of the nasopharynx, the development of viraemia on challenge or the development of microscopic lesions and cellular immunity may not prevent colonisation of the nasal epithelium.

Clinical signs

The clinical signs of Aujeszky's disease differ according to the infectious dose and the age of the animals affected. They are most severe in pigs aged 0-4 weeks in which morbidity and mortality may reach 100% in newborn animals declining to 40-60% in 4 week-old animals. Animals aged between 1 and 5 months are less severely affected (mortality up to 15%) and in adults the disease may produce few clinical signs.

Piglets newborn - 4 weeks of age

Clinical signs begin 3-7 days after infection in natural outbreaks and affected piglets may vomit or show diarrhoea and then become depressed, with trembling, incoordination (including circling), the adoption of a dog-sitting position, spasms of opisthotonus and prostration followed by death after at least 12 hours. Body temperature rarely exceeds 41.5°C, 107°F. The course of the disease is longer in older piglets and it may be accompanied by constipation. Mortality is less common in older piglets and death takes longer from the onset of clinical signs. Skin lesions resembling those of human cold sores may be present on the snout, lips and face.

Weaned pigs 4 weeks - 5 months of age

Clinical signs begin 5-7 days after infection with a rise in temperature to 40.6-41.7°C, 105-107°F, which may continue for 4-8 days. Anorexia with occasional vomiting occurs within 3 days of the onset of fever and is accompanied from the 4th day by nervous signs which begin with tremor and incoordination, in particular of the hind limbs, and progress to tonoclonic spasms of various muscle groups and to convulsions which may last only 45 seconds. These nervous signs are usually followed by prostration and death. The course of the disease usually takes 4-8 days from the onset of clinical signs. Finishing periods may be extended by 10-14 days. In outbreaks in Northern Ireland, and in growing and finishing pigs elsewhere, severe pneumonia has been recorded in addition to the nervous signs described above.

Adults

Infection may be asymptomatic or consist only of anorexia but is usually followed by a rise in temperature accompanied by coughing, salivation and other upper respiratory signs, anorexia, constipation and depression which may lead to recovery after 4-5 days or, rarely, to central nervous involvement and death (2%). Up to 50% of affected pregnant animals abort or give birth to mummified or macerated foetuses. Reproductive failure may follow these abortions or the early weaning consequent upon death of a litter. Boars may be affected and semen quality may decline from 10-14 days post-infection for a period of 1-2 weeks. Some sperm abnormalities may occur.

Humane endpoint: Animals which are ataxic or undergoing convulsions should be killed as should those with acute respiratory distress.

Pathological findings

Gross changes

Few gross changes are seen. There may be small haemorrhages and congestion of lymph nodes and petechiation of the kidney cortex. Where nervous involvement has occurred, there may be congestion of the meninges and excess cerebrospinal fluid may be present. Congestion of the nasal mucosa with necrotic foci and pulmonary oedema are common. Necrotic foci on the tonsil are a common finding and give it a "speckled" or white appearance. In the pneumonic form, large areas of the apical and cardiac lobes of the lung were consolidated and dark red with oedema of the interlobular septa. Necrotic foci in liver and small intestine may also occur, particularly in young piglets. Lesions in boars include changes in the seminiferous tubules of the testis and local lesions in the prepuce and penis. Aborted foetuses may have scattered 2-3 mm yellow-white necrotic foci in liver, spleen and lung. The placenta is often grossly normal, but necrotic lesions may be present. There may be mild endometritis and the wall of the uterus may be thickened and oedematous.

Histological findings

The major histological lesions occur in the C.N.S. and consist of a diffuse, non-suppurative meningoencephalitis which is most intense in the cerebral and cerebellar cortices. Neuronal necrosis, glial cell degeneration and lymphocytic accumulation occur about the blood vessels. Intranuclear inclusion bodies of the Cowdry Type A variety are rarely found in nervous tissue, but may be present in necrotic areas in tongue, muscle, adrenal or tonsil. Widespread necrosis with necrotising bronchitis, bronchiolitis and alveolitis and the exudation of fibrin were found in the pneumonic variant. In one study, infected cells in pulmonary necrotic foci were characterised by a thickened nuclear membrane and an amphophilic ground-glass appearance to the nucleus. Lymphoid hyperplasia, haemorrhages and intranuclear inclusions may be found in lymph nodes. In aborted foetuses, foci of coagulation necrosis may be seen in the liver and spleen. Inclusion bodies may be present in cells at the edges of the lesion. Necrotic lesions may also be found in the placenta and inclusion bodies may be seen.

Epidemiology

The disease is important in densely-stocked areas, particularly where rapid expansion of the pig population and unrestricted movement occurs between herds. The widespread use of vaccination in many countries has made the epidemiology of the disease difficult to monitor by conventional means and the presence of infection with wild type virus can only be followed where the vaccine types used can be complemented by an appropriate ELISA system e.g., gE(gI), TK deleted vaccine and gE(gI) ELISA.

Spread within a herd occurs by direct oronasal contact with affected animals, carriers or those shedding virus from reactivated latent infections, at service or during artificial insemination and by vertical transmission. Infected pigs produce large quantities of virus in nasal secretions and where these exceed 10^3 TCD50/100 mg mucus, aerosols are generated and spread the virus within the unit. Indirect spread within the unit may be by aerosol, by survival on concrete, clothing, soil, in slurry, in flies and other animal species such as birds (pigeons) mice, rats and sheep.

Spread within a unit depends upon its immune status and the nature of the introduction. Single serological reactors may not spread the virus, but those with latent infections often do (3/4 in one study). Widespread clinical disease may be followed by little or no disease for 2-3 years. Active disease may be restricted to a particular house or age group (e.g. finishers) and infection may die out in herds with fewer than 200 sows. Risk factor analysis suggests that high herd sizes, breeder-finisher units, indoor housing and density of the pig population all predispose to transmission and that low age at weaning, all-in-all-out housing reduce it. Vaccine use has affected the epidemiology, but wild-type virus persists in herds where replacement breeding stock are home produced or where vaccination of finishers is inadequate.

Spread between units or areas, or after depopulation may, in order of importance, be by -

1)   the introduction of carrier pigs - shedding virus for 7-14 days after clinical recovery or latently-infected for up to 170 days (exceptionally to 19 months)
2)   travelling boars and semen from affected animals. Unwashed embryos have caused seroconversion in recipient sows.

3)   aerosol for short distances of up to 2 km. Distances of 17 km overland and 60-70 km over water have been recorded (maximum halflife of 43 minutes at 4°C and 55% relative humidity).

4)   fomites on which infection persists (clothing, feed, straw and in faeces) for 2-4 days at 25°C, longer at 4°C, long enough to allow transmission between units.

5)   ivectors such as rodents (rats and mice) carnivores such as cats, dogs and foxes, sheep and cattle which cannot infect others of their species but may infect pigs, birds such as pigeons and flies which may carry the virus for up to 6 hours at 20°C.

6)   wild boar or feral pigs which may represent a reservoir of domestic pig virus (Poland, US) or a circulating adapted virus (Hawaii, Florida) spread chiefly by venereal means. Adults are most frequently antibody positive.

7)   survival in buildings which may remain infective for 4-7 weeks. Infection persists in animals (see above) on soil, fixtures and fittings, feed, straw, in slurry for 3-4 weeks and, potentially in the carcases of dead animals in cold conditions.

8)   in meat products. This is unlikely as the virus dies out within 35 days even when frozen at -18°C and does not survive processing for swill or meat and bone meal.

Risk to man. Transient seroconversions have been recorded but virus has not been re-isolated.

Diagnosis

Abortion, neonatal deaths, nervous signs in piglets and coughing and listlessness in finishing pigs spreading through a non-immune herd should suggest Aujeszky's Disease. Clinical signs may be slight or undetectable in vaccinated, partially immune herds or those with breeding herds or finishers only. Pruritis and death in other species in contact may be of value in reaching a diagnosis in pigs and death in farm cats and dogs, cattle or sheep is a common early sign. Where eradication has been completed in domestic pigs, these may result from wild boar contact. Gross pathological findings may be of little use in diagnosis but the presence of necrotic tonsils or a necrotic nasal septum and turbinates may indicate Aujeszky's disease. The presence of the characteristic intranuclear inclusion bodies is diagnostic, but they may be found in histological sections of less than half the field cases examined. Laboratory confirmation may be obtained using a fluorescent antibody test to detect the presence of virus in the tonsil, olfactory bulb or pons. Tissue should be frozen. Virus can be demonstrated in fixed tissue using immunoperoxidase with monoclonal antibodies directed against antigens present in wild type and/or vaccine viruses. Radio- or digoxigenin-labelled DNA probes directed against individual genes , in situ hybridisation and PCR may also be used in fixed tissue or tissue samples such as nasal swabs, brain or tonsil.

Virus can be isolated from the brain, spleen and lung of acutely-affected pigs. Material should be refrigerated or frozen at -70°C. Virus isolates may be subjected to monoclonal antibody panels, gene probes or restriction endonuclease fragment analysis and this information may be used to confirm whether an isolate is wild or vaccine type and may be of value in deciding its origin.

Serological testing is the most widely used method of identifying infected herds or recovered animals and meat juice can also be used. Virus neutralisation, complement fixation and gel diffusion tests, latex agglutination tests and ELISAs may be used on wild-type virus infections. To distinguish wild-type antibody from antibody from deletion mutants vaccines, ELISAs using recombinant proteins made in baculoviruses (e.g. gE), blocking ELISAs using monoclonals or indirect ELISAs can also be used. Commercial ELISA kits are available for use with most recombinant or deletion vaccines. Significant levels of antibody are determined for each test using positive and negative control sera.

Control

No treatment is possible at present. In some countries, prophylactic administration of hyper-immune serum may be given to piglets less than 4 weeks old.

Vaccination

Killed whole virus vaccines

A number of adjuvanted killed virus vaccines have been produced and have been used in many parts of the world. They may be prepared from wild type virus or from gene-deleted virus. Oil adjuvanted vaccines are intended for sows and may give protection for a year to the sow and to her litters for up to 9-10 weeks. A double injection 4 weeks apart may be necessary for initial immunisation. Finishing pigs may be vaccinated using alum adjuvanted vaccines.

Subunit vaccines

Subunit vaccines have been shown to be effective experimentally and in the field. They have been prepared from viral envelopes from both wild type and gE (gI)-deleted virus. Baculovirus recombinant protein gE (gI), gB (gII), gC (gIII) and gp50 subunit vaccines have all been prepared and have been given conventionally and intradermally. New adjuvants such as ISCOMS have been used.

Live vaccines

The original live vaccines were produced by attenuation in tissue culture or other host species and have been widely used (e.g. Bartha K61). More recently, a series of gene-deleted mutants have been produced. Thymidine kinase (TK) and gE(gI) deletion mutants have been used and a number of other combinations (TK⁻gC (gIII)⁻, TK⁻, gE (gI)⁻, gC (gIII)⁻) have been described. Some live vaccines have been found to be more effective if emulsified in oil. Live vaccines may be given parenterally or intranasally and, experimentally, by aerosol. Most vaccination programmes use live gene deleted vaccines.

Recombinant vectored vaccines

Vaccinia virus recombinants expressing gD (gp50), gB (gII) and gC (gIII) alone or together have been prepared and shown to be effective in pigs. Adenoviruses incorporating gD (gp50) have also been prepared. Neither type of vaccine is yet available commercially.

DNA vaccines

Plasmids containing gD (gp50) genes have been given by intramuscular injection and produce long-lasting immunity with antibody class switching. Not available commercially.

Vaccination is an effective means of protecting a herd against the economic consequences of Aujeszky's Disease infection. All vaccines are considered to be effective if they prevent reduction in weight gain in the face of challenge with wild type virus, prevent mortality and prevent reproductive loss. Few, if any, vaccines prevent infection by wild type virus, its colonisation of the nasal mucosa and the development of latent infections, but they reduce the period of viral shedding and its level, and have a similar effect on reactivated latent infections, often by preventing full nervous system colonisation.

Protection of the sow requires repeated vaccination, usually three times annually. Successful protection has been afforded by vaccinating the whole sow herd at the same time. All vaccines and natural infection in the sow give rise to maternal immunity in the piglet. This maternal immunity lasts for a variable length of time, from 9-10 weeks and sometimes to 14 weeks. Its presence in neonates, sucking piglets and weaners interferes with vaccination and live vaccines may have to be given on 3 successive occasions, at 10, 14 and 27 weeks in order to ensure that protective immunity of weaned animals lasts until slaughter. Vaccination with live vaccines at 4 and 10 weeks has been found to protect when vaccinal antibody is present, but not when wild-type antibody is present. This problem can be overcome by intranasal vaccination at 4 weeks followed by intramuscular vaccination at 10 weeks. Killed adjuvanted vaccines, DNA vaccines, and vector vaccines have been shown experimentally to improve the response to the first vaccination, but there is no general agreement on reliable protection.

Serum profiling

Serum antibody levels can be plotted against age in a farm or within a single building in order to identify the most economic point for administering vaccine. A single dose of live vaccine administered when maternal antibody has disappeared and prior to the rise in active antibody, may be sufficient for control. Serum profiling should be repeated annually.

Recombination

Live virus vaccines may recombine with others or with wild type virus and revert. Genes from other herpesviruses may be incorporated.

Distinction between vaccinal virus infection and wild type virus infection

ELISAs prepared with antigens missing from the vaccine in use can detect antibody to wild type virus and the two types of virus may be distinguished in tissue or in culture by the use of probes, PCR or restriction endonuclease fragment length polymorphism (RFLP). Reagents may be chosen with regard to the deletions present in the vaccine used in a herd or region.

(a) The Slaughter of positive herds and repopulation. This expensive option was used in Great Britain and, subsequently in Denmark. In Great Britain, the disease was made notifiable under the Aujeszky's Disease Order 1979 and the movement of affected pigs controlled under the Aujeszky's Disease of Swine Order 1982. A producer funded eradication campaign began in March 1983 and was substantially complete by September 1983 with 447 herds slaughtered and compensation paid. The campaign was carried out in stages: Phase 1, herds positive between May 1982 and March 1983, Phase 2, those positive between August 1979 and May 1982 and, finally, Phase 3, those prior to August 1979. Infected herds were slaughtered and normal animals sent for human consumption. Movement and neighbourhood tracing and 2 km (or later, 5 km) patrols examined nearby farms. A national serum survey and a survey of culled sow sera has continued and was extended to boars in 1988. 470 herds were slaughtered in the first year (to March 1984). Subsequently herds with 10+ reactors or active infection were slaughtered, but where less than 10 reactors were found with no subsequent transmission only the reactors were slaughtered.

Seven infected herds were identified in 1989 and slaughter or partial slaughter was carried out. Since that time Great Britain has remained free from Aujszky's Disease. A total of 523 herds was found to be infected, of which 82 were treated by removal of reactors and the remainder slaughtered completely. 440,190 pigs were slaughtered and the whole exercise cost £37,490,000 at 1995 prices.

In Denmark the disease reappeared as a result of aerosol spread from Schleswig Holstein. The risk of further recrudescence was reduced by vaccination in the border zone but the German eradication has now eliminated this risk.

b)   Test and removal.   The removal of all pigs which are seropositive from a herd has been shown to reduce the incidence of seroconversion and clinical disease and some serologically negative herds have resulted. Danish, British and US results suggest that this approach works, particularly in herds with low seroprevalence or in small herds..

c)   Isolation. Isolation of herds appears to be a satisfactory method of control although spread by aerosol or vectors may occur. In infected small herds (50 sows or less) the disease may die out once isolation is practised. It is unlikely to be successful in herds of 200 sows.

d)   All-in, all-out husbandry. This technique may prevent infection if piglets are weaned at 10-20 days and reared in isolation (contrary to legal commitments to EU welfare codes). This is particularly useful for the reduction of disease in finishing pigs.

e)   Early weaning to different sites. This increases the effects of early weaning.

f)   Vaccination alone. Northern Ireland, US, French and Belgian experience suggests that herds may become seronegative after continued vaccination. This does not occur in every case and does not appear to apply to herds with more than 200 sows. U.S. experience suggests that vaccination in the early stages of an outbreak, coupled with the removal of clinically-affected pigs, may succeed.

g)   Vaccination with serological testing and removal of pigs infected by wild virus can eliminate infection and is in use in a number of European countries and the US. This policy depends upon the widespread use of a single gene deleted (usually live) vaccine in an area and the use of complementary ELISAs for wild type antigens such as gE (gl) when gE (gl) deleted vaccines are in use. All pigs in the herd are vaccinated. Pigs with antibody to wild type virus are removed. Movement from infected farms can only be to slaughter. It is the method of choice in current control and eradication programmes.

h)   Vaccination and hysterectomy. Successful eradication from infected herds has been reported following the production of piglets by caesarian, hysterectomy or even snatching from vaccinated sows and rearing on separate premises. (g) is cheaper and easier.

i) Washing embryos. Genetic transfer may be carried out from infected herds by washing harvested embryos with an intact zona pellucida in 0.25% trypsin to remove any adsorbed virus.

Supportive measures

The success of all these measures presupposes a supply of clean breeding stock for repopulation (such as the nucleus herds of the UK breeding companies in the 1980s) and the removal of infection by disinfecting buildings and slurry (by adding lime at 30 kg per m^3 of slurry to give a pH of 11.5 or by heat treating at 62°C for 3 minutes) if depopulation is practised.. The entry of pigs should be monitored and quarantine practised. Entry of potentially infected personnel or vehicles should be prevented and clean units should be sited outside the range of aerosol transmission of the virus if at all possible.

References

Banks, M. and Cartwright, S. (1983). Comparison and evaluation of four serological tests for detection of antibodies to Aujeszky's Disease virus. Vet. Rec. 113, 38-41.

Banks, M. (1993). DNA restriction fragment length polymorphism among British isolates of Aujeszky's Disease Virus: use of the PCR to discriminate amongst strains. Br.Vet.J. 149, 155-163.

Basinger, D. (1990). The politico-economic aspects of Aujeszky's Disease control in Great Britain from 1955-1989. Pig Vet J. 24, 102-121

Beran, G.W. (1993). Understanding the transmission of pseudorabies virus (Aujeszky's virus). Vet.Med. 88, 70-79.

Botner, A. (1991). Survival of Aujeszky's Disease virus in slurry at various temperatures. Vet.Microbiol. 29, 225-235.

Bourgueil, E., Hutot, E., Cariolot, R., Vannier, P.(1992) Air sampling procedures for evaluation of viral excetion level by vaccinated pigs infected with Aujeszky's Disease (pseudorabies) virus. Res.Vet.Sci. 52, 182-186.

Brown, T.T. (1981). Laboratory evaluation of selected disinfectants as virucidal agents against porcine parvovirus, pseudorabies virus and transmissible gastroenteritis virus. Am.J.Vet.Res. 41, 1033-1036.

Brown, T.T., Shin, K.O., Fuller, F.J. (1995). Detection of pseudorabies viral DNA in tonsillar epithelial cells of latently-infected pigs. Am.J.Vet. Res. 56, 587-594.

Christensen, L.S., Mousing, J., Mortenson, S., Sorenson, K.J., Strandbygaard, S.B., Henriksen, C.A., Andersen, J.B. (1990). Evidence of long-distance airborne transmission of Aujeszky's Disease (pseudorabies) virus. Vet. Rec. 127, 471-474.

Christensen, L.S. (1988). Comparison by restriction fragment pattern analysis and molecular characterisation of some European isolates of Suid herpesvirus I : a contribution to strain differentiation of European isolates. Arch.Virol. 102, 39-47.

Donaldson, A.I., Wardley, R.C., Martin, S. and Harkness, J.W. (1984). Influence of vaccination on Aujeszkys Disease: virus and disease transmission. in Yorkshire 1981-82: the possibility of airborne disease spread. Vet. Rec. 115,121-124.

Fischer,L., Barza, S., Andreoni, C. Buisson, N., Brun, A., Audonnet, J.C. (2003). DNA vaccination of neonatal piglets in the face of maternal immunity induces humoral immunity and protection against virulent pseudorabies virus challenge. Vaccine 21, 1732-1741.

Gerdts, V., Jons, A., Makoschey, B., Visser, N., Mettenleiter, T.C. (1997). Protection of pigs against Aujeszky's Disease by DNA vaccination. J.Gen. Virol. 78, 2139-2146.

Gloster, J., Donaldson, A.I. and Hough, M.N. (1984). Analysis of a series of outbreaks of Aujeszky's Disease. Vet. Rec. 114, 234-239.

Harris, D.L. (1992). Producing pseudorabies-free swine breeding stock from an infected herd. Vet. Med. 87, 166-170.

Henderson, L.M., Levings, R.L., Davis, A.J., Sturtz, D.R. (1991). Recombination of pseudorabies virus vaccine strains. Am.J.Vet.Res. 52, 820-825.

Hoblet, K.H., Miller, G.Y., Bartter, N.G. (1987). Economic assessment of a pseudorabies epizootic breeding herd removal/repopulation and downtime in a commercial swine herd.). J.Am.Vet.Med.Assn. 190, 405-409.

Kit, S. (1990). Genetically engineered vaccines for the control of Aujeszky's Disease (Pseudorabies). Vaccine 8, 420-424.

McCullough, S.J. and Todd, D. (1988). Subclinical Aujeszky's disease virus infection a a pig herd and characterisation of the strain of virus isolated. Vet.Rec. 122, 77-81

82

Maes, R.K., Kanits, C.L., Gustafson, D. (1983). Shedding patterns in swine of virulent and attenuated pseudorabies virus. Am.J.Vet.Res. 44, 2083-2086.
Martin, S., Wardley, R.C. (1987). Local humoral and cellular responses in Aujeszky's disease virus infections in pigs. Res.Vet.Sci. 42, 170-174.
Medveczky, I., Solti, L., Haraszti, J., Ronay, G., Ekes, K., Belak, S., Tury, E., Seregi, J., Varga, J. (1996). Transmission of Aujeszky's Disease (Pseudorabies) virus is blocked by trypsin treatment of transferred embryos. Theriogenology 46, 1357-1365.
Mengeling, W.L. (1989). Latent infection and subsequent activation of pseudorabies virus in swine exposed to pseudorabies virus while nursing immune dams. Am.J.Vet.Res. 50, 1658-1664.
Mengeling, W.L., Brockmeier, S.L., Lager, K.M., Vorwald, A.C. (1997). The role of biotechnologically-engineered vaccines and diagnostics in pseudorabies (Aujeszky's Disease) eradication strategies. Vet. Micro. 55, 49-60.
Mellencamp, M.W., Pfeiffer, N.E., Sutter, B.T., Harness, J.R., Beckenhauter, W.H. (1989). Identification of pseudorabies virus-exposed swine with a gI glycoprotein enzyme-linked immunosorbent assay. J.Clin.Micro. 27, 2208-2213.
Miry, C., Pensaert, M.B. (1989). Sites of virus replication in the genital organs of boars inoculated in the vacum vaginale with pseudorabies virus. Am.J.Vet.Res. 50, 345-348.
Nes, A.van, DeJong, M.C.M., Verheijden, J.H.M. (1998). Experimental quantification of transmission of pseudorabies virus in conventional finishing pigs. Proc. IPVS 15, 180.
Oirschot, J.T. van. (Ed.) (1988). Vaccination and Control of Aujeszky's Disease, Dordrecht, Netherlands, Kluyver Academic Publishers.
Oirschot, J.T. van., Waal, C.A.H. de., (1987). An ELISA to distinguish between Aujeszky's disease vaccinated and infected pigs.). Vet.Rec. 121, 305-306.
Oirschot, J.T. van, Wismuller, J.M., Waal, C.A.H. de., Lith, P.M. van (1990). A novel concept for the control of Aujeszky's Disease: experiences in two vaccinated pig herds. Vet.Rec. 126, 159-163.
Paul, S., Mengeling, W.L., Pirtle, E.E. (1982). Differentiation of pseudorabies (Aujeszky's disease) virus by restriction endonuclease analysis. Arch.Virol. 73, 193-198.
Poitier, M.F.Le, Fournier, A., Houdayer, C., Hutch, E., Auvigne, V., Hery, D, Sanaa, M., Toma, S.B. (1998). Use of muscle exudates for the detection of antigE antibodies to Aujeszky's Disease virus. Vet.Rec.143, 385-387.
Riviere, M., Tartaglia, J., Perkus, M.E., Norton, E.K., Bongermino, C.M., Lacoste, F., Duret, C., Desmettre, P., Paoletti, E. (1992). Protection of mice and swine from pseudorabies virus conferred by vaccinia virus based recombinants. J.Virol. 66, 3424-3434.
Romero, C.H., Meade, P.N., Homer, B., Shultz, J.E., Lollis, G. (2003). Potential sites of virus latency associated with indigenous peudorabies viruses in feral swine. J.Wildlife Dis. 39, 567-575.
Rziha, H.J., Mittenleiter, T.C., Ohlinger, V., Wittmann, G. (1986). Herpesvirus (pseudorabies virus) latency in swine: occurrence and physical state of viral DNA in neural tissues.). Virology 155, 600-613.
Schoenbaum, M.A., Beran, G.W., Murphy, D.P. (1990). Pseudorabies virus latency and reactivation in vaccinated swine. Am.J.Vet.Res. 51, 334-338.
White, A.K., Ciacci-Zanella, J., Galestra, J., Ele, S., Osorio, F.A. (1996). Comparison of the abilities of serologic tests to test pseudorabies-infected pigs during the latent phase of infection. Am. J. Vet. Res. 57, 608-611.
Wittman, G. and Hall, S.A., Eds, 'Aujeszky's Disease' A seminar in the Animal Pathology Series of the E.E.C. Programme of Co-ordination of Agricultural Research held at Tubingen, Federal Republic of Germany, June 9-10, 1981. Martinus Nijhoff the Hague Netherlands (1982).
Wittmann, G., Ohlinger, V. and Rziha, H.J. (1983). Occurrence and reactivation of latent Aujeszky's disease virus following challenge in previously vaccinated pigs. Arch.Virol. 75, 29-41.
Zimmerman, J.J., Hallam, J.A., Beran, G.W. (1989). The cost of eradicating pseudorabies from swine herds in Iowa. Prev.Vet.Med. 7, 187-189.

Classical Swine Fever (Hog Cholera)

Definition

Classical Swine Fever (CSF) or Hog Cholera (HC) is a highly contagious viral disease of pigs characterised clinically by rapid spread, fever, high morbidity and mortality in a susceptible herd and by characteristic haemorrhagic lesions at post mortem. Chronic and mild forms of the disease exist.

Incidence

Swine fever is a notifiable disease in the EU, US, Canada, Australia and many other areas of the world (OIE List A). It was eradicated from Britain in 1966.

Since then, small outbreaks of swine fever have occurred in Britain in 1971, 1986, 1987 and 2000 (16 herds in East Anglia). The United States, Canada and Australia are free from the disease. The EU countries are officially free from the disease but outbreaks have occurred in several countries in recent years. Austria, Greece, Denmark, Sweden, Finland, Ireland, Portugal, France and UK are free from disease, but Germany has suffered repeated outbreaks, 4 (1996) 46 (1997) as has Italy 49 (1996), 55 (1997), The Netherlands was affected by a major outbreak of German origin in 1997 (424 herds) which overflowed into Belgium (8 outbreaks) and Spain suffered 78 outbreaks. Ten million pigs were slaughtered in the Dutch outbreak and direct costs reached 2 billion euro and indirect costs another 2 billion. Wild boar are a source of infection in Germany and other Central European countries. The disease is still present in South East Asia, Latin America and China.

Aetiology

Swine fever is caused by an ether-sensitive RNA virus belonging to the Pestivirus subgroup of the Flavoviridae. The virus varies in size but is mostly 40-50 nm in diameter with a 29 nm cubic nucleocapsid and spikes 8 9 nm in length on the envelope. The RNA genome is 12 kilobases in size and has been sequenced. Genes for a number of proteins have been identified and cloned. Important protein constituents of the virus include envelope glycoproteins of 33 kDa (E1), 55 kDa (E2) and 44-48 kDa and a number of core proteins of 36 kDa, 23 kDa and 14 kDa. The genome can now be distinguished from those of related pestiviruses, Bovine Viral Diarrhoea Virus (BVDV) and Border Disease Virus (BDV) which can cause mild disease in pigs and which are covered here. It multiplies in cell cultures prepared from pig tissues (including leucocyte cultures) but the vast majority of strains do so without producing C.P.E. It can persist in cell cultures.

Swine fever virus is acid resistant (pH 5) and relatively heat stable. One hour at 66°C is required for total inactivation of the virus in blood, but it survives in frozen pork for at least 1,500 days and in chilled meat and in carcases preserved by pickling, salting or smoking for 3-6 months or more. It can survive in Parma ham for 313 days.

Exposure of hams to 70°C for 1 minute and 65°C for 90 minutes eliminates virus. The bone marrow is frequently the site of persistence. In conditions where putrefaction occurs, the virus is rapidly destroyed and rarely survives for more than 2 days in faeces or infected pens at 37-65°C but may survive for 4 weeks in winter. Use of Antigen ELISA and RT-nPCR show that antigen and RNA may persist for longer, especially in carcase organs where it can be demonstrated for at least 28 days. It is rapidly destroyed by 2% sodium hydroxide, ether, chloroform or bile and at pH 3.

Swine fever virus occurs as a single major antigenic type although minor differences in antigens have been recorded. Monoclonal antibody typing systems suggested that at least three major groups, 5 subgroups and individual ungrouped isolates exist. More recent analysis of the sequences of the E2 and other genes confirm this. Isolates have been shown to differ in pathogenicity for pigs and to share a soluble antigen with BVDV to a varying extent. Swine fever virus can replicate in sheep and cattle although it does not produce clinical signs and BVDV can infect pregnant sows and may initiate antibody response. Swine fever virus isolates of high pig pathogenicity seem to be less closely related to BVDV than those of low pathogenicity. Border disease virus may also infect pigs.

Pathogenesis

The virus enters the body through the upper digestive tract or through the upper respiratory tract. It appears to be taken up by macrophages and reaches local lymph nodes, e.g. the tonsils and the pharyngeal and submandibular lymph nodes in which it multiplies. Twenty four hours after the initial multiplication, a transient viraemia occurs during which the virus becomes localised in the endothelial cells of the blood vessels and lymphatics. It reaches parenchymatous organs after 3-4 days. A secondary viraemia follows 5-6 days after infection as the clinical signs develop and the virus reaches its peak titre in the blood on the 7th day after infection. The pathological findings are related to the fact that the virus primarily attacks (1) the endothelial cells of small blood vessels and (2) reticuloendothelial cells. The blood vessels become occluded by proliferation of the vascular endothelium. The gross and microscopic changes are produced by a combination of direct infection and cytokine release from infected monocytes and endothelial cells (IL 1, 6 and 8) and the persistence of the virus is partly explicable by its ability to block some defences.

Virus spreads to epithelial surfaces such as salivary gland and bladder where it is shed. It reaches the testis where the spermatogonia are infected and from which virus can be shed in semen. It reaches the ovary, but does not appear to infect the follicle. Infection is followed by a rise in antibody levels but may also be accompanied by widespread depletion of the lymphoid system and effects on body defences such as those of the lung and intestine. The sequence of lymphoid cell depletion is still being elucidated. Virus may cross the placenta in pregnant sows and lead to abortion, the birth of pigs with persistent viraemia (up to 90 days) and no antibody. Foetuses infected after 65-67 days' gestation may develop antibody, be aborted or born with haemorrhagic lesions or become mummified.

Clinical signs

Acute, chronic and mild forms of swine fever occur in countries where the disease is enzootic, and, although outbreaks in swine-fever-free countries are usually of the classic, acute type, outbreaks in susceptible pigs in Australia and the US have been caused by low virulence virus which has produced less striking clinical signs. Some recent European outbreaks have been difficult to identify by their clinical signs and infection in adults and wild boar may be mild. The disease has an incubation period of 5-10 days (range 2-30 days) after which the following signs may be observed:

Hyperacute disease. One or two young pigs may be found dead and others may show signs of the acute type when examined.

Acute disease. Affected animals are dull, lethargic, anorexic and show fever of 40.5-41.5°C, 105-107°F at first. These signs are followed by conjunctivitis, in which the eyelids may be stuck together by exudate, and constipation followed by diarrhoea with occasional vomiting. The animals often huddle in piles in the bedding, walk reluctantly with a swaying movement of the hindquarters and may seek the support of walls or posts. Erythema and blotching of the skin and dyspnoea occur and may be present until death. Nervous signs, in particular, convulsions, occur early in the disease and are followed by circling, incoordination and ataxia. Death normally occurs within 4-8 days of infection in hyperacute cases, 9-19 days in acute cases and in some cases a chronic disease may occur in which death occurs between 30 and 95 days after onset. Emaciation, with blotching and necrosis of the ears may occur. Adult sows may abort in the acute stage of the disease, foetal resorption may occur, or weak and trembling piglets may be born (Congenital Tremor Type A1 Myoclonia Congenita).

Leucopaenia is a prominent finding and levels as low as 3-9,000/µl may be found (normal >18,000) within 2-6 days of infection.

Chronic disease. Few clinical signs may be observed. Fever may appear within 4-5 days of infection and persist accompanied by leucopaenia. Temporary recovery may be followed by death in 30-95 days. In some infected herds individual affected litters may be the only clinical signs of infection. Pigs may remain carriers

Low virulence virus. Infections often resemble chronic disease but may be less severe. Transient pyrexia and inappetence with no clinical signs other than leucopaenia may occur. Posterior ataxia has been recorded 4 months after birth in pigs born to sows infected with low virulence virus. There may be reproductive signs such as abortion and the birth of mummified or stillborn piglets.

Humane slaughter of affected animals should be carried out as soon as diagnostic criteria have been met.

Pathological findings

Gross lesions

In hyperacute cases there may be no gross lesions, but in acute cases the skin may be reddened and haemorrhages may be widespread. Enlarged haemorrhagic "strawberry" lymph nodes are commonly found, in particular in those of the pharyngeal, submandibular and abdominal regions. The haemorrhage is distributed peripherally in the nodes. Petechiation and ecchymoses are found in the kidney (80% of cases) as the "turkey egg" kidney (also seen in other septicaemic conditions), in the skin (50%) and in the bladder and lung (30%).

Infarction of the spleen occurs in 20% of cases and is due to thrombosis of small end-arteries in the spleen and ischaemia of the areas supplied. "Button ulcers", circular ulcers 1-2 cm in diameter with a necrotic centre are commonly found in the proximal portion of the colon but can occur elsewhere in the intestine. They result from damage to mucosal arteries with infarction distal to the occluded, damaged part and occur later in the disease.

In chronic or persistent infections, atrophy of the thymus and general lymphoid atrophy are common. Adrenal cortical hyperplasia and chronic rib lesions with a band of calcification proximal to the costochondral junction are present.

Cerebellar hypoplasia may be present in newborn trembling pigs (see Congenital Tremor Type AI or Myoclonia Congenita).

The basic lesions are the hydropic degeneration and proliferation of the vascular endothelial cells leading to occlusion of blood vessels. A marked non-suppurative encephalitis is present in most cases.

Epidemiology

Infection takes place as a result of the ingestion of virus-contaminated feed or litter or through abrasions, but can be venereal and follow artificial insemination. Virus is present in all body secretions, especially in the urine, and close contact between infected and susceptible pigs is necessary for transmission to occur. It is present in all tissues of affected pigs and ingestion of meat or other tissues frequently results in infection. Virus may be present in semen from 5-11 days post infection and possibly longer (RT-PCR data). Animals housed in pens separated by pig-proof partitions may remain uninfected during outbreaks of the disease on a farm, although aerosol transmission over short distances within piggeries has now been demonstrated.

Transmission between farms is normally by:-

1. The purchase of infected pigs direct from an infected farm. A number of recent European outbreaks have resulted from the purchase of such animals.

2. Direct contact between infected and susceptible pigs at markets or in transport

3. Feeding improperly boiled swill containing infected pork products (1971 and 1986 UK outbreaks). In some cases infected meat has been fed to pigs, particularly in the 1993 outbreaks and 1996/7 Paderborn outbreak in Germany. The survival time of the virus in some meat products is given above. Studies suggest that virus may survive for up to 5 months in meat fragments in silage and that such material is not safe until 9 months after production.

4. The purchase of infected pregnant sows. These may show few clinical signs of the disease after recovery, but the virus may cross the placenta and the resulting litter may show "trembling" or myoclonia congenita and may excrete virulent virus for up to 56 days after birth. Horizontal transmission amongst the offspring appears to result in seroconversion but not clinical disease because of maternal immunity. Low virulence virus may persist as a viraemia but does not appear to be shed under these circumstances.

5. Indirect transfer. This mechanism of spread is relatively unimportant and includes the use of contaminated vaccines, sera, semen or embryos. One outbreak in Belgium was traced to a veterinarian and spread in this way is always possible. Thirty of over 1600 farms at risk became infected following AI from an infected boar stud in the 1997/98 Dutch outbreak.

6. Spread from wild boar. Eradication of the disease from domesticated pig populations in Europe has revealed that wild boar are an important reservoir of infection. Infection has spread from wild boar in Germany, France and Italy. Disease has been identified in wild boar in Sardinia and Tuscany. Recent studies with monoclonal antibodies to envelope proteins and sequence data from the E2 gene have confirmed that wild boar and domestic pig isolates are similar.

7. Other local means of spread may have been involved in the recent (1997) Dutch outbreaks and studies suggest that herds within 500m of an infected herd are at particular risk.

Tracing of disease movement has been enhanced by international databases holding E2 sequences.

Diagnosis

The clinical signs accompanied by the findings of a high fever in large numbers of pigs, and some deaths should lead to suspicion of swine fever, particularly if the herd affected is swill-fed or if animals have been recently bought in. Trembling piglets with cerebellar hypolasia must also be considered possible cases of congenital infection. If the disease is suspected, it should be notified to the Competent Authority immediately. Diagnosis is confirmed by:

1. Post mortem findings - the haemorrhagic lymph nodes and petechial haemorrhages in the acute form, splenic infarcts and button ulcers in more chronic cases.

2. Clinical Pathology - A white blood cell count of less than 10,000 cells/µl in affected pigs more than 5 weeks of age and affected for less than 6 days

indicates swine fever. Leucopaenia is a prominent clinical pathological finding in early cases.

3. Demonstration of virus

(a) Fluorescent antibody test. Frozen sections of tonsil, nictitating membrane, kidney, spleen or ileum, mandibular, maxillary and mesenteric lymph nodes from animals which have been affected for between 5 and 10 days may be used for the highly specific fluorescent antibody test for the virus. Specific cytoplasmic fluorescence is considered diagnostic.

(b) Immunoperoxidase has been used in similar circumstances. Peroxidase-linked monoclonal antibodies are more sensitive and can be more specific than polyclonal antibody.

(c) Virus isolation may be attempted in pig kidney cells (PK 15) using spleen or leucocytes as a source of infectious material. Positive from 8 days post-exposure.
Infected cells are identified by immunofluorescence or immunoperoxidase using monoclonal antibodies at 22-72 hours post-inoculation (pi). The tissues listed above, and the blood in EDTA should be submitted.
Panels of monoclonal antibodies and DNA probes have been developed to distinguish isolates of swine fever virus from other pestiviruses isolated from pigs. The E2 gene is often sequenced.

(d) Immunoassay for antigen. An antigen-capture ELISA for virus antigen in peripheral blood, leucocytes and spleen cells has been described and is available commercially. Positive from Day 8 pi.

(e) Polymerase chain reaction. Reverse transcriptase-PCR (RT-PCR) using primers for pestivirus in general and classical swine fever in particular is now commonplace. RT-nested PCR (RTnPCR) using sequences from the E2 gene have been used and may detect virus longer than isolation. The use of Real Time RT-PCR (ReTi RT-PCR) allows results to be obtained within 2 hours

Monoclonal antibodies, DNA primers and probes capable of distinguishing between BVDV, BDV and swine fever virus have been used for (a) (b) and (e) and are important because of the possibility that clinical signs or pathology resembling CSF may be associated with these viruses.

4. Serology

Serum antibody may be detected by:

(a) Serum neutralisation tests. Cytopathogenic virus or non-cytopathogenic virus detected by immunofluorescence of immunoperoxidase neutralisation peroxidase-linked assay (NPLA) or the fluorescent antibody virus neutralisation test. The presence of higher titres to CSFV than to BVDV or BDV confirms that the antibody is to CSFV.

(b) Complement fixation tests have been used.

(c)   ELISAs.   Whole virus may be used to identify antibody to CSF presumptively but monoclonal antibody blocking ELISAs or BVDV or BDV ELISAs are necessary to confirm the antibody as being CSF.
A specific ELISA based on gpE2 and a complex trapping blocking ELISA have also been described. Antibody using these ELISAs may be detected from 20 days post exposure. Wild type virus

5.   Animal transmission - The final definitive test for swine fever in newly affected areas.   The use of controls immunised against swine fever is of value in separating the disease from African Swine Fever.

The disease may be differentiated from acute African Swine Fever in countries where both are present by the persistent high temperature in Swine Fever (it falls prior to the clinical signs in African Swine Fever), the appearance of the disease in pigs vaccinated against swine fever and the lack of button ulcers, laryngeal haemorrhages and turkey-egg kidney in African Swine Fever.   Lesions occurring in the latter but not in Swine Fever include oedema of the lung and gall bladder and massive infarction of the hepatic lymph node.   Haemorrhages on the heart are more common.   Laboratory tests confirm.
BVDV and BDV infections may be distinguished from classical swine fever using the tests described above.
A recent outbreak (England 2000) was initially confused with PDNS and PDNS cases should always be examined carefully to ensure the absence of CSF.
Acute erysipelas, salmonellosis, thrombocytopaenic purpura, congenital tremor and some types of abortion and foetal mummification may all lead to suspicion of swine fever.

Control

Swine fever is controlled in the EU at present by a slaughter policy in which all pigs in contact with confirmed cases are slaughtered and buried or burned on the affected farms or removed safely for rendering. Farms are disinfected and left depopulated for a period. Restocking begins with sentinel pigs and follows when these are unaffected. All markets in the affected area are closed until danger of further infection has passed and pig movements in the affected areas are strictly controlled. Movement is banned in the 3km protection zone around an outbreak and in the 10km surveillance zone. Tracing of contacts is carried out, and herds in the protection and surveillance zones are screened for disease. Large numbers of progeny have had to be slaughtered to maintain animal welfare on the movement-restricted units. Studies of the efficacy of these procedures suggest that slaughter of all pigs within 1000m of the outbreak as soon as possible would significantly reduce local spread. Swill feeding has been banned in an attempt to prevent the recurrence of Foot and Mouth Disease and this benefits the control of swine fever.   UK legislation dealing with swine fever includes the Swine Fever Orders 2003 putting EU legislation into domestic form. EU regulations to control swine fever within the Community include agreement on the diagnostic criteria to be used in the Community. Current diagnostic tests in use for international trade are given by OIE.

Vaccination

In countries in which the disease is enzootic, live attenuated (lapinised) virus vaccine (LPC - China virus) or the cell culture attenuated Japanese GP strain can be given either before colostrum is taken by newborn piglets or at 30-60 days of age. Vaccination should be repeated at 9 month intervals and does not eliminate infection but reduces multiplication of virus in the tonsil. Vaccine virus may be present in the semen of recently-vaccinated boars and cross the placenta. Maternal vaccinal titres may be differentiated from swine fever wild type antibody. Antibody titres of 1:32 or less allow LPC vaccine to provide protection, those greater than 1:32 do not and animals with that level of passive immunity at vaccination later become susceptible. At 5-6 weeks 11% piglets respond to vaccine, 42% at 7-8 weeks and 77% at 10 weeks in vaccinated herds.

A number of vector vaccines have been developed, using vaccinia virus, adenovirus or pseudorabies virus expressing proteins such as envelope proteins E1 and E2. None are yet available commercially. DNA vaccines have also been shown to be protective. Recombinant E2 protein has also been shown to protect experimentally. C strain viruses have been engineered to incorporate BVD genes.

Marker vaccines based on recombinant E2 antigens have been widely evaluated and protect against clinical disease for at least 6 months but do not prevent vertical transmission. An ELISA based on the E^{rns} protein has been used to distinguish wild type and vaccine responses.

Control in Wild Boar

Freeliving wild boar in several countries of Europe are infected and reduction in infection has been carried out by hunting bans followed by culling of young animals or by vaccination campaigns. These use C type live virus vaccine in baits and are administered twice over infected areas in each of spring, summer and autumn. Infection has been eliminated in some areas with consequent reduction in spread to domestic pigs.

Disinfection

An important part of the control of swine fever is disinfection between farms in infected areas, disinfection of implements and vehicles and disinfection of infected premises. Infected premises should be disinfected, cleaned and finally disinfected once more. The concentrations appropriate for use are given in the UK in the lists of approved disinfectants under the UK Diseases of Animals (Approved Disinfectants) Order 1978 updated at intervals. Sample dilutions include phenols at 1:50-80 and Antec Farm Fluid S 1:160. Virkon S is also effective.

References

Collin, E.D., Bloemraad, M., Wensvoort, G. (1997). An improved ELISA for the detection of serum antibodies directed against classical swine fever virus. Vet Micro. 59, 15-25.

Dahle, J., Liess, B. (1992). A review of classical swine fever infection in pigs: epizootiology, clinical disease and pathology. Comp.Immunol.Microbiol. and Infectious Disease 15, 203-211.Dewulf, J., Laevens, H., Koenen, F., Mintiens, K., Kruif, A.de (2000). Airborne transmission of classical swine fevervirus under experimental conditions. Vet. Rec. 735-738.

Dijkhuizen, A.A. (ed) The 1997-1998 outbreak of classical swine fever in the Netherlands. Special issue, Prev.vet.med. 39, (4)

Edwards, S., Moennig, V., Wensvoort, G. (1991). The development of an international reference panel of monoclonal antibodies for the differentiation of hog cholera virus from other pestiviruses. Vet.Micro. 29, 101-108.

Elbers, A.R.W., Stegeman, J.A., Jong, M.C.M. de (2001). Factors affecting the introduction of classical swine fever virus into pig herds in the central area of the 1997-1998 epidemic in The Netherlands. Vet.Rec. 149, 377-382.

Elbers, A.R.W., Stegeman, J.A., Moser, H., DeJong, M.C.M., Ekker, H.M., Smak, J.A., De Leeuw, P.W. (1998). Effectiveness of preventive culling of pig herds during the Dutch CSF Epidemic in 1997. Proc IPVS 15, II, 271.

Harkness, J.W. (1985). Review: Classical swine fever and its diagnosis. Vet.Rec. 116, 288-293.

90

Hooft van Iddeking, B.J.L., Wind, N.de, Wensvoort, G., Kimman, T.G., Gielkens, A.L.J., Moormann, R.J.M. (1996). Comparison of the protective efficacy of recombinant pseudorabies viruses against pseudorabies and CSF in pigs: influence of different promoters on gene expression and on protection. Vaccine **14**, 6-12.

Kaden, V., Lange, E., Fischer, U., Strebelow, G. (2000). Oral immunisation of wild boar against classical swine fever: evaluation of the first field study in Germany. Vet.Micro. **73**, 239-252.

Koene, F., Vanderhallen, H., Laevans, H., Deluyker, H. (1998). Serological and virological evolution of classical swine fever diagnosis after experimental infection simulating field conditions. Proc IPVS **15**, II, 191

Laevens, H., Koenen, F., Deluyker, H., Kruif, A.de (1999). Experimental infection of slaughter pigs with classical swine fever virus, transmission of the live virus, course of the disease and antibody response. Vet. Rec. **145**, 243-248.

Le Forban, Y., Cariolet, R. (1992). Characterisation and pathogenicity for pigs of a hog cholera virus strain isolated from wild boars. Annales de Recherche Veterinaire **23**, 93-100.

Liess, B. Ed. (1988). Classical Swine Fever and related viral infections. Martinus Nijhoff in the series 'Developments in Veterinary Virology.

Meyers, G., Rumenapf, T., Thiel, H.J. (1989). Molecular cloning and nucleotide sequence of the genome of hog cholera. Virology **171**, 555-567.

Moennig, V. (1992). The Hog Cholera Virus. Comp. Immunol. Microbiol. Infect. Dis. **15**, 189-201.

Paton, D., Edwards, S. (eds) Special Issue: Clasical swine fever. Vet. Micro. **73**, 91-252.

Pearson, J.E. (1992). Hog cholera diagnostic techniques. Comp. Immunol. Microbiol. Infect. Dis. **15**, 213-219.

Robertson, I., Owen, J. (1994). Notifiable Diseases of Pigs. In Practice **16**, 110-128.

Rumenapf, T., Stark, R., Meyers, G., Thiel, H.J. (1991). Structural proteins of hog cholera virus expressed by vaccinia virus: further characterisation and induction of protective immunity. J.Virol. **65**, 589-597.

Sharpe, K., Gibbens, J., Morris, H., Drew, T. (2001). Epidemiology of the 2000 classical swine fever outbreak in East Anglia: preliminary findings. Vet.Rec. **148**, 91.

Shannon, A.D., Morrisy, C., Mackintosh, S.G., Westbury, H.A. (1993). Detection of hog cholera virus antigens in experimentally-infected pigs using an antigen capture ELISA. Vet.Microbiol. **34**, 232-248.

Smit, A.J.de, Bouma, A., Terpstra, C., Oirschot, J.T.van (1999). Transmission of classical swine fever virus by artifical insemination. Vet. Micro. **67** 239-249.

Terpstra, C., Wensvoort, G. (1988). Natural infections of pigs with Bovine Viral Diarrhoea Virus associated with signs resembling swine fever. Res.Vet.Sci. **45**, 137-142.

Wirz, B., Tratschin, J.D., Muller, H.K., Mitchell, D.B. (1993). Detection of hog cholera virus and differentiation from other pestiviruses by polymerase chain reaction. J.Clin.Microbiol. **31**, 1148-1154.

Wood, L., Brockman, S., Harkness, J.W., Edwards, S. (1988). Virulence and tissue distribution of UK 1986 viruses. Vet.Rec. **122**, 391-394.

Williams, D.R., Matthews, D. (1988). 1986 UK outbreak and its control. Vet.Rec. **122**, 479-483.

African Swine Fever

Definition

African Swine Fever is a highly contagious often highly fatal viral disease of pigs characterised by clinical signs and gross lesions which may be difficult to distinguish from European Swine Fever. It is caused by an unrelated virus.

Incidence

African Swine Fever has never occurred in Britain and was confined to Africa until 1957 when infection spread through Portugal, Spain, Southern France and Italy. Infection persists in Sardinia, Italy, with 198 cases (2005) but has been eradicated from the Italian mainland, France, Belgium, Malta, Cuba, the Dominican Republic,

Brazil and The Netherlands in all of which countries small numbers of outbreaks have occurred. Infection was finally eradicated from the Iberian Peninsular in 1994 when there were 13 outbreaks in Spain. A last outbeak occurred in Portugal in 1999. Outbreaks have occurred in domestic pigs in a number of African countries outside the areas commonly reporting disease. New areas of Mozambique (1994), Cote d'Ivoire (1996) and Benin (1997) have been affected with spread to Togo and Nigeria. Madagascar has reported outbreaks.

Aetiology

The African Swine Fever virus is a large ether-sensitive DNA iridovirus which is icosahedral in form, enveloped and 175-215nm in diameter. Restriction endonuclease analysis can distinguish between different field isolates and between these and tissue-culture adapted strains. Up to 113 viral proteins have been described, one of which, Vp73, may be useful as an antigen in ELISA tests but is unrelated to protection. Protein P12 is associated with adsorption to cells and antibody to it can prevent adsorption *in vitro*. The genome of the virus has been sequenced, and some proteins cloned and expressed in *E.coli* or in baculoviruses. There is molecular biological evidence of a relationship to pox viruses. Isolates of African swine fever virus from Africa are very variable although one RFLP type (ESAC-WA) was involved in the European, American and West African outbreaks.. The variation in the DNA is reflected in antigenic differences between strains and primers for PCR have to be chosen from non-variable regions of the genome.

The virus grows in cultures of porcine bone marrow and buffy coat with the production of syncytia. In kidney cell cultures some strains produce C.P.E. preceded by haemadsorption. It has been grown in some arthropod cell lines. In the field the virus is found in pigs, multiplies in ticks and pig lice and is found in the blood of wild pigs in Africa, in particular in wart hogs. The virus is very resistant and survives conditions of putrefaction and sunlight which would destroy swine fever virus.. It can survive 2 hours at 56°C, survive for 6 months in carcases held at 4°C, for 2 years when dried at room temperature and almost indefinitely when frozen in meat at -20°C. It is stable between pH 3 and pH 10 but is inactivated by 1% formaldehyde in 6 days and by 2% NaOH in 24 hours.

Pathogenesis

The main route of infection is via the upper respiratory tract and initial virus replication occurs within 24 hours of infection in the lymphoid tissue draining the nasal mucosa and in the pharyngeal tonsil. Viraemia follows and the virus affects the vascular endothelium and causes lymphopaenia. Thrombin clotting times increase from day 4 post-infection and thrombocytopaenia occurs from day 6 post-infection. After 4-5 days the sub-endothelial lesions involve basement membranes and death ensues due to pulmonary oedema.

Virus multiplies in monocytes, macrophages, hepatocytes, endothelial cells and some epithelial cells throughout the body. Virus may be shed within 24 hours of the onset of fever. Surviving animals are persistently infected and viraemia persists in spite of the presence of high levels of circulating antibody, apparently because of interference from incomplete antibody. This may result in immune glomerulonephritis. Antibody may be detected first at 11 days post-infection and from that time virus levels in the plasma fall to disappear by day 46 post-infection. Haemadsorption of red cells to infected cells occurs *in vitro* and 95% infectivity in the blood of infected pigs is in the form of virus adsorbed on erythrocytes. Reduction in levels of virus is related to the presence of antibody. Protection against re-infection appears to be related to cellular immunity which may develop within 7-10 days of infection and be antibody-dependent cell-mediated cytotoxicity (ADCC).

Clinical signs

The incubation period averages 1 week (5-15 days) and is followed by pyrexia (40-42°C, 104-108°F) for a period of 48 hours during which affected animals remain bright and continue eating. Clinical signs begin as the temperature drops and consist of dullness, anorexia, huddling together, incoordination, dyspnoea and coughing (30% of cases), skin cyanosis and occasional vomiting or diarrhoea, sometimes with serous mucopurulent or bloody ocular and nasal discharges. Death occurs within 7-10 days of the onset of clinical signs and in classic outbreaks the mortality rate is 95-100%. Chronic cases appear emaciated with lameness, swollen joints and skin ulceration. Mild forms may occur in herds or areas in which the disease is enzootic. Abortion may occur in sows in all stages of pregnancy 5-8 days after infection or 1-3 days after fever develops. A high proportion of such mildly affected animals may recover.

Affected pigs should be slaughtered humanely.

Pathological findings

Severe haemorrhages are widespread throughout the body. The lymph nodes are so haemorrhagic that they resemble pieces of spleen, the ecchymoses on serous membranes are severe and those on the epicardium may lead to haemopericardium and those on the pleura and peritoneum may stain the peritoneal and pleural effusions with blood. Haemorrhages may also be found in the myocardium, lung, liver, kidney and bladder. The gall bladder is oedematous and the hepatic lymph node is haemorrhagic even in cases of mild disease. There may be oedema of the lung. Haemorrhagic ulceration may develop in the large intestine, but button ulcers are rare and the laryngeal haemorrhages and turkey egg kidney found in swine fever are uncommon. In chronic cases, pericarditis, pleuritis, pneumonia, arthritis and cutaneous ulcers are seen. Some African isolates may only cause petechiation of the kidney and visceral lymph nodes with an increase in abdominal fluid. Aborted foetuses have ecchymotic placental and petechial cutaneous haemorrhages.

Histological findings include congestion, lymphoid infiltration of the letptomeninges of the brain and nuclear changes in lymphocytes in all tissues. There is thickening of blood vessels and severe damage to vascular endothelium with perivascular haemorrhages. A fall in the number of lymphocytes is common. The use of peroxidase-linked monoclonal antibodies to the virus or its subunits can demonstrate virus in phagocytes, hepatocytes, endothelial cells and some epithelia throughout the body.

Epizootiology

Infected pigs have a persistent viraemia and the virus is present in all body fluids, secretions and excretions. Virus is shed for 7-10 days after the onset of fever, can form aerosols but is present in greatest amounts in faeces. It persists in blood for up to 8 weeks and in lymphoid tissues for 12 weeks or more and carriage has been recorded for up to 21 weeks. Virus has been demonstrated in blood for more than 500 days by PCR. Animals which have recovered are immune to challenge with homologous virus but can succumb to other strains of virus. Maternal immunity may protect for up to 7 weeks.

Transmission in Europe was by the following routes in order of importance:

a)   direct contact with pigs excreting virus

b)   the ingestion of infected meat products (often improperly cooked swill)
c)   the bites of biological vectors such as *Ornithodoros erraticus* (Iberia) (and *O.moubata* or *O. porcinus porcinus*, Africa). Ticks remained infective in disused piggeries for 5 years (Iberia).
d)   the bites of mechanical vectors such as biting flies, lice etc.
e)   parenteral inoculation which allows infection from low titres of virus.

In Africa infection may be derived from carrier wart hogs which are the source of infection for ticks or occur as a warthog-independent infection in domestic pigs. The disease persists on infected premises for long periods of time. Where the disease has become enzootic in Sardinia, the clinical signs are less dramatic and chronic infection may occur so that carrier pigs are important in the spread of the disease. Onward transmission from recovered animals is not inevitable as many antibody-positive animals are virus-negative. Wild boar are infected in Sardinia, and in 1990 1.5% of wild boar sampled were seropositive. Free range pigs are most commonly affected in Sardinia. The relationship between infected ticks, boar and domestic pigs is not clear in some areas. In the Caribbean outbreaks, spread within a farm was slow and from pen to pen. Adjacent buildings were unaffected for a long period. The virus is introduced to countries in pig products and then spread by the methods noted above. In Belgium (1985) spread by fomites was particularly important.

Diagnosis

African Swine Fever should be suspected where a highly infectious syndrome causes 95-100% mortality in pigs of all ages with clinical signs resembling those of swine fever. A point of difference is the fall in temperature before the onset of clinical signs. Mild forms of the disease may be more difficult to diagnose. At post-mortem examination, findings of multiple haemorrhages, petechiated kidneys, haemorrhagic lymph nodes (especially the hepatic, in chronic or wild cases) and splenic infarcts also suggest one of the swine fevers. Laboratory confirmation should always be sought. The actual techniques used are to be found in the current O.I.E. handbook, but material for investigation should include clotted blood and blood in EDTA, lymph node, kidney, spleen and lung. In abortion from African Swine Fever, infection is more easily demonstrable in the sow rather than the foetus. Placenta is the best product of abortion for diagnosis.

The tests used are as follows:

a)   Demonstration of antibody in tissue or body fluids. Classically by indirect immunofluorescence on infected tissue culture monolayers, immunoperoxidase can improve results. ELISAs have been described using whole virus, p73 or p30 (recombinant or tissue-culture-derived) as antigen. Other tests such as complement fixation, immunoblotting, radioimmunoassay, radio-immune-precipitation have all been used.

b)   Demonstration of virus in tissue. Classically by immunofluorescence on frozen tissue sections, immuno-peroxidase may be of equal value. ELISA using monoclonal antibody may also be used but may be of reduced value where antibody complexes mask antigen. Electron microscopy may reveal virus on red cells or macrophages The polymerase chain reaction (PCR) has been used with primers from non-variable regions on extracts from tissue and body fluids and can detect 10 pg of virus. It does not require live virus.

c) Virus isolation in cultures of buffy coat leucocytes or macrophages. Cytopathic effects may be seen, but the presence of virus is usually demonstrated primarily by the haemadsorption test in which infected cells are ringed by erythrocytes. The presence of virus can be confirmed by ELISA, neutralisation, PCR, immunofluorescence, immunoperoxidase or gel diffusion, immunoblot etc.

d) Animal transmission. The ultimate confirmation, especially of new introductions and to distinguish it from classical swine fever.

Carrier pigs may be identified by serological tests. These include a commercial ELISA or indirect tests using infected monolayers and fluorescent antibody to pig immunoglobulins. Monoclonal antibodies can be used to detect IgM or IgG antibody. Immunoelectrophoresis and immunoradial diffusion can also be used. PCR can also detect virus in blood.

Control

African Swine Fever is currently controlled by restrictions on movement of pigs or meat from infected areas. In all EC countries and most American countries it is a notifiable disease (African Swine Fever Orders, 2003, UK). Measures such as the prohibition of swill feeding and the import of infected pigs or meat have safeguarded the UK but infected meat has caused outbreaks in Belgium and The Netherlands. Outbreaks of the disease are controlled by slaughter of all pigs on the infected farm and any farms in direct contact. Affected farms are disinfected and sentinel pigs introduced prior to restocking depopulated farms. Movement is prohibited in the surrounding areas.

Disinfectants with specific claims for use in ASF outbreaks include Farm Fluid S (1:160) and Virkon S (1:100); Antec International. In enzootic areas, education, restriction of animal movement and prompt and generous compensation have reduced the levels of disease to low levels.

Vaccines have been studied experimentally.

References

Bech-Nielsen, S., Fernandez, J., Martinez-Perez, F., Espinosa, J., Perez-Bonillas, Q., Sanchez-Vizcario, J.M. (1995). A case study of an outbreak of African Swine Fever in Spain. Br. vet J. 151, 203-214.
Beeker, Y. (Ed.) (1987) . African Swine Fever, Martinus Nijhoff Publishers. Developments in Veterinary Virology series.
Biront, P., Castryck, F., Leunen, J. (1987). An epizootic of African Swine Fever in Belgium and its eradication. Vet.Rec. 120, 432-434.
Galo, A. (1993). Agriculture: Coordination of Agricultural Research, African Swine Fever: Proceedings of a workshop of agricultural research, Lisbon, Portugal 7, 8, 9 October 1991. Luxembourg, Commission of the EC.
King, D.P., Reid, S.M., Hutchings, G.H., Grierson, S.S., Wilkinson, P.J., Dixon, L.K., Bastos, A.D.S., Drew, T.W. (2003). Development of a TaqMan® PCR assay with internal amplification control for the detection of African Swine Fever Virus. J.Virol. Methods 107, 53-61.
McVicar, J.W. (1984). Quantitative aspects of transmission of African swine fever virus. Am.J.Vet.Res. 45, 1535-1541.
Oleaga-Perez, A., Perez-Sanchez, R., Encinas-Grandes, A. (1990). Distribution and biology of Ornithodoros erraticus in parts of Spain affected by African swine fever. Vet.Rec. 126, 32-37.
Pastor, M.J., Arias, M., Escribiano, J.M. (1990). Comparison of two antigens for use in an ELISA to detect African swine fever antibodies. Am.J.Vet.Res. 51, 1540-1543.

Perez-Sanchez, R., Astigarraga, A., Oleaga-Perez, A., Perez-Sanchez, R., Encinas-Grandes, A. (1994). Relationship between the persistence of African swine fever and the distribution of Ornithodorus erraticus in the province of Salamanca, Spain. Vet. Rec. 135, 207-209.

Petit, F., Boucraut-Baralon, C., Py, R., Benazet, F., Picavet, D.P., Chantal, J. (1991). Detection of African swine fever virus by a biotinylated DNA probe: assay on cell cultures and field samples. Annales de Recherche Veterinaire 22, 201-209.

Rodriguez, F., Fernandez, A., Perez, J., Martin de las Mulas, J., Sierra, M.A., Jover, A. (1996). African swine fever: morphopathology of a viral haemorrhagic disease. Vet. Rec. 139, 249-254.

Schlafer, D.H., McVicar, J.W., Mebus, C.A. (1984). African swine fever convalescent sows: subsequent pregnancy and the effect of colostral antibody on challenge inoculation of their pigs. Am.J.Vet.Res. 45, 1361-1366.

Schlafer, D.H., Mebus, C.A. (1984). Abortion in sows experimentally-infected with African swine fever virus: clinical features. Am.J.Vet.Res. 45, 1353-1360.

Schlafer, D.H., Mebus, C.A. (1987). Abortion in sows experimentally-infected with African swine fever virus: pathogenesis studies.Am.J.Vet.Res. 48, 246-254.

Schlafer, D.H., Mebus, C.A., McVicar, J.W. (1984). African swine fever in neonatal pigs: passively acquired protection from colostrum or serum of recovered pigs. Am.J.Vet.Res. 45, 1367-1372.

Steiger, Y., Ackerman, M., Mettraux, C., Kihm, M. (1992). Rapid and biologically safe diagnosis of African swine fever using polymerase chain reaction. J.Clin.Microbiol. 30, 1-8.

Robertson, I., Owen, J. (1994). Notifiable Diseases of Pigs. In Practice 16, 110-128.

Wardley, R.C., Norley, S.G., Wilkinson, P.J., Williams, S. (1985). The role of antibody in protection against African swine fever virus. Vet.Immunology and Immunopathology 9, 201-212.

Wilkinson, P.J. (1980). Pig News and Information 1, 17-20.

Wilkinson, P.J. (Ed.) (1983). African Swine Fever: Proceedings of an EC Seminar, Sardinia 1981 Eur 8466.

Swine Vesicular Disease

Definition

Swine vesicular disease is an infectious disease of pigs clinically indistinguishable from foot and mouth disease and is caused by an enterovirus.

Incidence

A vesicular disease of pigs was first observed in Italy in 1966 and then in Hong Kong in 1971. In December 1972, an outbreak occurred in swill-fed pigs in Staffordshire, UK and was thought to be Foot-and-Mouth disease. Similar outbreaks also occurred in Poland, Austria, France and Italy within a few weeks of each other. It occurred sporadically in Britain, particularly in Humberside, from 1979-82. It has recently occurred in several EC countries. Outbreaks were identified only in Italy in 2005 (14) and 2004 (125) and in Portugal in 2004 (1).

Aetiology

The disease is caused by a picornavirus 30-32 nm in size (as opposed to 24-25 nm for that of Foot-and-Mouth Disease. The virus is fatal to newborn mice, a character of the Coxsackie group of enteroviruses and is related to, and apparently derived from, the human strain Coxsackie B5 on the basis of virus neutralisation tests and the nucleotide sequences of the 3 capsid genes. Its genome is closely (90%) related to that of coxsackie viruses B1, B3, B4, B5, A9 and A16 and it is regarded by some as a porcine coxsackie virus.

The virus has been named Porcine Enterovirus England/72. Swine vesicular disease virus is stable at pH 5 and more resistant to acid and alkaline conditions than F.M.D. virus. A pH below 2.5 or above 12.5 is necessary to destroy the virus. It is destroyed by moist heat at 60°C within 30 minutes, but in cool, humid conditions it can persist for more than 4 months and it survives indefinitely in infected refrigerated pig tissues. A number of antigenic types (7 at present) have been identified using polyacrylamide gel electrophoresis. The 1979 strain, UK 1/79, differed from those found here previously and from those present at that time in Europe and RT-PCR has now shown that 4 groups of virus have been present in Europe: 1, the earliest viruses; 2, 1972-1981 (Europe and Japan); 3, Italy 1988-1992 and 4, Rumania and all Western European isolates 1987-1994

Pathogenesis

The exposure of susceptible pigs to infected animals results in infection through the tonsil in 90% of cases. Virus may also enter through the skin of the head, tongue and especially the foot, and also through the gut. It then multiplies in the draining lymph node and subsequently gives rise to a viraemia within a day followed by clinical signs within two days. The gastrointestinal tract may be exposed to $10^{7.5}$ particles without the occurrence of infection but the dose required to infect the coronary band is only $10^{3.6}$ viable virus particles. Infections from swill may, therefore, have taken place through the skin. There is field but little experimental evidence for transplacental infection. IgM antibody can be detected at 3 days post infection and neutralising antibody at 7 days after infection. Antibody peaks at 28 days post-infection, .

Clinical signs

The disease in the field is indistinguishable from foot and mouth disease in pigs but does not affect sheep or cattle although the virus may be present in these animals.

The development of lesions is accompanied by fever (40-41°C, 104-106°F) and by 1 or 2 days' inappetence. Lameness or tenderness of the feet is apparent and affected pigs may be disinclined to move and may arch their backs or group their feet beneath themselves. In severe cases, they may scream or walk on their knees, although the lesions are said to be less painful than those of F.M.D.

The lesions first appear as blanched areas of skin or epithelium which develop into vesicles within 2-4 hours and then rupture a few hours later to leave clean ulcers with, at first, a ragged periphery. Healing by granulation may be complete within 4 days. The incubation period varies with the weight of infection but is usually 2-4 days for local, primary lesions, 5-6 days after viraemia and 7-11 days after ingestion.

The lesions are most commonly found on the coronary band of the feet and the supernumerary digits but also extend into the inter-digital space. Under-running of the horn and sloughing of the claw may occur. Vesicles also occur on the skin of the limbs, the mammary glands and in about 5% of animals, on the snout and in the mouth, especially on the dorsum of the tongue. In many cases, especially in sows, the lesions may be mild and may pass unnoticed until later cases have been traced.

In some outbreaks, nervous signs have been recorded. They include head-pressing and disturbances of gait and may result in death following convulsions. From 25-70% of pigs may be affected, mainly those over 3 months of age. Mild cases occur and there is little mortality except when CNS involvement occurs. Some animals show no clinical signs but develop neutralising antibody.

The humane endpoint is when severe lameness is accompanied by loss of digital horn and when nervous signs lead to paralysis or convulsion.

Epidemiology

The incubation period is 2-7 days and virus may be shed as early as the second day after infection and shedding usually ceases 8-15 days after the appearance of the lesions. Subclinically-infected pigs can transmit the disease to others after mixing; virus is excreted in the faeces. The carrier state does not occur with most strains, although some Italian strains appear capable of persisting for 120 days. Virus is shed in vesicular fluid and spread on the farm appears to be largely by pig-pig contact.

The ability of the virus to survive in pig faeces (138 days in moist faeces stored between 12 and 17°C) means that environmental contamination may be a significant cause of the persistence of disease on premises and is important in the spread of the disease by lorries and by human carriage (on clothing, footwear, etc.). The 5 primary UK outbreaks appeared in pigs fed swill containing pork products of foreign origin and the secondary outbreaks appear to have resulted from direct movement of pigs from infecting premises, movement through markets (including contact infections) and transport on contaminated lorries. Swill-fed pigs have proved to be responsible for many outbreaks. At first, disinfection measures were inadequate and some recrudescence of infection occurred.

Examination of sera from slaughter pigs for antibodies to S.V.D. in 1974 showed that there was no widespread undisclosed disease in the most heavily infected areas, Lancashire and Yorkshire, although one farm was found to have evidence of active infection and significant antibody levels were found on 3 others out of 369 surveyed. Serological surveys in EC countries show that the UK, Greece, Denmark and Portugal were free in 1995. In The Netherlands antibody was not present in the general pig population. The situation in Italy was less clear and active infection was identified in that country in 2003 and 2004.

Diagnosis

The clinical signs only allow a diagnosis of a vesicular condition to be made unless the case is linked to a confirmed outbreak of S.V.D. Laboratory tests carried out at reference laboratories (Pirbright UK) in confirmation include complement fixation tests, virus isolation and, in long-standing cases, serum virus neutralisation tests and double immunodiffusion tests. Counter-immuno electrophoresis tests can used and ELISA tests are useful for widespread screening and distinction between Foot-and-Mouth and S.V.D. Recent developments include a liquid phase blocking sandwich ELISA for screening and a monoclonal based competitive ELISA (MACELISA) with 0.45% false positives False positives in some ELISAs may result from antibody to other enteroviruses and neutralisation tests may be necessary to confirm their identity.

RT-PCR and nested RT-PCR have been developed using primers from the 2B region of the genome and can distinguish SVD virus from foot and mouth virus and other vesicular viruses at levels of 0.1 TCD_{50} (better than isolation) in nasal swabs, tissues and faeces from day 7 to day 176 post infection. Contamination may be important with this method. The recent development of real time RT-PCR has allowed the automation of testing.

Diagnosis is most difficult where seropositive herds or single antibody-positive pigs occur with no contact with clinical signs of SVD (singleton reactor pigs/herds).

Control

Swine Vesicular Disease is controlled under the Swine Vesicular Disease Order 1972 which resembles the F.M.D. Orders, but only applies to pigs. The

Diseases of Animals (Waste Foods) Order 1974 made the installation of adequate swill treatment mandatory for swill feeders. The recent ban (2001) on swill feeding represents a major step in the control of the disease. Movement of pigs is controlled under the Movement and Sale of Pigs Order 1975. This order slows down pig movement which can only be made under local authority licence except for pigs going direct to slaughter. Swill-fed pigs were licensed only to move to a slaughter house.

Pigs going to market or other farms must be licensed and come from farms on to which no pigs have been moved within the preceding 21 days and be free from notifiable disease. Markets for pigs of 21 day status and those for slaughter pigs cannot be held on the same premises. Strict rules for disinfection of lorries and premises are in force.

Clinically affected pigs must be reported and are slaughtered under the S.V.D. Order 1972. Disinfection with 1% sodium hydroxide and flame guns is carried out, although certain other disinfectants, e.g. iodophors may be used. A full list is given in the Disease of Animals (approved disinfectants) Order 1978, amended 2005.

In spite of apparent eradication, the disease reappeared in Autumn 1976, Winter 1977 in 5 swill-fed herds and a reservoir of infection may have existed in frozen pork. The origin of the 1979 outbreak was not clear, particularly in view of the different antigenic nature of the virus. There were only 14 outbreaks of swine vesicular disease in 1982 and no evidence of infection has been found since in spite of widespread serum surveys. Recent studies of Group III enteroviruses which are epitheliotropic suggest that they could cause vesicular diseases. Similar methods are used in other countries.

References

Anon., Vet. Rec. (1973), 92 , 234-235.
Armstrong, R.M., Barnett, J.T.R. (1989). An ELISA for the detection and quantitation of antibody against swine vesicular disease virus. J.Virol.Methods 25, 71-79.
Brocchi, E., Berlinzani, A., Gamba, D., Simone, F.de, (1995). Development of two novel monoclonal antibody-based ELISAs for the detection of antibodies and the identification of swine isotypes against swine vesicular disease. J. Virol. Methods 52, 155-167.
Dekker, A., Moonen, P., Boer-Luutze, E.A. de, Terpstra, C. (1995). Pathogenesis of SVD after exposure of pigs to an infected environment. Vet. Micro 45, 243-250.
Ferris, N.P., Dawson, M. (1988). Routine application of ELISA in comparison with complement fixation for the diagnosis of foot-an-mouth and swine vesicular diseases. Vet.Microbiol. 16, 201-209.
Herniman, K.A., Medhurst, P.M., Wilson, J.N. and Sellers, R.F. (1974). Vet. Rec. 93, 620-625.
Lin, F., Mackay, D.K.J., Knowles, N.J. (1997). Detection of swine vesicular disease RNA by reverse transcription polymerase chain reaction. J. Virol. Methods 65, 111-121.
Lowes, E. Vet. Annual 1973 pp, 51-54.
Mann, J.A. and Hitchings, G.H. (1980). Swine vesicular disease: pathways of infection. J.Hygiene 84, 355-363.
Mowat, G.N., Darbyshire, J.H., Huntley, J.F. (1972). Differentiation of a vesicular disease of pigs in Hong Kong from Foot and Mouth Disease. Vet.Rec. 90, 618-621.
Reid, S.M., Ferris, N.P., Hutchings, G.H., King, D.P., Alexandersen, S. (2004). Evaluation of real time RT-PCR assay for the detection of swine vesicular disease virus. J.Virol. Methods 116, 169-176.
Robertson, I., Owen, J. (1994). Notifiable Diseases of Pigs. In Practice 16, 110-128.
Seechum, P., Knowles, N.J., McCauley, J.W. (1990). The complete nucleotide sequence of a pathogenic swine vesicular disease virus. Virus Research 16, 255-274.
Sellers, R.F. (1982). Swine vesicular disease. Pig News and Information, 3, 21-24.
Zhang, A., Wilsden, G., Knowles, N.J., McCauley, J.W. (1993). Complete nucleotide sequence of Coxsackie B5 virus and its relationship to SVDV. J.Gen.Virol. 74, 845-853.

Foot and Mouth Disease

Foot-and-Mouth Disease in pigs is an acute and very contagious viral disease characterised by fever, the formation of vesicles on the coronary band and less frequently, on the snout, lips and tongue. Morbidity is high but mortality is low, except amongst young pigs in which sudden death commonly occurs. It is an OIE List A Disease.

Incidence

Foot-and-Mouth Disease is normally absent from Britain, Ireland and most EU countries. It has occurred from time to time in most of Europe as isolated outbreaks or as epizootics, which occurred in Britain in 1967-68 when 113, 800 pigs were slaughtered and most recently in 2001 when a major outbreak arose in pigs and then spread to ruminants in Great Britain, Ireland, France and The Netherlands The disease is present in South America, in some parts of Eastern Europe, in Africa, in many parts of Asia, but is not present in Australia and North America.

Aetiology

Foot-and-Mouth Disease virus is an aphthovirus with a particle size of 23 nm and a cubical capsid containing 32 capsomeres. Four polypeptide chains and occasionally a fifth are present in the virion. The virus may be cultivated in bovine or pig kidney cells, calf thyroid cells or bovine lingual epithelium. Baby hamster kidney cells are widely used. The virus is highly cytopathic for porcine cell lines and, unlike swine vesicular disease virus, for bovine thyroid cultures. It is inactivated below pH 6 and above pH 8. 0 and is rapidly destroyed by sunlight.

Infectivity is lost within a few days at 37°C but remains for many months at 4-7°C and for years when frozen, particularly at temperatures as low as -30 to -70°C. Under natural conditions, the virus can remain infective for years in tongue epithelium stored at +4°C, in blood or vesicular fluid, for 4 weeks on hair, 15 weeks on leather and 20 weeks on hay or straw at room temperature, and for up to 6 days in milk. Pasteurisation by the flash process (72°C for 15 seconds) may not inactivate the virus completely and it may be present in milk powder for years. Survival in meat products varies. The virus is rapidly destroyed by lactic acid formation in muscle but may persist for up to 6 months in bone marrow and 4-5 months in parenchymatous organs and lymph nodes. In pickled meats, the virus may survive for 1-2 months and in Parma ham for 3-5 months.

Seven serotypes exist. They are: 3 European (A, 32 subtypes; O, 11 subtypes and C, 5 subtypes), 3 South African Territories (S.A.T. 1, 7 subtypes - S.A.T. 2, 3 subtypes - S.A.T. 3, 4 subtypes) and Asian (Asia 1 , 3 subtypes) . Only types A, O and C have been recorded in Europe. There is no cross-immunity between types and only partial immunity between subtypes within a type. All 3 were identified in one Italian outbreak. Recent studies suggest that the RNA polymerase genes of all types are high conserved.

Pathogenesis

Infection takes place by inhalation and ingestion and can also result from the infection of abrasions on the skin and other body surfaces. The pig may be relatively resistant to infection. Under 100 Tissue Culture Infective Doses (TCID50) will not infect, 300 TCID50 cause short term subclinical infection and 800 TCID50 are required for typical disease. Initial virus multiplication takes place in the pharyngeal region (soft palate, tonsil and floor of the pharynx) or at the point of inoculation and spread to regional lymph nodes is followed by viraemia and then multiplication in epithelial surfaces. Local spread to the tongue may occur. Secondary vesicles appear on the coronary band, back of the snout and on the udder of suckling sows, often within 24 hours of the appearance of lesions in the mouth. Maximum shedding of virus by aerosol occurs at this time (much of it from early replication in the upper respiratory tract and the trachea) and $10^{5.8}$-$10^{6.4}$ TCID50 may be shed per hour. Vesicles rupture and if uncontaminated, heal rapidly. Those on the feet may result in destruction of growing horn and loss of the hoof. Immunity to the type and subtype of the infecting virus develops within 3-7 days of the clinical signs but may last for only 6 months. Piglets can be protected by colostral antibody.

Clinical signs

The sudden onset of severe lameness is the commonest finding in affected pigs, the feet of which are obviously painful. The back may be arched, reluctance to move is common and movement may be accompanied by squealing. Vesicles appear as raised white areas 0.5-1 cm in diameter on the dorsum of the tongue, on the snout and on the teats of the sow and rupture readily to leave small ulcers. Ulcers heal relatively quickly unless infected. Frothy saliva may be present and vesicles develop on the coronary band of the feet, particularly towards the heel, in the interdigital space, and on the supernumerary digits. Vesicles on the coronary band may disturb horn growth and lines of damaged horn may be seen on the hoof, moving towards the tip with time. When severe, they cause "thimbling" as the damaged horn is shed. Fever (up to 41°C-106°F) accompanies the earliest stages of the disease. Affected animals are depressed, anorexic and lose condition. Mortality rarely exceeds 5%, but it may reach 50% or more in piglets in which sudden death may occur before vesicles develop in either piglets or the sows. Animals with loss of horn or acute lameness and piglets suffering from severe heart failure should be killed humanely.

Pathology

Apart from the presence of vesicles and the appearance of a fevered carcase, patchy necrosis or even haemorrhage of the heart muscle may be seen in young pigs which have died suddenly. The latter may not have vesicles.

Epidemiology

The incubation period is 2-7 days and virus is shed even before the appearance of the lesions, particularly from the upper respiratory tract. Shorter incubation periods are seen when infection with high concentrations of virus occur or there are large numbers of pigs exposed. As there is no carrier state, the ability of the virus to survive under various conditions is important and has been listed above. Foot-and-Mouth disease in pigs is a major source of virus for other species. The high concentration of virus produced in early stages of the disease, coupled with the large numbers of pigs in an airspace and forced ventilation, can give rise to virus aerosol plumes which can travel long distances. Infection results from direct or indirect contact with affected animals, carcases or animal products. Passive human carriage occurs, but virus cannot be demonstrated in nasal washings and carriage is prevented by washing hands and change of outer clothing and showering. Transmission may be by the aerosol route, by contact with other species of affected livestock, by fomites and from infected material of animal origin in incompletely cooked swill. Milk, either skim or whole, may be a source during outbreaks. Pigs do not remain carriers and viral genome sequences cannot be found 28 days post infection. The speed and severity of the spread of the disease is emphasised by the 1997 outbreak in Taiwan where between March and July 4,658,515 animals were destroyed. The first 3 herds infected 1100 within 10 days and ultimately 24.2% herds were infected (4395) with a 21.7% morbidity rate, a 3.95% mortality rate and an 18.2% case fatality rate. The virus appeared to be pig adapted. The 2001 UK outbreak began in pigs fed on contaminated swill, was detected at abattoir where local spread occurred, but had already been transmitted locally to sheep and then spread largely through animal movements within the UK , to Ireland, France and The Netherlands.

Diagnosis

The clinical signs only allow a diagnosis of a vesicular condition to be made but Foot-and-Mouth disease may be suspected if the case is linked to a confirmed outbreak of F.M.D. Laboratory diagnosis is based on the examination of fresh lesion material taken from suspected clinical cases. Material for examination should be transported in 50/50 glycerol/phosphate buffer pH 7.2-7.6 and kept at 4°C or lower. Virus may be detected by the complement fixation test using lesion material as antigen against antibody to all 7 serotypes or by antigen ELISA using monoclonal antibody to all 7 types of virus. Recombinant integrin $\alpha v \beta 6$ has been used for this purpose in ELISAs. A variety of RT-PCR tests have been described to detect viral RNA using primers from the 2B gene and a reverse transcriptase. Real Time and TaqMan RT-PCR tests have allowed automation of testing and some tests can be read 3 hours after arrival of the sample. Isolation in tissue culture may be performed and virus can be detected using ELISA and radioimmunoassay. Passage through baby mice has been used. Acid sensitivity distinguishes the virus from S.V.D. virus. Serum from recovered cases and populations or even blood dried on paper discs may be tested by virus neutralisation, but more frequently by ELISAs, especially by liquid and solid phase blocking ELISAs. Serological tests increasingly use recombinant peptide antigens. Penside tests have been developed as have latex agglutination tests
Tests in current use for international trade are constantly under review and the OIE website should be consulted for details.

Prophylaxis and control

Control in the EC is based on early recognition, followed by slaughter, incineration or rendering of animals on affected farms and of dangerous contacts, disinfection and strict control of movement by the competent authority. UK legislation is based on EU Directives and the Foot and Mouth Disease Order, 1983 as amended. The disease is kept out of the EC by control over the import of animals and animal products and by the UK policy, under the Animal Byproducts Order 1999 and the Movement and Sale of Pigs Order 1975. A ban on feeding swill to pigs was introduced in 2001 and will reduce the possibility of infection by this route. The Transport and Cleansing and Disinfection Orders (2003) govern hygiene and Approved disinfectants should be used.

In future outbreaks, vaccination may be used strategically in areas surrounding an outbreak in combination with the existing slaughter and surveillance policy, but in the UK this can only be carried out with EU approval and regulations have been incorporated in domestic legislation (2006). This combination of using vaccination and slaughter has been used with success elsewhere. In countries where the disease is enzootic, annual vaccination is practised.

Inactivated vaccines are made from virus growth in bovine tongue epithelium or other suitable cells, inactivated with formalin, acetylethyleneimine (AEI) and other ethyleneimines and incorporated with oil, saponin or aluminium hydroxide adjuvants. Pigs are not readily immunised and require high concentrations of virus, although immunity has been demonstrated for up to 9 months using oil-adjuvanted vaccines. These cause granulomatous reactions and should be given into the pinna of the ear or intraperitoneally. One or more different serotypes may be included. Protection may take 7-20 days to develop and re-vaccination is required every 6-8 months. IgG appears to be the important protective antibody. Emergency vaccines using Montanide ISA 206 adjuvant may give a more rapid response. It is clear from experiment that transmission may still occur if vaccination takes place within 7 days of challenge but not at 14 days. To overcome maternal immunity, vaccination should be given at 10 and 14 weeks, but timing is farm dependent.

ELISAs which detect wild type virus exposure but not vaccinal antibody have been developed using recombinant peptides 2C and 3ABC. They have been evaluated in countries where vaccination has been used for control and appear useful.

Attenuated live vaccines are not used in pigs but are continuously under review.

Subunit vaccines are being developed by genetic engineering and direct synthesis from viral polypeptides but are not commercially available. Subunits as small as 3 amino acids have been shown to provide some protection. Recent constructs include some using FMD peptides and adenovirus recombinant IFNα to provide short term protection.

DNA vaccines have only been used experimentally.

References

Alexandersen, S., Brotherhood, I., Donaldson, A.I. (2002). Natural aerosol transmission of Foot and Mouth Disease virus to pigs: minimal infectious dose for strain O1 Lausanne. Epidemiology and Infection 128, 301-312.

Alexandersen, S., Kitching, R.P., Mansley, L.M., Donaldson, A.I. (2003). Clinical and laboratory investigations of five outbreaks of Foot and Mouth disease during the 2001 epidemic in the United Kingdom. Vet. Rec. 152, 489-496.

Alexandersen, S., Oleksiewicz, M.B., Donaldson, A.I. (2001). The early pathogenesis of Foot and Mouth Disease in pigs infected by contact: a quantitative time course study using TaqMan PCR.. J.Gen.Virol. 82, 745-755.

Armstrong, R.M., Crowther, J.R., Denyer M.S. (1991). The detection of antibodies against FMDV in filter paper eluates from pig sera or whole blood by ELISA. J.Virol.Methods. 34, 181-192.

Barteling, S.J., Vreeswick, J. (1991). Developments in Foot-and-Mouth vaccines. Vaccine. 9, 75-88.

Chung, W.B., Liao, C. (2003). Monitoring of Foot and Mouth Disease Virus non-structural protein 3AB antibody in intensive pig farms after a severe outbreak of Foot and Mouth Disease. Vet.Rec. 153, 273-275.

Dunn, C.S., Donaldson, A.I. (1997). Natural adaptation to pigs of a Taiwanese isolate of foot and mouth disease virus. Vet. Rec. 141, 174-175.

Donaldson, A.I., Ferris, N.P. and Wells, G.A.H. (1984). Experimental foot-and-mouth disease in fattening pigs, sows and piglets in relation to outbreaks in the field. Vet.Rec. 115, 509-512.

Ferris, N.P., Dawson, M. (1988). Routine application of ELISA in comparison with complement fixation for the diagnosis of FMD and SVD. Vet.Microbiol. 16, 201-209.

Meyer, R.F., Brown, C.C., House, C., House, J.A., Molitor, T.W. (1991). Rapid and sensitive detection of FMDV in tissues by enzymatic RNA amplification of the polymerase gene. J.Virol.Methods. 34, 161-172.

Morgan, D.O., Moore, D.A. (1990). Protection of cattle and swine against FMD using biosynthetic peptide vaccines. Am.J.Vet.Res. 51, 40-45.

Robertson, I., Owen, J. (1994). Notifiable Diseases of Pigs. In Practice 16, 110-128.

Vesicular exanthema

A calicivirus disease which caused vesicular lesions resembling those of foot-and-mouth disease and S.V.D. in California. Not seen since 1959, the virus is present in fish and sea lions (San Miguel Sealion Virus) and these might at any time form a source for pigs. The virus is spread by contact and fomites, but primary cases followed the feeding of contaminated uncooked swill.

Reference

Berry C.S., Skilling, D.E., Barlough, J.C., Vedros N.A., Gage, L.J., Smith, A.W. (1990). New marine calicivirus serotype infective for swine. Am.J.Vet.Res. **51**, 1184-1187.

Vesicular stomatitis

Another vesicular disease of the Western Hemisphere caused by two RNA vesiculoviruses (members of the rhabdoviridae) and rarely found in pigs. The virus also affects cattle, horses and man, possibly from a wild life or insect reservoir and probably transmitted by the sand fly *Lutzomyia shannoni* associated with maritime live oaks. It is transmitted in flies by the transovarial route. Transmission to pigs has been demonstrated by infected blackflies, *Simulium vittatum*. It is enzootic in Mexico and other parts of Central America and occasionally occurs in the Southern and South Western US e.g. 1995 and 1997. It is seasonal, occurring in the summer. Antibody levels in the South Eastern US. can vary from 12-60%. Once in pig populations the virus may be transmitted by contact and fomites. It may cause mild clinical signs in humans and the similarity of the lesions to those of Foot and Mouth Disease means that it is Notifiable in the USA
Control should include disinfection and protection from insects. Movement of stock from infected farms should not take place for 30 days after recovery.

References

Howerth, E.W., Stallknecht, D.E., Dorminy, M., Pisell, T., Clarke, G.R. (1997). Experimental vesicular stomatitis in swine. Effects of route of inoculation and steroid treatment. J. Vet. Diag. Invest. **9**, 136-142.
Mead, D.G., Gray, E.W., Noblet, R., Murphy, M.D., Howerth, E.W., Stallknecht, D.E. (2004). Biological transmission of VSV (New Jersey serotype) by *Simulium vittatum* (Diptera, Simuliidae) to domestic swine (*Sus scrofa*). J.Med Entomol.**41**, 78-82.
Stallknecht, D.E., Greer, J.B., Murphy, M.D., Mead, D.G., Howerth, E.W. (2004). Effect of strain and serotype of VSV on viral shedding, vesicular lesion development and contact transmission in pigs (Am.J.Vet. Res. **65**, 1233-1239.

Rabies

A rare, fatal viral disease of pigs in rabies-infected areas characterised by sudden onset, nervous signs and death.

Incidence

Less than 0.05% of rabies cases notified in Europe occur in the pig (1-10 p.a. in domestic pigs and a similar number in wild boar). It is equally rarely diagnosed in pigs in other parts of the world in which rabies is present.

Aetiology and pathogenesis

Caused by an RNA lyssavirus (rhabdoviridae), 75 x 180 nm with a characteristic shape. Exposure from bites or aerosol infection results in passage of the virus up nerves to central nervous system.

Clinical signs

Sudden onset, loss of coordination, twitching of the nose, excessive salivation and muscular spasm followed by prostration and death within 72-96 hours. Incubation period 50-120 days. Affected pigs should be killed, but pigs known to be exposed can be treated.

Pathological findings

No gross changes; central nervous system changes may include the presence of Negri bodies. Other changes are very variable but may include diffuse meningitis

Diagnosis

Clinical signs and history of exposure to rabies. Presence of rabies antigen in brain using specific immunofluorescence or animal inoculation. PCR may also be used.

Control

General control of other rabid animals. Successful vaccination has been reported from China. Wild boar exposed to vaccinia recombinant and attenuated vaccine viruses in baits intended for foxes in Europe can seroconvert. Exposed (bitten) pigs have been vaccinated and given hyperimmune serum.

Not Present in UK or Eire, notifiable (Rabies (Control Order) 1974) and transmissible to man as a fatal disease.

References

Hazlett, J. and Koller, M.A. (1986). Small outbreak in housed pigs exposed to a rabid cat. Canadian Vet.J. **27**, 116-118.
Mitmoonpitak, C., Limusanno, S., Khauplod, P., Tepsumethanon, V., Wilde, H. (2002). Post exposure rabies treatment in pigs. Vaccine **20**, 2019-2021.

Japanese B. Encephalitis

Definition

A viral infection of pigs in Eastern Asia, India and Queensland in Australia, transmitted by mosquitoes and responsible for reproductive failure in pigs.

Aetiology

A flavivirus (RNA) 40 nm in diameter. It has been defined antigenically and by restriction endonuclease techniques into at least 3 genotypes. It is extremely labile and rapidly inactivated by disinfectants, heat and extremes of pH. It grows well in most cell types.

Pathogenesis

Infection results from mosquito bites and viraemia results. The central nervous system may be affected but the major effects result from infection of the testis and the development or orchitis and multiplication in the foetus between 40 and 60 days' gestation to cause foetal death. Virus may persist in spleen macrophages and has been demonstrated by RT-PCR during winter when virus cannot be isolated.

Clinical signs

Clinical signs may follow infection in piglets but it is normally asymptomatic. The major effects are on numbers born alive which are reduced. Mummified foetuses, stillborn and weak pigs are produced. Boars lose libido, develop abnormal semen and azoospermia.

Pathology

Largely restricted to affected foetuses or stillborn pigs where there may be oedematous changes and neuronal changes.

Epidemiology

Transmitted by mosquitoes, principally *Culex tritaeniorhynchus* but other mosquito species may be involved (*C. vishnui*, India, C. annulirostris, *C. sitiens* Torres Straits). Pigs are a major host and can allow survival through the winter in Taiwan. Wild birds may be a reservoir and infection can be transmitted to man. Infection may be transmitted in semen.

Diagnosis

Antibody can be detected by haemagglutination inhibition tests, latex agglutination tests and by ELISA (especially an IgM capture ELISA). RT-PCR and nested RT-PCR can detect sequences even when virus cannot be isolated. Presence in an area may be confirmed from pooled mosquito material or by the use of sentinel pigs which seroconvert.

Control

Live attenuated virus vaccines should be given to breeding stock twice 2-3 weeks before the start of the mosquito season. Killed, oil adjuvanted vaccines have been described. Semen from affected boars should not be used.

Reference

Habu, A. (1991). Studies on the disorders of spermatogenic function in boars infected with Japanese Encephalitis Virus and its prevention. Bull.Nippon Veterinary and Animal Science University **40**, 107-108.

Getah Virus Infection

A haemagglutinating virus causing viraemia and foetal death in sows one week after infection. Described from Japan and South Korea and confirmed serologically by ELISA and haemagglutination Inhibition tests and by isolation from viraemic pigs. CPE produced on PK15 cells. Antibody is present in 10-25% feeding pigs and 21-73% sows in South Korea particularly during August-October. Also present in the Shanghai area of China.

Reference

Izumida, A., Takuma, H., Inaga, S., Kubota, M., Hirahawa, T., Kodama, K., Sasaki, N. (1988). Experimental infection of Getah virus in swine. Japanese J.Vet.Si. **50**, 679-684.

Other Arthropod-Transmitted Viruses

Other arthropod-transmitted viruses have been identified in pigs.

In Asia these include Apoi, Akabane, Ibaraki ,Batai (Japan and India), Dengue, West Nile and Chikungunya (India) and in Europe, West Nile virus and tickborne encephalitis (Rumania) and Louping III (Scotland). Rift Valley Fever has now been identified in pigs in Nigeria while Eastern Equine Encephalitis has occurred in the United States.

Louping III

Louping III is transmitted by ingestion and by the tick *Ixodes ricinus* and has caused nervous signs including hydrophobia. A non-suppurative meningo-encephalitis with neuronal necrosis, neuronophagia and lymphoid perivascular cuffing has been described in the brain stem. Virus has been demonstrated in, and is isolated from, the brain.
Prevention by the use of the oil-adjuvanted killed vaccine would be possible subject to local reaction.
Louping III is a zoonosis and a Category 3 agent. Advice should be sought if suspected..

Reference

Ross, H.M., Evans, C.C., Spence, J.A., Reid, H.W., Krueger, N. (1994). Louping III in free ranging pigs. Vet.Rec. **134**, 99-100.

Eastern Equine Encephalitis

Outbreaks of disease may occur in pigs in areas where this disease occurs (South Eastern US, Gulf of Mexico coasts) following mosquito infestation. Mortality may be high (280/350 in feeder pigs in one US outbreak) with growth retardation in survivors. Casualty animals had brain lesions typical of EEE, and multifocal necrosis and inflammation in the myocardium, but survivors had only mild brain lesions and antibody to EEE.

Reference

Elvinger, F., Liggett, A.D., Tang, K.N., Harrison, L.R., Cole, J.R., Baldwin, C.A., Nessmith, W.B. (1994). Eastern Equine Encephalitis in swine. JAVMA. **205**, 1014-1016.

Rinderpest

Identified in European pigs in India, this morbillivirus infection may occur in pigs in contact with diseased animals of other species. It is a Notifiable Disease. Virus can be identified in nasal discharge and carcase lymph nodes particularly 10-15 days post infection. Mortality of 7% has been reported

Reference

Govindarajan, R., Muralimanohar, B., Kotteeswaran, A., Venugopalan, A.T., Varalakshmi, P., Shaila, M.S., Ramachandran, S. (1996). Occurrence of rinderpest in European Pigs in India. Vet. Rec. **139**, 473.

Hepatitis E

Early reports of Hepatitis E in pigs came from experimental infection of pigs in Russia with faeces from an affected human case which resulted in jaundice 3-4 weeks post-infection, histological evidence of hepatitis and was of particular relevance to human health in areas with street pigs and poor sanitation. Infection of this type was also found in Nepal. The specific pig virus was later (1997) found in pigs in the USA and is now known to be present in pigs worldwide.

Hepatitis E virus infection is clinically inapparent in pigs but may cause microscopic lesions. It is of most importance as a zoonosis as the virus can infect humans and closely resembles human Hepatitis E viruses and can infect humans to cause clinical hepatitis.

The virus is an RNA virus belonging to the Hepeviruses (Hepeviridae) and was formerly considered a calicivirus. It cannot be grown at present in tissue culture and its presence is demonstrated by RT-PCR and by antibody detection. It occurs in at least 4 genotypes worldwide, shared by human Hepatitis E.

Infection is faecal oral and experimental infections result in hepatic inflammation and hepatocellular necrosis in experimental pigs. A more severe infection can be produced when human isolates are used. Changes peak at 20 days post infection and are still present at 55 days pot infection. Studies of the distribution of virus in tissues using DNA probes have demonstrated it in hepatocytes and bile duct epithelium most commonly, but it is also present in tonsil, lymph nodes, spleen, kidney and both small and large intestinal mucosa. The virus is present in the faeces which are infective as is raw liver. Infection did not cross the placenta in experimental pregnant gilts. Neonates may have maternal antibody but do not begin to seroconvert until about 2 months of age, increasing slightly to 3 months, peaking at 4 months and then declining slightly by slaughter. Sows may be seropositive. Viraemia parallels this distribution with piglets being free, weaners and growers being positive and finishers being negative for virus. As exposure is variable, the actual time course of infection will also vary.

Human infection results from exposure to pigs and is most common in pigkeepers or from the consumption of undercooked pig liver. Clinical disease has followed consumption of wild boar meat and is in the form of a sporadic hepatitis. Virus RNA and antibody closely resembling or identical to the local pig virus can be demonstrated in the plasma of contacts and cases. There is an association between this virus and abortion in pregnant women

References.

Banks, M., Heath, G.S., Grierson, S., King, D.P., Gresham, A., Girones, R., Widen, F., Harrison, T. (2004). Evidence for the presence of hepatitis E virus in pigs in the UK. Vet.Rec **154**, 222-237.

Halbur, P.G., Kasorndorkbua, C., Gilbert, C., Guenette, D., Potters, M.B., Purcell, R.H., Emerson, S.U., Toth, T.E., Meng, X.J. (2001). Comparative pathogenesis of infection of pigs with hepatitis E viruses recovered from a pig and a human. J.Clin Microbiol. **39**, 918-923.

Meng, X.J., Purcell, R.H., Halbur, P.G., Haynes, J.S., Bruna, J.D., Royer, R.L., Emerson, S.U. (1998). Experimental infection of pigs with swine hepatitis E virus (swine HEV) but not with human strains of HEV. Proc IPVS **15**, 177.

Meng, X.J., Purcell, R.H., Halbur, P.G., Lehman, J.R., Webb, D.M., Tsareva, T.S., Haynes, J.S., Thacker, B.J., Emerson, S.U. (1997). A novel virus in swine is closely related to the human hepatitis E virus. Proc. Natl. Acad. Sci. **94**, 9860-9865.

Retrovirus

Retroviruses have been identified in porcine cell lines but clinical disease has not been reported. Particles have been seen in myeloid leukaemias. Complete and incomplete sequences of the virus have been demonstrated in a variety of pig tissues and the possibility of their transfer to man in transplanted organs has been a matter of considerable discussion.

Reference

Phanh Thanh, L., Kaeffer, B., Bottreau, E. (1992). Arch.Virol. **123**, 255-265. Porcine retrovirus: optimal conditions for its biochemical detection.

Porcine Spongiform Encephalopathy

Bovine spongiform encephalopathy has been experimentally-transmitted to a pig by inoculation of bovine brain. Depression, inappetence, aimless biting and ataxia developed after 69 weeks. Spongiform lesions of the mid-brain were identified. Disease has not been transmitted by feeding either bovine brain or scrapie material.

Reference

Dawson, M., Wells, G.A.H., Parker, B.N.J., Scott, A.C. (1990). Primary parenteral transmission of bovine spongiform encephalopathy to the pig. Vet.Rec. **127**, 338.

BACTERIAL DISEASES

Diseases caused by bacteria, mycoplasmas, rickettsiae, chlamydia and eperythrozoon are all considered in this section. The identification of an infectious syndrome caused by bacteria is subject to the criteria already outlined for viral diseases with two important differences:

1) Many bacterial diseases respond to appropriate antimicrobial treatment.

2) A few bacteria may produce toxins in the feed which can be ingested to cause disease.

Bacterial diseases may be recognised by the identification of clinical signs, post-mortem findings or epidemiological features with those of the diseases described below and under Differential Diagnosis at the end of the book. These diseases can then be confirmed by the demonstration of the agent, its DNA, its products or antibody to it. Some bacterial diseases are enzootic in pig herds (enzootic pneumonia, *Mycoplasma hypopneumoniae* and *E.coli* post-weaning diarrhoea) and it should be realised that the disease may behave very differently in a herd with enzootic infection when compared with the same disease in a non-immune herd. It is important to identify cases where more than one agent is present in a lesion because bacteria are capable of colonising lesions caused by other agents. This problem is particularly acute when considering enteric lesions which may be initiated by viruses, parasites or bacteria and then colonised by other bacterial pathogens. In these complicated syndromes associated with bacteria, a decision has to be made about the most significant agent or agents present and these can then be controlled. Successful identification of the initiating agent can only be confirmed by a favourable response to a specific vaccine, a particular control measure or therapy in a controlled split herd study or by laboratory confirmation..

Minor pathogens or opportunists are described here in order to provide some ideas about possible causes of, or contributions to, bacterial disease.

When disease fails to respond to control measure expected to be effective, consider that:

a) antimicrobial may be ineffective because it is given too late, in too low levels (inactivated in water, by pelleting, by settlement in feed) or may be given by a route inappropriate to the body system affected. It may also fail because the wrong antimicrobial was chosen for the organism concerned due to innate or acquired resistance.

b) Vaccine may be inappropriate because a different serotype of the organism is involved in disease or antibody/cellular immune levels are too low.

c) Re-infection is taking place because of mixing of stock or survival of the agent in the environment.

If none of these factors account for the problem, reconsider the diagnosis.

Leptospirosis

Definition

Infection with one of the serovars of the eight *Leptospira* species may be inapparent, or may cause fever, meningitis, icterus and death in piglets and abortion and stillbirth in sows. *Leptospira interrogans* serogroup Canicola, serogroup Icterohaemorrhagiae and serogroup Australis serovar *bratislava* are the major causes of the syndrome in Britain. *L.interrogans* Seroroup Pomona is most important worldwide, perhaps followed by *L. borgpetersenii* Serogroup Tarassovi and *L.interrogans* serovar *bratislava* for all of which the pig is the maintenace host.

Incidence

Leptospirosis occurs in pigs worldwide. The range of serogroups and serovars reported from each country varies. Reporting depends upon a) those actually present and b) those sought (which can vary according to the strains used as antigens and the ability of laboratories to isolate and identify them). Infection is more common in animals kept outside, but infection with serovar *bratislava* occurs in housed pigs and serogroups Canicola and Icterohaemorrhagiae have occurred in housed pigs in Britain in the past. In a serological survey of pig herds in Britain, antibody to the following serovars of *L.interrogans* was found: Australis 23%, Cynopteri 12%, Icterohaemorrhagiae 4%, Ballum 3% and others 3%. Studies in Northern Ireland have shown that serovars *bratislava* and *muenchen* of the Australis serogroup were present in 71% of aborted piglets and on 68% farms examined. Infection with Australis serovars has been identified in the US and Canada as well as many European countries, Australia and South America. Infection rates vary. In many countries serogroup Pomona and Tarassovi infections may be present in up to 30% of herds and outbreaks of Canicola and Icterohaemorrhagiae infection may occur.

Aetiology

Leptospira are fine spiral bacteria (spirochaetes),10 µm in length and 0.2 µm in diameter with a central body which is hooked at each end and surrounded by an envelope. Within this lies a single axial filament arising from each end and overlapping centrally. They may be grown in complex media such as EMJH and E medium, and are aerobic. Primary isolation from tissue takes 2-6 weeks and 5-fluorouracil, rifampicin, amphotericin B or cycloserine are included in isolation media. The 9 species are defined by DNA-DNA homology (70%) and divided into serogroups by the production of antisera which are then absorbed with organisms of other groups. The serogroups have been shown to be associated with the possession of particular combinations of envelope antigens. Each serogroup consists of a number of serovars which are distinguished using monoclonal antibodies. Serovars have been sub-divided in their turn by the use of factor analysis with monoclonal antibodies and more recently by restriction endonuclease analysis and 16SrRNA gene analysis. Individual subdivisions of serovars have been associated with particular syndromes such as *L. interrogans* serogroup Australis serovar *bratislava* genotype B2b and serovar m*uenchen* M2 in abortion and serovar *bratislava* B2a in meningitis.

Leptospirae are sensitive *in vitro* to many antimicrobials such as penicillin and streptomycin and are sensitive to most disinfectants, to soaps, detergents and are rapidly destroyed by drying. They may, however, persist for weeks or months in water.

Antibodies to serogroups Pomona, Canicola, Tarassovi, Icterohaemorrhagiae, Sejroe, serovar *hardjo*, Ballum, serovars *bratislava* and *autumnalis* have all been found in pigs. Infections with Pomona and Tarassovi are an important cause of morbidity in the United States, Australia and Europe, but in Britain, Canicola, Icterohaemorrhagiae and Australis are the most important serogroups. Serovars *muenchen* and *bratislava* are the two most common Australis serovars. Serogroup Pomona serovar *mozdok* has been identified in Dorset but serovar *kennewicki*, the classic pig adapted Pomona has never been found in the UK.

Pathogenesis

Infection is by ingestion, direct contact and entry through abrasions, transplacental transmission or by the venereal route. The organisms multiply to produce a septicaemia which may produce clinical signs. They may cause damage in the liver and elsewhere in the body and penetrate basement membranes into sites protected from circulating antibody which normally limits leptospiraemia within 7-10 days of infection. In Pomona infections, organisms penetrate from the blood vessels through the interstitial tissue of the kidney to the basement membrane within 3-5 days of infection and cause swelling of the tubular epithelial cells. By 7 days post-infection they are present within the tubular epithelial cells and macrophages are prominent in the interstitial tissue and by 14 days after infection are restricted to the microvilli of the lumenal surface. Plasma cells and lymphocytes are prominent in the interstitial tissue. Leptospirae are shed in the urine from time to time during a period of months after clinical recovery. Localisation may also occur in the pregnant uterus, cause foetal invasion and abortion 10 days to 4 weeks after infection and may also occur in the fallopian tubes and seminal vesicles. Penetration into the central nervous system may result in meningitis and damage to the liver in the acute stage may result in jaundice. The pathogenesis of *muenchen* infections in sows appears to be similar with few detectable clinical signs and a shorter period of leptospiruria (30 days) Leptospirae may enter the genital tract from systemic infection or from venereal infection. Embryos and foetuses must be infected prior to 50 days of gestation for death to result. The organisms may persist in the genital tract of both sows and boars.

Clinical signs

Three main clinical syndromes are associated with leptospira infection in pigs.

1.   Subclinical infection

Serological evidence of infection (see above) is widespread in pig populations in Britain, especially in finishing pigs and gilts reared extensively in which clinical signs of disease are rarely seen. Leptospirae may be isolated from the kidneys and genital tracts of these animals

2.   Acute or subacute infection

Fever to 40°C (105.8°F) for 3-5 days has been recorded in serogroup Canicola and Icterohaemorrhagiae infection in piglets and in Pomona and Tarassovi infections. Affected pigs become dull, anorexic, show diarrhoea and rarely develop icterus with or without haemoglobinuria. Heavy mortality may occur. Nervous signs may be seen, e.g. weakness of the hindquarters, meningitis or tremor if leptospirae enter nervous tissue. Animals with severe jaundice, haemorrhagic disease or nervous signs such that prostration occurs, should be killed humanely if treatment is ineffective.

3. Reproductive disorders

Abortion, stillbirth and neonatal mortality accompanied by fever, loss of milk and jaundice in the sows are common consequences of leptospiral infection in breeding herds. Serovars *muenchen* and *bratislava* and serogroup Canicola are often implicated in Britain, but Pomona is an important cause worldwide. In experimental infections, abortion occurred 4-7 days after infection with Canicola in sows less than 4-5 weeks pregnant. In sows which were infected later, weak piglets were born. Mummified and macerated foetuses also occur commonly amongst the litters of sows with leptospirosis. Abortion in the last trimester of pregnancy is common. Infertility associated with venereal spread in non-immune herds may be responsible for returns to service, particularly with the Australis serovars *bratislava* and *muenchen.*

Pathology

Death from leptospirosis only occurs infrequently in Britain, so post-mortem findings are mainly incidental, e.g. at slaughter, or as a result of the examination of aborted foetuses. In acute cases, signs of generalised septicaemia occur, often coupled with jaundice and signs of liver damage. Kidney lesions may be present. In leptospiral abortions, associated with Pomona and Icterohaemorrhagiae, affected foetuses may be mummified, or have uniformly pale organs with or without jaundice. Freshly aborted foetuses often have petechiae on the skin and haemorrhages in kidney, lungs and liver. Excess straw-coloured fluid is often present in the serous cavities. In other cases few distinctive changes may be present. In Australis abortions mummification is not a feature and abortions take place in the last third of gestation or litters of stillborn piglets are produced at full term. Renal lesions are the most common finding, and often occur in clinically-normal pigs. The basic lesion is a greyish-white focus 1-3 mm in diameter in the cortex. This lesion may be surrounded by an area of congestion, and is seen when the capsule is stripped. Petechiation may be present. Histological findings in the early stages include the presence of the organism in silver-stained sections, especially in the kidney tubules. Tubular damage and mononuclear cell infiltration may be seen in sections of affected kidneys. Leptospirae may also be demonstrated by immunofluorescence and immunoperoxidase in tissue. Antigen demonstrated by these means remains detectable after whole organisms have disintegrated and can no longer be cultured or recognised in silver-stained sections. DNA probes have also been used and may detect 10^2 organisms/g tissue.

Epidemiology

Infection with *Leptospira* may arise from the organisms shed in the urine of carrier animals, from organisms shed by carrier rodents or by venereal spread. Rat infestation is a common source of infection due to Icterohaemorrhagiae and in Europe and other countries, Pomona infections may be associated with infections in field mice. Dogs may be infected and act as sources of infection. The organisms may persist in clean water for periods up to 30 days and infections may be water borne from a source upstream or from drinking water contaminated with rodent urine. Pomona infections due to serovar *kennewicki* may be enzootic in herds. In such a herd, the prevalence of serum antibody in young piglets is high, falls to a low point by 6-10 weeks of age and rises rapidly thereafter to a high prevalence. In herds with sporadic infection in which infection is contracted from rodents or by venereal spread, the prevalence of specific antibody rises gradually with age. Many animals with localised infections may not have serum antibody levels and thus escape detection.

Pigs infected with leptospira may act as sources of infection for man and leptospirosis is a zoonosis, affecting farm workers, abattoir staff and butchers.

Diagnosis

Clinical signs such as abortion in the last trimester of pregnancy, reduced conception, vulval discharge, the birth of weak piglets, and fever with icterus and mortality in older piglets and weaners may suggest leptospirosis. The post-mortem findings, especially the kidney lesions, may also be suggestive. Diagnosis is usually confirmed by demonstration of the organism or by antibody to it.

The organism may be demonstrated by dark ground microscopy of the urine of aborting sows or in urine, semen, aborted foetuses and the organs of slaughtered pigs by culture. Culture requires specialist media and is most reliable when the tissue concerned is fresh and uncontaminated. Contamination may be reduced by using fresh urine, kidneys with the capsule intact, or the anterior chamber of the eye in aborted foetuses. Liver, lung, brain, the blood, exudates and reproductive organs and secretions may all be examined. Samples should be submitted in a transport medium similar to the isolation medium and isolation can be carried out by a specialist laboratory but may take 6-12 weeks. Isolation is one of the most sensitive methods of confirmation of diagnosis.

The organism, its antigens or products may also be demonstrated in tissue by silver staining of fixed tissue, by immunofluorescence or immunoperoxidase, and by DNA probes.

Serological tests are widely used. Antibodies to leptospira appear in the serum with 1-2 weeks of infection and reach titres of 1:10,000-1:30,000 (Microscopic Agglutination Lysis Test, MAT) which may persist for some weeks. The MAT, using live organisms, is the most sensitive test and detects rising titres which follow infection particularly well. Microscopic agglutination tests can be carried out using killed antigen but are less sensitive (94.%). An IgM Enzyme Immunoassay (EIA) with 82% sensitivity and whole cell ELISA and axial filament ELISAs with 97% sensitivity have also been described. A competitive ELISA has been produced for serovar *bratislava* and is safe and effective.

Serum antibody can only be used as a herd test. Antibody levels suggestive of chronic infection are 1:100 (MAT) but infected animals may be seronegative. Antibody occurring in thoracic exudates in stillborn foetuses is diagnostic. Cross reaction between serogroups and serovars may occur and accurate serology is best carried out using local serovars.

Treatment

The parenteral administration of a number of antibiotics such as penicillin, semisynthetic penicillins, streptomycin and tiamulin is of value in acutely ill animals. Abortions may be prevented and renal carriers eliminated by parenteral treatment with streptomycin (25 mg/kg) as a single dose or for 3-5 days. Treatment 1 week before service and 2 weeks before farrowing has been found to be most satisfactory in preventing reproductive losses.   Feed or water medication with tetracyclines at 800 g/tonne may be of value or parenterally (40 mg/kg for 3 or 5 days) and both tylosin (44mg/kg for 5 days) and erythromycin (25mg/kg for 5 days) have been shown to be effective. Re-infection should be prevented by hygiene and isolation.

Control

Vaccination of uninfected sows with killed vaccines containing the appropriate serotype or serotypes before service may prevent abortion. Piglets should be vaccinated before the period of risk (6-10 weeks of age), but if protection does not result, confirm the point at which infection is occurring by preparing a herd serum antibody profile and vaccinate prior to exposure. Only Icterohaemorrhagiae, Canicola and *hardjo* vaccines are available in the UK, but elsewhere Pomona, Tarassovi, *hardjo*, *bratislava* and Grippotyphosa have been used either alone or in various combinations. Vaccination may not prevent renal colonisation and is unlikely to eliminate it if it is already established. Serovar *bratislava* vaccine has been shown to produce significant improvements in numbers born in the face of *bratislava* infection. Regular revaccination is advisable.

Transmission of infection may be eliminated by hygiene, vaccination, treatment or slaughter of carriers or a total slaughter policy combined with disinfection, elimination of rodents and restocking. As leptospirae can survive freezing, the practice of feedback of foetal material for SMEDI control may predispose to leptospiral infection and should be avoided.

References

Alt, D.P., Bolin, C.A. (1996) Preliminary evaluation of antimicrobial agents for treatment of *Leptospira interrogans* serovar *pomona* infection in hamsters and swine. Am. J. Vet. Res. **57**, 59-62

Baker, T.F., McEwen, S.A., Prescott, J.F. and Meek, A.H. (1989). The prevalence of leptospirosis and its association with multifocal interstitial nephritis in swine at slaughter. Can.J.Vet.Res. **53**, 290-294.

Barlow, A.M. (2004) Reproductive failure in sows associated with Leptospira Mozdok from a wildlife source. Pig J. **54**, 123-131.

Chappel, R.J., Prince, R.W., Mullar, B.D., Mead, L.J., Jones, R.T. and Adler, B. (1992). Comparison of diagnostic procedures for porcine leptospires. Vet.Micro. **30**, 151-163.

Ellis, W.A. (1989). *L.australis* infection in pigs. Pig Vet.J. **22**, 83-92.

Ellis, W.A., McParland, P.J., Bryson, D.G. and Cassells, J.A. (1986). Prevalence of leptospira infection in aborted pigs in Northern Ireland. Vet.Rec. **118**, 63-65.

Ellis, W.A., McParland, P.J., Bryson, D.G. and Cassells, J.A. (1986). Boars as carriers of leptospires of the Australis serogroup on farms with an abortion problem. Vet.Rec. **118**, 563.

Ellis, W.A., McParland, P.J., Bryson, D.G., Thiermann, A.B. and Montgomery, J. (1986). Isolation of leptospires from genital tract and kidneys of aborted sows. Vet.Rec. **118**, 294-295.

Ellis, W.A., Montgomery, J.M. and McParland, P.J. (1989). An experimental study with an *L.interrogans* serovar *bratislava* vaccine. Vet.Rec. **125**, 319-321.

Ellis, W.A., Montgomery, J.M. and Thiermann, A.B. (1991). Restriction endonuclease analysis as a taxonomic tool in the study of pig isolates belonging to the Australis serogroup of *L.interrogans*. J.Clin.Microbiol. **29**, 957-961.

Franz, J.C., Hanson, L.E. and Brown, A.L. (1989). Effect of vaccination with a bacterin containing *L.interrogans* serovar *bratislava* on the breeding performance of swine herds. Am.J.Vet.Res. **50**, 1044-1047.

115

Frizzell, C., Mackie, D.P., Montgomery, J.M., Ellis, W.A. (2004). Development of a competitive ELISA for the detection of serum antibodies of Leptospira serovar Bratislava. Pig J. **53**, 195-199.
Hathaway, S.C., Little, T.W.A. and Stevens, A.E. (1981). *Leptospira hardjo* in pigs. A new host - parasite relationship in the UK. Res. Vet. Sci. **31**, 169-173.
Kingscote, W.F. (1986). Leptospirosis outbreak in a piggery in Southern Alberta. Can.Vet.J. **77**, 188-197
Michna, S.W. and Campbell, R.S.F. (1969). Leptospirosis in pigs: Epidemiology, microbiology and pathology. Vet.Rec. **84**, 135-138.

Actinobacillosis

Definition

Actinobacillus suis and *A.equuli* may cause fatal septicaemia, endocarditis and arthritis in pigs 1-6 weeks of age. In older animals, skin lesions may be seen and a focal necrotising pneumonia may occur.

Incidence

Present in many countries but reported from few. First identified in UK in 1971, it is not uncommon. It has been studied most extensively in Canada in recent years.

Aetiology

Actinobacillus suis and *A.equuli* have both been reported. Both produce 2 mm translucent circular colonies on blood agar and small pink colonies on MacConkey agar after 24 hours' incubation. *A.suis* produces alpha-haemolysis on horse blood agar and B-haemolysis on sheep blood agar. *A.suis* also hydrolyses aesculin, produces acid from arabinose, cellobiose and salicin and is pathogenic for mice. All isolates (Canada) appear to belong to one antigenic and REF group but another (O1K1 appears to be more common further south, in the USA. *A. suis* has been shown to possess the ApxI and ApxII also found in *A.pleuropneumoniae*.

Pathogenesis

Infection appears to occur via the upper respiratory tract in young pigs and results in septicaemia. The animal may die at this stage or the infection may localise to give vegetative endocarditis or arthritis. In older pigs infection may be by the respiratory route and result in pneumonia.

Clinical signs

Sudden death may occur in sucking piglets and can be attributed to crushing or still birth in neonates. Piglets may be found to be febrile (39-40.5°C, 102.5-105°F) with multiple haemorrhages on the skin, particularly of the ears and abdomen. Swollen carpal and hock joints and septic or necrotic lesions of the skin may also be seen alone or together. Recovering animals remain unthrifty. Adults may have round or rhomboid cutaneous haemorrhages later becoming subcutaneous abscesses, particularly on the neck, withers and flanks.

Lesions may resemble those of erysipelas. Finishers usually die suddenly but may have pyrexia, dyspnoea and cyanosis prior to death. Adults are rarely affected but deaths have been reported following the introduction of the disease into high health herds.

Mild cases respond to antimicrobial treatment, but animals with chronic arthritis, vegetative endocarditis or cyanosis should be killed humanely.

Pathology

Animals which have died from actinobacillus infections may have discoloured areas, purpura or necrosis of the skin. The carcases may appear normal apart from the presence of petechiae on lung, the kidney and an excess of pleural fluid. Histological lesions in the lung are characteristic as they consist of a microcolony of bacteria surrounded by necrosis and inflammatory cells. The skin lesions contain thromboemboli in both superficial and deep vessels surrounded by infarcted dermal and epidermal tissue. Chronic cases may have vegetative endocarditis, fibrinous pericarditis, pneumonia or polyarthritis. Lesions resembling those of pleuropneumonia in fattening pigs have yielded *Actinobacillus spp. A.equuli* or, more commonly, *A.suis*, may be isolated in pure culture from the kidney, liver, or heart blood and from localised lesions.

Epidemiology

There are some reports of contact with horses in *A.equuli* cases and outbreaks of *A. suis* infection may occur following the introduction of carrier animals to the farm, giving rise to an increase in preweaning mortality of 1 pig per litter. Studies of enzootically-infected herds show that antibody to the 104 kDa toxin is present in colostrum and that active antibody appears at 6-8 weeks of age. *A.suis* can be recovered from the tonsils of sucking pigs, from sow vaginas and from the preputial diverticula of boars. Human wound infection has been recorded.

Diagnosis

The clinical signs and post-mortem lesions are not specific, although the skin lesions are suggestive of this disease, particularly when fever and purpura are found, erysipelas should be ruled out. Isolation of the organism will confirm. *Pasteurella haemolytica* septicaemia usually follows contact with sheep. Serological cross reactions with *A. pleuropneumoniae* occur in the C.F. test for the latter and ELISA tests using the 104 kDa toxin may also cross-react but neutralisation tests are specific. The organism should be distinguished from *A. pleuropneumoniae* Biotype II.

Treatment

Tetracyclines, ampicillin, trimethoprim sulphonamide, ceftiofur and enrofloxacin may be given parenterally or orally if appropriate in small pigs. Recovery is normally complete after 2-5 days' treatment. Resistance to tetracyclines, amoxycillin, ampicillin and tetracyclines has been recorded. Treatment of sows prior to farrowing with trimethoprim sulphonamide has been used to eliminate carriage in control programmes.

References

Jones, J.E.T. and Simmons, J.R. (1971). Endocarditis in the pig caused by *Actinobacillus equuli*. A field and experimental case. Brit.Vet.J. **127**, 25-29.

Miniats, O.P., Spinato, M.T. and Sanford, S.E. (1989). *Actinobacillus suis* septicaemia in mature swine. Two outbreaks resembling erysipelas. Can.Vet.J. **30**, 943-947.

Ostaaijen, J.van, Frey, J., Rosendal, S., MacInnes, J.I. (1997). *A. suis* strains isolated from healthy and diseased swine are clonal and carry *apx*1CABD$_{\text{var suis}}$ and *apx*IICA$_{\text{var suis}}$ toxin genes. J.Clin. Micro. **35**, 1131-1137.

Sanford, S.E., Josephson, G.K.A., Rehmtulla, A.J., Tilker, A.M.E. (1990). *Actinobacillus suis* infection in pigs in south western Ontario. Can.Vet.J. **31**, 443-447.

Actinobacillus ureae

This organism, formerly *Pasteurella ureae* has been recorded in placentitis and abortion. There is no experimental evidence for its causal role.

Reference

Orr, J., Chirino-Trejo, M., Saunders, B., Kumor, L., Sawatsky, J. (1990). Association of *A.ureae* with porcine abortion. Can.Vet.J. **31**, 42.

Brucellosis

Definition

Brucella suis infection may be inapparent or may result in stillbirths, abortions and infertility in both sexes. In the boar, infection of the testicles and accessory sex glands is common.

Incidence

Brucellosis does not occur in pigs in Britain or Ireland but still occurs in many countries in Europe, Asia and Australia with wild or feral pigs and in half the states of the US. It appears to be absent from Canada. In most countries with developed pig industries the incidence is declining.

Aetiology

B.suis biotype 1 (worldwide), biotype 2 (West Central Europe), biotype 3 (US., S. America, S.E. Asia) is the causal agent. It is a small, slender, aerobic gram-negative bacillus and forms 1-2 mm domed colonies on blood agar after 2-4 days' aerobic incubation. *B.abortus* and *B.melitensis* have been found to infect pigs. The species *B. suis* is currently classified as *B.melitensis* biovar Suis and then the biotype e.g.2, but is referred to here as *B. suis*

Pathogenesis

Infection by the oral or venereal route is followed by multiplication in local lymph nodes. After 1-7 weeks a bacteraemia develops and persists for at least 5 weeks (up to 34 weeks). The organisms remain in lymph nodes, joints bone marrow and the genital tract. Invasion of the foetus may lead to abortion. Infection may persist for at least 64 months and, in boars, for life. Antibody usually develops 6-8 weeks after infection.

Clinical signs

Early abortion (returns to oestrus 5-8 weeks after service) results from infection at service, but infection later in pregnancy gives rise to litters with mummified, stillborn or weak pigs. Copious bloody vulval discharge, retention of foetal membranes and endometritis occur. Testicular swelling, orchitis and epididymitis may occur in boars within 7 weeks of infection and testicular atrophy may be present within 19 weeks. Bones and joints may be involved in both sexes and posterior paralysis and lameness may occur. Lame animals and those with paralysis should be destroyed on humane grounds.

Pathology

Necrotic or abscessed testicles may be seen in boars and there may be marked enlargement or atrophy of these organs. In the sow there may be oedema, haemorrhage and necrosis of the uterine lining and the presence of miliary white 2-3mm lesions. There may be a purulent arthritis in both sexes. Granulomatous lesions may be present in the liver, kidney, spleen and reproductive tract.

Epidemiology

Infection is introduced to a herd by live infected pigs or contact with infected hares (Europe) or, less commonly, by contaminated meat products and semen or ova. Infection is often oral. Infected boars form a major source of infection within a herd and transmit the disease by natural service or artificial insemination. Sows may remain carriers, shed organisms in milk and uterine discharges and up to 10% of their progeny may contract infection which they retain until adulthood. Lateral spread may also occur amongst weaners. Infection may persist in dried secretions in cold conditions for up to 2 years and reservoirs of infection in the European brown hare and Wild Boar are important in Europe while infected feral pigs are important in Australia and the South Eastern US. The infection occurs in outdoor herds of domestic pigs where infected hares and wild boar are found. The organism infects man to cause brucellosis, usually through contact with infected wild boar meat but the organism survives up to 126 days in sausage, can occur in cows' milk and cause laboratory infection (Category 3) .

Diagnosis

Clinical signs may suggest brucellosis but diagnosis is often made by isolating the organism by culture of the mandibular, gastrohepatic and external iliac lymph nodes on a regular basis and from other organs affected in the particular outbreak. A PCR using the omp2b gene has recently been described. Serological tests are also important but may be misleading. Some infected animals are antibody-negative. B.abortus standard antigen is used for tests as the same antigens are present in B.suis. Tube and plate agglutination tests can be used but the brucellosis card test and the Rose Bengal Plate Test are widely used for large scale surveillance. Indirect and competitive ELISA tests have recently been shown to be 98% sensitive and 100% specific. Antibody to Yersinia enterocolitica type O9 may cause cross reaction and false positives in Rose Bengal and SAT tests.

Control

Slaughter followed by restocking is the most successful method of control. Separation of outdoor pig populations from wild or feral pigs by effective fencing is essential. Disinfection is a vital part of control. International trade is safeguarded by the export of seronegative pigs and the testing of boars upon entry to AI stations. Vaccination with attenuated strains such as the Chinese S2 strain and treatment have been described but are not 100% effective. The oral vaccination of pigs with the RB51 strain of *B. abortus* has been described.

References

Cornell, W.D., Chengappa, M.M., Stuart, L.A., Maddux, R.L., Hail, R.I. (1989). *Brucella suis* biovar 3 infection in a Kentucky swine herd. J.Vet. Diagnostic Investigation 1, 20-21.

Done, S.H., Wrathall, A.E., Broughton, E.S., Spencer, S. (1998). Brucellosis in swine. Pig J. 41, 113-120.

Edmonds, M.D., Samartino, L.E., Hoyt, P.G., Haguis, S.D., Walker, J.V., Enright, F.M., Schurig, G.G., Elzer, P. (2001). Oral vaccination of sexually mature pigs with Brucella abortus vaccine strain RB51. Am J.vet Res. 62, 1328-1331.

Wrathall, A.E., Broughton, A.E., Gill, K.P.W., Goldsmith, G.P. (1993). Serological reactions to Brucella species in British pigs. Vet.Rec. 132, 449-454.

Listeriosis

Infection with *Listeria sp.* is common in pigs. Studies in Denmark, Japan and Yugoslavia suggest that about 10% of slaughter pigs may be contaminated in life and that the organisms, principally *L.monocytogenes* and *L.innocua* are present in tonsils and in faeces. Carriage rate increases when liquid feed or silage are fed.

L.monocytogenes is a Gram-positive bacillus 1.2 µm by 0.5 µm which grows from 4°C to 37°C. Colonies on blood agar are beta-haemolytic, greyish and opaque with a narrow zone of haemolysis.

Infection rarely causes disease, but sudden death in piglets, septicaemia and nervous signs have all been recorded. Abortion, stillbirths and the birth of weak piglets may all occur in sows. Lesions in piglets may include necrotic lesions in the liver, patchy lesions in the lung and hydrothorax. Histological lesions include meningitis, perivascular cuffing and microabscess formation in the brain. The bacteria may be seen in these.

Listeria infection in pigs is a potential source of infection for man. Up to 30% of minced pork products may be contaminated and preservatives such as sodium chloride 3%, dextrose 1% and phosphate 0.04% have been shown to enhance resistance to heating. Diagnosis is based on isolation of the organism but serum antibody may be present in infected pigs, especially in sows after abortion. A wide range of enrichment and PCR methods based on listeriolysin gene detection are available for use in meat.

The organism is sensitive to a number of antimicrobials and may be treated in piglets if caught in time. Paralysed pigs should be destroyed.

Reference

Lopez, A. and Bildfell, R. (1989). Neonatal porcine listeriosis. Can. Vet. J. 30, 828-829

Mycoplasma haemosuis infection (Eperythrozoonosis)

Definition

Infection results in anaemia, fever and icterus in pigs of 0-5 days of age. Poor growth may result in weaners and growers and sows may also be affected.

Incidence

Present in the US (16-40% herds), Germany, France, China, Taiwan and many other pig-rearing countries. Reported in the UK (26.4%, 1995). The use of tetracyclines may reduce the incidence of disease.

Aetiology

Clinical disease is associated with *M. haemosuis* (formerly *Eperythrozoon suis*). Another organism, *E.parvum*, was originally described but differed only in size and lack of clinical disease. *M. haemosuis* is rod-shaped, coccoid or ring-like, 0.8-1 µm in diameter and is located on the erythrocyte membrane.

Pathogenesis

After infection by parenteral or oral transmission the organisms begin to multiply and to cause disease in as little as 5-6 days. Most studies have been carried out in splenectomised pigs which are sensitive indicators. At the onset of clinical signs, up to 80% of erythrocytes are infected. They cause increased fragility of the red cell membranes leading to breakdown, anaemia and icterus. Hypoglycaemia occurs because the consumption of blood glucose exceeds gluconeogenesis. Liver enzymes and bilirubin levels rise and intravascular coagulation occurs.

Antibody levels rise to a peak lasting 2 months and cold (IgM) agglutinins may also affect red cell integrity. PRRS may be a predisposing factor.

Clinical signs

Pallor and icterus has been described in neonatal pigs 0-5 days of age and then resolves leaving the animals uneven in size. In weaned pigs, varying degrees of unthriftiness, jaundice (bilirubin values 46-68 µ.mole/l.) and anaemia occur. The tips of the ears may be cyanotic and mottled. In sows these signs are accompanied by fever (40-41.5°C, 104-107°F) and oedema with effects on reproduction such as abortion and an increase in stillbirths. Infection may be subclinical.

Pathology

Anaemia, watery blood, icterus of the carcase, enlargement of liver and spleen and fluid in all cavities with reddening of the bone marrow may be seen.

Epidemiology

Related at present to PRRS, infection can be transmitted to non-immune pigs by bites from lice (*Haematopinus suis*), infected needles, rough handling (nasal snares) and the ingestion of blood, urine or secretions containing it. *In utero* transmission has been described but not venereal transmission. Infection is usually introduced with carrier pigs.

Diagnosis

Based on clinical signs and confirmed by demonstrating the organisms on erythrocytes in blood smears stained by Giemsa or acridine orange, particularly at the onset of clinical signs. Blood films should be made at sampling for best results. DNA probes and PCR have recently been described. Antibody can be detected by Indirect Haemagglutination and indirect immunofluorescence but recently ELISAs, using whole organisms, have been described. Serology detects herd infection and is unreliable for individuals.

Treatment

Tetracyclines given by injection (to affected animals) or orally for 14 days will eliminate disease. Symptomatic treatment may also be required.

Control

Reduction in exposure of susceptible pigs to blood of infected animals.

References

Gresham, A., Rogers, J., Tribe, H., Phipps, L.P. (1994). *Eperythrozoon suis* in weaned pigs. Vet.Rec. **134**, 71-72.
Gwaltney, S.M., Hays, M.P., Oberst, R.D. (1993). Detection of *Eperythrozoon suis* using the polymerase chain reaction. J.Vet.Diagnostic Investigation **5**, 40-46.
Henderson, J.P., O'Ilagan, J., Hawe, S.M., Pratt, M.C.H. (1997). Anaemia and low viability in piglets infected with *Eperythrozoon suis*. Vet. Rec. **140**, 144-146
Hoelzle, L.E., Adelt, D., Hoelzle, K., Heinritzi, K., Wittenbrink, M.M., (2003). Development of a diagnostic assay based on novel DNA sequences for the detection of Mycoplasma suis (Eperythrozoon suis) in porcine blood. Vet Micro. **93**, 185-196.
Hsu, F.S., Liu, M.C., Chou, S.M., Zachary, J.F., Smith, A.R. (1992). Evaluation of an ELISA for the detection of *Eperythrozoon suis* antibodies in swine. Am.J.Vet.Res. **53**, 352-354.
Oberst, R.D., Hall, S.M., Jasso, R.A., Arndt, T., Wen, L. (1990). Recombinant DNA probe detecting *Eperythrozoon suis* in swine blood. Am.J.Vet.Res. **51**, 1760-1764.
Smith, J.E., Cipriano, J.E., Hall, S.M. (1990). *In vitro* glucose consumption in swine eperythrozoonosis. J.Vet.Med. Series B. **37**, 587-592.

Clostridium perfringens Type C

Clostridium perfringens type C produces a fatal necrotic and haemorrhagic enteritis in piglets less than 7 days of age and may cause chronic infection in older piglets.

Incidence

The disease occurs in most pig keeping countries. In Britain, 3-4 litters or part of a litter in a herd may be affected by severe disease. In other countries up to 50 litters have been reported to be affected in outbreaks.

Aetiology

Clostridium perfringens type C is a large Gram-positive rod which only occasionally forms spores. It bears attachment factors and produces toxins the most important of which is the protease/trypsin-sensitive β toxin. A second toxin the β2 toxin has been identified in animals with necrotic enteritis but its function and role in diarrhoea is as yet unclear. The organism grows readily on blood agar on which it forms 3 mm greyish colonies with an irregular edge and varying degrees of B-haemolysis after 24 hours. It is capable of forming spores and in this form is very resistant to heat although it can be killed by formalin. Varying amounts of alpha, beta and delta toxin are produced by porcine type C. *C. perfringens* type B has also been isolated.

Pathogenesis

C.perfringens type C colonises the neonatal bowel within 12-24 hours of birth on contaminated farms, and, in the absence of specific colostral immunity multiplies to cause damage to the cells of the epithelial cells of the villi of the jejunum and ileum by means of the beta toxin. Toxic damage is rapidly followed by penetration of the damaged epithelium by organisms which then adhere to the basement membrane of the villi. Necrotic damage to the core of the villus follows and the villi are shortened and covered in necrotic debris. The sensitivity of the toxin to trypsin means that disease is most likely when antitryptic factors such as those in colostrum are being ingested i.e. in the neonatal period and in the piglets of non-immune sows. Systemic absorption of the toxin occurs.

Clinical signs

Affected pigs are normal at birth and may sicken on the first or second day of life and usually die within 12-24 hours of the onset of clinical signs. A dramatic, profuse diarrhoea occurs and rapidly becomes claret-coloured. The hindquarters may be soiled with bloody faeces. Affected piglets become weak, collapse and die. Some may be found dead. In more chronic cases, shreds of necrotic material may appear in the reddish-brown watery faeces. Affected animals become very thin and pale before death. Depression of growth rate may be a feature in chronically-infected piglets.

Piglets with abdominal discolouration, subnormal temperatures or severe blood-stained diarrhoea do not recover and should be killed.

Post-mortem findings

The jejunum of affected piglets is a swollen, angry purplish-red colour and if death has been sudden, is usually full of pasty, blood-stained contents. In more chronic cases, a diptheritic layer forms and the contents are more watery. Shedding of the villi of the jejunum and the presence of Gram-positive rods at the bases of the crypts may be seen in histological sections.

Epidemiology

Outbreaks often follow the introduction of infected breeding stock and disease persists in herds for up to 2 months, but where new stock is constantly introduced, outbreaks may continue for up to 15 months. Farrowing houses or areas may become heavily contaminated and some organisms may sporulate. Transmission of vegetative organisms occurs in faeces. Other animal species

123

may be infected and may theoretically represent a source of infection for pigs. Organisms of pig origin have caused disease in man.

Diagnosis

The clinical signs and the post-mortem findings of haemorrhagic enteritis in the jejunum of piglets of this age are suggestive. Mouse protection tests may confirm the presence of *C.perfringens* type C toxin in filtrates of intestinal contents and the organism may be demonstrated in smears of the small intestinal contents. Beta toxin may be demonstrated by ELISA in intestinal contents and in culture filtrates. Clostridia may be isolated in profuse culture from the lesions in anaerobic conditions but culture filtrates must be shown to contain type C toxin or the gene for B toxin must be demonstrated in cultures or the gut before the organism can be said to be involved. Multiplex PCR tests for the toxin genes of clostridia are available.The organism may be present in lesions of other diseases such as T.G.E. in older pigs and may occur when antitryptic factors are present in the diet of weaned pigs.

Treatment and control

Affected animals die, but prophylactic injection of 2 ml hyperimmune antiserum to type C toxins gives complete protection to animals protected at birth, and usually protects animals which have not yet developed clinical signs. Oral ampicillin can be used to treat the survivors of an affected litter and, when given soon after birth may reduce the mortality in litters at risk or prevent the occurrence of the disease completely. It may be necessary to give more than one daily dose.

These measures, coupled with improved hygiene, may stop an outbreak but more permanent control is obtained by vaccination. Alum adjuvanted vaccines containing the toxoids of *C.perfringens* type C, or killed cultures of the organism, may be used alone or in combination with other vaccines such as *E.coli*. Sheep vaccines may also be used if no other licensed product is available. Sows should be vaccinated 6 and 2 weeks prior to farrowing and piglets will be protected provided they ingest colostrum. Levels of antibody in colostrum may vary considerably. Very low levels of protection may allow the development of chronic disease.

References

Arbuckle, J.B.R. (1972). The attachment of *Clostridium welchii* (*Cl.perfringens*) type C to intestinal villi of pigs. J.Pathology **106**, 65 -72.
Bergeland, M.E. (1972). Pathogenesis and immunity of *C.perfringens* type C enteritis in swine. J.Am.Vet.Med.Ass. **160**, 658.
Gasmory, H.S., Chanter, N., Frech, N.P., Bueschel, D., Songer, J.G., Titball, R.W. (2000). Occurrence of Clostridim perfringens β2 toxin in animals determined using genotyping and subtyping PCR assays. Epidem. and Infect. **124**, 61-67.
Mackinnon, J.D. (1989). Enterotoxaemia caused by *C.perfringens* type C. Pig Vet.J. **22**, 119-125.
Moller, K., Ahrens, P. (1996) Comparison of toxin neutralisation, ELISA and PCR tests for typing of Clostridium perfringens and detection of the enterotoxin gene by PCR. Anaerobe **2**, 103-110.
Ripley, P.H. and Gush, A.F. (1983). Immunisation schedule for the prevention of infectious necrotic enteritis caused by *C.perfringens* type C in piglets. Vet.Rec. **112**, 201-202.

Clostridium perfringens Type A

Definition

Causes a syndrome in piglets resembling that caused by *C.perfringens* type C but less severe. Involved in and able to cause diarrhoea in weaned pigs.

Incidence

Syndromes of the type described here appear to be present in many countries and to be fairly common in Britain. They have been identified in the Netherlands, Belgium, France, Germany, Rumania and Japan.

Aetiology

C.perfringens type A vegetative cells produce alpha toxin as the major toxin. This, with the theta toxin, enables colonies to be identified by the double zone of haemolysis on blood agar and by its lecithinase effect on egg yolk agar. Sporulation is rare in *C.perfringens* type A but sporulating strains have been isolated from weaned pig and piglet diarrhoeas and enterotoxin, produced during sporulation, has been demonstrated in intestinal contents and faeces. In some cases, the $\beta2$ toxin may be present.

Pathogenesis

Oral infection leads to multiplication in the small intestine but attachment to the villi is not commonly demonstrated. In neonatal piglets the same factors appear to operate as in *C.perfringens* type C disease with colostrum from immune sows protecting against clinical signs but not colonisation. Organisms multiply in the gut lumen of the unprotected piglet and reach high numbers in the ileum, caecum and colon. Lesions of mild villous atrophy, mucosal hyperaemia and mild necrosis develop. The reason for the enteritis is not clear as antibody to pure alpha toxin protects piglets against infection with vegetative forms. Infection with sporulating strains producing enterotoxin appear capable of causing diarrhoea within 24-72 hours of infection and enterotoxin can be demonstrated in terminal ileum, large intestine and faeces. It can be demonstrated adsorbed to colonic epithelial cells and its action may persist in this site. Enterotoxin from pig strains of *C.perfringens* type A can cause fluid production and transient diarrhoea when introduced into the small intestine. Serum antibody to alpha toxin can be demonstrated in some older pigs. Antibody to enterotoxin is passed in the colostrum and falls to levels of 1:4 (counter immunoelectrophoresis) at 4-6 weeks of age to rise again thereafter to adult levels. Many sows and finishing pigs in the UK have demonstrable antibody to enterotoxin. Other agents are frequently present.

Clinical signs

Vegetative strains may cause sudden death within 48 hours of infection or birth in non-immune piglets or may cause diarrhoea. Affected diarrhoeic sucking piglets appear dull with sunken flanks and evidence of loss of condition. The perineal area is heavily pasted with yellowish faeces. The faeces present on the pen floor frequently contains some mucus but is often creamy or pasty containing flecks of fresh blood or of a pinkish tinge. Marked depression of growth occurs. Sporulating strains may produce a transient watery diarrhoea with no mortality. In weaned pigs immunity is common but non-sporulating strains can induce transient nervous signs and minor faecal changes, sometimes accompanied by loss of condition in experimental infection. Sporulating strains cause a greyish, sometimes mucoid diarrhoea lasting 3-7 days or more after the onset of clinical signs. Inappetance and reduction in weight gain occur. Loss of condition and faecal staining of the perineum and coat are common.

Affected pigs rarely die, but piglets with low rectal temperatures and discoloured abdomens will not survive and should be killed.

Pathology

The small intestine of dead piglets is often congested and its contents creamy or watery but not blood filled as in type C infections. Necrotic areas may be seen on the mucosal surface of the jejunal and ileal mucosa with a dissecting microscope and villous atrophy is obvious. Few changes apart from congestion and darkening of the carcase are seen outside the gut. Similar findings may be seen in chronically infected piglets and C.perfringens may contribute these changes to syndromes initiated by other agents. Histological changes include widespread shedding of villous epithelial cells and destruction of the villi.

C.perfringens type A may be seen in direct smears and isolated in profuse culture from the small intestine, its contents and from the faeces of live affected piglets. Spores may be identified in direct smears where enterotoxigenic strains are involved. In weaned pigs it is present in the small intestines which are flaccid and often contain mucopus and bubbles of gas and in the uniform, fluid, bubbling contents of the flaccid large intestines which have macroscopically-normal mucosa. The histological changes described above are present to a lesser extent. C.perfringens type A may be isolated in profuse culture from the small intestines of animals with enteritis caused by a number of agents such as T.G.E. virus, rotavirus and cryptosporidial infections. Lesions are those of the most important contributor to the syndrome present.

Epidemiology

The organism is ubiquitous, being present in soil, intestinal contents and faeces. C.perfringens type A sporulating strains have been identified in meat and may cause food poisoning in man. Antibody to both alpha toxin and enterotoxin is widespread in pig populations and levels often rise with age.

Diagnosis

Requires the demonstration of C.perfringens type A by direct culture or immunofluorescence and the elimination of other causes of similar disease of piglets, such as type C disease and coccidial infections. A marked response to penicillin therapy may be suggestive of a clostridial condition. Diagnosis of uncomplicated C.perfringens type A disease in older pigs relies on the clinical signs of greyish diarrhoea or soft motions, and loss of condition in pigs aged from 5-6 weeks onwards. The presence of enterotoxin in faecal filtrates can be confirmed using commercial Reversed Passive Latex Agglutination tests, counter immunoelectrophoresis, ELISA and Vero cells. Sporulating strains may be isolated by dilution of faeces in ethanol for 1 hour or by heating at 80°C for 10 minutes and then culturing anaerobically. The genes for the toxins concerned can be detected by PCR, but only confirm the involvement of the organism.

126

Treatment

Penicillin, ampicillin or antibiotics other than aminoglycosides given orally can treat the disease in neonates. Antimicrobial treatment in the feed may reduce the effects of disease. A vaccine containing toxoided α toxin has been produced and tested but is not available in the UK. Some protection may be afforded by other clostridial vaccines, but not against enterotoxin.

References

Estrada Correa, A., Taylor D.J. (1986). Enterotoxigenic *C.perfringens* type A as a cause of diarrhoea in pigs. Proc.IPVS. **9**, 171.

Estrada Correa, A., Taylor, D.J. (1988). Enterotoxigenic *C.perfringens* type A as a cause of diarrhoea in weaned pigs. Proc.IPVS. **10**, 138.

Jestin, A., Popoff, M.R., Mahe, S. (1985). Epizootiological investigations of a diarrhoeic syndrome in fattening pigs. Am.J.Vet.Res. **46**, 2149-2151.

Nabuurs, M.J.A., Haagsma, J., Molen, E.J. van der. and Heijden, P.J. van der (1983). Diarrhoea in 1-3 week-old piglets associated with *C.perfringens* type A. Annales de Recherches Veterinaire **14**, 408-411.

Taylor, D.J., Estrada Correa, A. (1988). Avoparcin in the prevention of enterotoxigenic *C.perfringens* type A infections and diarrhoea in pigs. Proc.IPVS. **10**,139.

Taylor, D.J., Olubunmi, P.A. (1982). Enteric disease in sucking and weaned pigs initiated by and associated with *C.perfringens* type A. Proc.IPVS. **7**, 66.

Clostridium difficile typhlocolitis

Definition

C.difficile has occasionally been isolated from the intestines of individual pigs with chronic or haemorrhagic diarrhoea, but large scale outbreaks in piglets in Canada, the USA and France and experimental studies confirm that the organism can cause disease. These outbreaks have allowed the disease to be distinguished clinically and pathologically following post-mortem examination. It is not clear to what extent the condition follows routine treatment of neonatal pigs with antimicrobial, but their use could contribute to the development of this disease and there have been recent antimicrobial associated deaths from this condition in sows.

Aetiology

C. difficile is a toxigenic clostridium readily cultivated on blood agar in anaerobic conditions, recognisable by its flat, elongated grey colonies and safety-pin-shaped sporulating cells. It produces two toxins, A and B which are involved in its pathogenicity. It colonises the large intestines of many species which have been exposed to antibiotic, and those of neonates to cause necrosis and colitis. It is a potential zoonosis.

Clinical Signs

The onset of this disease is anywhere between 1 and 7 days after birth. Affected piglets develop dyspnoea, emaciation, mild abdominal distension and scrotal oedema. Diarrhoea may develop and affected animals may appear dehydrated with sunken eyes and have perineal faecal staining. It can cause preweaning losses of up to 90% but mortality is usually less than 50%. Adults sows with mastitis have been affected when treated with fluoroquinolone. Clinically-affected piglets with abdominal distension are unlikely to recover and should be killed.

Pathology

Piglets which have died from *C. difficile* infection may be dehydrated and have perineal faecal staining. There may be distension of the abdomen. The findings include ascites, with more than 50 ml of fluid being present in the peritoneal cavity, oedema of the mesocolon, hydrothorax and urate deposits in the kidneys. There may be scrotal oedema. Affected piglets have full stomachs. The mesocolic oedema is accompanied by large intestinal lesions including necrosis of the mucosa. There is local exudation of mucus, fibrin and neutrophils into the lumen of the colon and caecum (volcano lesions) and deep ulcers may give rise to transmural necrosis.

The organism can be demonstrated in direct smears of the colonic wall, by isolation on Difficile agar and its preformed toxins can be demonstrated in colonic contents by Reverse Passive Agglutination Tests or ELISA and the presence of the B toxin gene detected by PCR. The samples required for this condition are portions of the large intestine rather than the small intestine as in the other conditions.

Epidemiology

Present in the USA, France and some other countries, but apparently absent from Belgium and UK. Spread of the organism within a farm results from faecal contamination and poor hygiene and antimicrobial treatment can precipitate.

Diagnosis

The clinical signs of diarrhoea between days 1 and 7 after birth are not particularly distinctive, but the presence of abdominal distension and scrotal oedema are unusual and would lead to suspicion of *C. difficile* disease. High mortality rates would also be suggestive, particularly if routine treatments with antimicrobials had been given early in life. The post mortem findings provide reinforcement of the provisional diagnosis as ascites, mesocolic oedema and colitis without major small intestinal involvement are unusual in piglets of this age group.

The organism can be demonstrated in direct smears of the colonic wall, by isolation on Difficile agar and its preformed toxins can be demonstrated in colonic contents by Reverse Passive Agglutination Tests, ELISA or commercial solid state immunoassay and the presence of the B toxin gene detected by PCR. The samples required for this condition are portions of the large intestine and its contents rather than the small intestine as in the other conditions.

Treatment and control.

Support affected piglets. No antitoxic or vaccine therapy has yet been shown to be successful in the pig. Vancomycin and metronidazole, the human therapeutic agents, are not available for the pig. Tylosin treatment has been suggested. Hygiene should be improved and environmental problems reduced.

References

Songer, J.G., Post, K.W., Larson, D.J., Jost, B.H. and Glock, R.D. (2000). Infection of neonatal swine with *Clostridium difficile*. Swine Health and Production **8**, 185-189

128

Waters, E.H., Orr, J.P., Clark, E.G., Schaufele, C.M. (1998). Typhlocolitis caused by *Clostridium difficile* in sucking piglets. Journal of Diagnostic Investigation **10**, 104-108.

Tetanus

Definition

Infection with *Clostridium tetani* causes stiffness and abnormal gait leading to tetanic spasms and death. The condition occurs sporadically in young pigs and may be associated with umbilical infections or with castration, especially when a contaminated knife has been used or where sheep have been lambed in the same accommodation.

Aetiology

C.tetani is a slender rod-shaped Gram-positive anaerobic bacillus 0.4 by 3-8 μ with terminal spherical spores and forming weakly haemolytic colonies with fibrils of growth extending over the medium from their edges. The clinical signs result from the peptide neurotoxin and not from the haemolysin.

Pathogenesis

Following inoculation into penetrating wounds or the umbilicus, spores germinate in the anaerobic, often contaminated tissue debris and form neurotoxin. This diffuses from the site of multiplication to neuromuscular junctions and travels in the axoplasm and sheaths of motor nerves to the central nervous system where it inhibits the release of inhibitory transmitters by inhibitory neurones. Recovery is associated with the development of circulating antibody to the toxin.

Clinical signs

Clinical signs appear a few days to weeks after wound infection and affected animals show abnormalities of gait and can be identified in this way in affected batches. Within 1-2 days the muscles stiffen, the ears are held erect and the tail straight and affected pigs finally lie on their sides in opisthotonus with fore and hind limbs rigidly extended and pointing backwards. Stimuli, e.g. noise, result in tetanic spasm of the muscles. Death normally results. Affected sucking pigs should be killed but affected weaners may recover with treatment. If severely affected and unable to stand they should be killed.

Epidemiology

Spores are present in soil and live for many years. Outbreaks in pigs have followed housing in sheep barns.

Diagnosis

Diagnosis is based on the characteristic clinical signs. Dead pigs may be rigid in the characteristic attitude, but no specific gross lesions are seen at post-mortem examination. A wound abscess or umbilical lesion may be present and a smear may be made from this and the diagnosis may be confirmed if the characteristic "drum-stick" bacilli and spores are seen.

Treatment and control

Severely affected animals rarely recover after treatment. Tetanus antitoxin may be given intramuscularly or intrathecally to mildly affected animals or intramuscularly to those at risk and antibiotic injections should also be given. Affected animals may also be given barbiturate as a relaxant, (in EU may not be appropriate for food animals), kept quiet and should be given an antibiotic such as penicillin. The disease is normally controlled by hygiene, particularly at castration, although vaccination either of sows or piglets may be carried out using tetanus toxoid alone given in divided doses of 1 or 2 ml subcutaneously with an interval of 4 weeks and gives complete protection. Tetanus toxoid is included in many sheep vaccines for protection against *C.perfringens* type C and other clostridia.

Clostridium novyi (*C. oedematiens* infection)

Definition

Clostridium novyi type B infection causes sudden death in large fattening pigs and sows.

Incidence

Sporadic, particularly in swill fed pigs and older sows. Worldwide.

Aetiology

C.novyi (oedematiens) type B a large clostridium 5-10 μm or more in length with oval, central or subterminal spores is a fastidious anaerobe and is difficult to isolate. It is responsible for most infections, although some cases have recently been shown to be caused by type A.

Pathogenesis

Unknown at present, but these organisms produce powerful toxins and multiplication in the liver appears to follow or be associated with decrease in liver oxygenation resulting from chronic pneumonia or enteritis.

Clinical signs

Often found dead.

Pathology

Rapid decomposition of the carcase is common. Carcase condition score 3 or more, findings include submandibular swelling, pulmonary oedema and tracheal froth, sero-fibrinous or bloody exudates in the pericardial and peritoneal cavities, and most frequently, the presence of excess gas in the liver which appears light in colour and resembles "Aero" chocolate or foam rubber.

Diagnosis

The post mortem findings described above suggest *C. novyi* infection in freshly dead animals. Other causes of death should be excluded and *C.novyi* type B (or A) identified in the liver by fluorescent antibody staining or PCR. The organisms are large Gram-positive rods with oval subterminal spores. 10^3-10^6 organisms per g of liver can be demonstrated by culture as opalescent colonies in anaerobic conditions on egg yolk agar. The diagnosis is complicated by post-mortem change.

Treatment and control

Treatment of predisposing conditions such as pneumonia or enteritis with appropriate antimicrobials reduces the mortality and protection with a vaccine containing *C.novyi* (oedematiens) type B antigens may prevent the disease if given before the period of risk, e.g. in weaners or store pigs. Vaccines intended for sheep have been used. Bacitracin zinc at 225-260g/tonne has been used in sow rations to prevent the disease.

Reference

Duran, C.O., Walton, J.R. (1998). Clostridium novyi sudden death in sows: description of 17 cases from indoor breeding herds. Proc IPVS **15**, 81.

Botulism

A rare, sometimes fatal flaccid paralysis of pigs resulting from ingestion of preformed toxin of *Clostridium botulinum* in food.

Incidence

Worldwide but rarely described.

Aetiology

C.botulinum is capable of multiplying in anaerobic decaying animal and plant material at temperatures of 25-30°C and producing toxin. Six toxin types (A-F) exist.

Pathogenesis

Preformed toxin is ingested with contaminated food and is absorbed, probably via the lymphatics, to fix to the neuromuscular junction and prevent muscular contraction.

Clinical signs

Flaccid paralysis may occur 8 hours to 3 days after exposure and begins with the forelegs, progresses to the hindlegs and results in lateral recumbency and death. Anorexia, blindness and inability to control salivation and micturition may occur.
Animals which have collapsed should be killed.

Pathology

No gross lesions other than those associated with paralysis.

Epidemiology

The organism is widespread and the pig is relatively resistant. Ingestion of sufficient toxin to cause clinical signs depends upon consumption of sufficient contaminated feedstuff such as fish, meat or possibly vegetation such as spoiled silage. There is a risk to man from the ingestion of meat from affected pigs.

Diagnosis

Based on clinical signs of progressive flaccid paralysis and the demonstration of the toxin in gut contents or affected muscle tissue by ELISA or biological means. The organism can be isolated from the normal gut or from tissue (3-4% livers in Denmark are positive), so isolation alone is not confirmatory.

Treatment and Control

Prevention of further ingestion of toxin is most useful. Technically, animals might be nursed, given milk containing magnesium sulphate (39g/L) and antitoxin of the appropriate type parenterally and orally or protected by vaccination, but the rarity of the condition makes this unlikely.

Other clostridia

C.septicum and *C.chauvoei* may be isolated from cellulitis and gangrene as may *C.perfringens* type A or other clostridia.

Escherichia coli infections

E.coli infection causes neonatal septicaemia, neonatal diarrhoea, postweaning diarrhoea, oedema disease, cystitis and mastitis in pigs and can colonise existing lesions elsewhere in the body. Some strains form part of the normal faecal flora, whilst others are pathogenic.

Infections occur at different ages:

Septicaemia

"Colisepticaemia" is commonest in the newborn piglet 0-4 days of age and may be associated with diarrhoea.

Enteritis (Enteric colibacillosis) is associated with diarrhoea at three main periods in the pig's life:

1.   Neonatal diarrhoea (0-4 days of age)
2.   Neonatal - weaning diarrhoea. Between the neonatal period and weaning i.e. 4 days - 3-4 weeks.
3.   Post-weaning diarrhoea or post-weaning enteritis associated with weaning.

Oedema disease usually occurs in pigs which have recently been weaned (see Bowel Oedema).

Mastitis and cystitis occur in adult sows.

E.coli disease in the young pig

Incidence

The organism occurs in every pig. Disease occurs when specific pathogenic strains enter a susceptible population or when management factors lead to an increase in challenge or a decrease in specific immunity. *E.coli* is identified as the cause of over 50% of all reported cases of pig enteritis in the UK and in many other countries.

Aetiology

E.coli is a normal inhabitant of the gut and is restricted to the lower small intestine and large intestine in mature healthy animals. The organism is a short Gram-negative rod or coccobacillus with flagellae, fimbriae or pili and sometimes a capsule. It grows aerobically and anaerobically on a wide variety of media to produce 3-5 mm colonies within 24 hours. Some are β haemolytic on sheep blood agar and most isolates ferment lactose. Its identity is confirmed by biochemical tests. Further classification is by serotyping based on 'O' or cell wall antigens, 'K' or capsular antigens 'H' or flagellar antigens and 'F' or fimbrial antigens. Monoclonal antibodies produced against pathogenic determinants and DNA probes or PCR primers containing sequences of genes for pathogenic determinants allow pathotypes to be identified. Organisms may be further classified within strains by antibiotic resistance patterns (antibiograms), plasmid profiles or genetic sequences of conserved genes for epidemiological purposes. Analysis by other systems such as multilocus enzyme electrophoresis and restriction endonuclease analysis may not agree with serotypes, but often agree with pathotyping/virotyping (the possession of recognised virulence factors).

E.coli can survive drying for months, is killed by heating to 66°C for 30 minutes and by most disinfectants. It is sensitive to a wide range of antimicrobials but resistance to most of them has been recorded.

Characters of pathogenic *E.coli* strains

Strains of *E.coli* with particular combinations of O and K antigens are associated with particular syndromes. Neonatal septicaemia strains are often non-haemolytic on sheep blood and include those such as 08 K87, K88 and 078 K80. They may be serum resistant due to the production of columinic acid but rarely cause disease at the intestinal epithelium.

E.coli strains involved in enteric disease possess a number of pathogenic features, and those found in enteric disease in species other than the pig are continually being identified in pig enteric isolates. Major determinants are:

a) Fimbriae

Fimbriae or pili are filamentous structures 2.1-7.0 nm in diameter which allow the organisms to adhere to the brush borders of intestinal epithelial cells. Fimbriae associated with enteric disease include F4(K88) in the ab, ac or ad forms, (MW 27.5 kDa), F5 (K99), F6 (987P), F41 F107 (15.1 kDa). Pili such as F165 (MW 18.5 kDa) are present on septicaemic strains and F18ab,ac on Oedema Disease strains. Genes for most fimbriae have been sequenced and the proteins have been defined. The genes may be located on transmissible plasmids (F4, F5 and F6) or the chromosome (F41). An *E.coli* strain may possess genes for more than one fimbrial type but some of these such as F6 and F41 may only be expressed in appropriate conditions.

b) Toxins

Toxins produced by enterotoxigenic *E.coli* and are: LTp or heat labile toxin, MW 91.5 kDa which is antigenic and occurs in two parts, LTA and LTB; STa and STb, heat stable toxins which are non-antigenic (STap, MW 1.8-2.0 kDa) or poorly antigenic (STbp, MW 5.0 kDa) and Verotoxin/Shiga-like toxin (VTIIe/SLTIIe) MW 70 kDa, and antigenic. The genes for these toxins are located on plasmids. Other toxins have been described such as EAST1 (related to STa) cytotoxins (Cytotoxic Necrotising Factors, CNF, cytolethal distending toxin (CDT)) and the haemolysin (Hly).

c) Outer Membrane Proteins

A 94 kDa outer membrane protein (intimin) has been associated with the *eaeA* gene and with attachment and effacement of ileal brush borders. The presence of many of these pathogenic determinants on plasmids means that they can occur in more than one strain. An adhesin involved in diffuse adherence (AIDA) is increasingly being identified and appears to be involved in biofilm formation on the large intestinal microvilli.

A typical diarrhoea-producing strain is Abbotstown, 0149 K91, F4 (K88) ac which produces LT and STa, others are 09 K103 (987P), 0147 K89, F4 (K88). F5 (K99) and F6 (987P) strains do not produce LT but produce STa (STb). Recent studies with DNA probes have demonstrated that various combinations of determinants such as F4 (K88) STb LT, F4 (K88), F6 (987P) STb, LT, STa, F5 (K99) F41 STa (STb) and F4 (K88)-ve LT+ve can occur. The verocytotoxin may also occur in some isolates. It is present in all oedema disease strains which include 0139 K82(B), 0138 K81(B), 0141 F18 (K85(B)) F4 (K88) ac and 041 K85(B).

Pathogenesis

The way in which *E.coli* causes disease has been the subject of considerable study. Oedema Disease will be treated separately but the factors affecting a) the production of lesions by *E.coli* and b) the factors which allow the organism to reach numbers high enough to cause disease are both outlined below.

a) Pathogenic strains of *E.coli* produce their effect in the young pig by:-

i) direct invasion of the upper respiratory tract or anterior small intestine in the non-immune piglet to cause septicaemia. Strains involved in this way include 08, K87, F4 (K88) and 078, K80. Both capsule and F165 have been shown to be necessary for septicaemia in 0115K F165. Many strains are serum-resistant. Other enterobacteria may contaminate the umbilicus and cause septicaemia.

ii) attaching to the brush borders of the cells of the mucosal epithelium by their adhesive antigens or to the overlying mucus. The brush border and mucus receptors for several fimbrial types have been characterised and the genetics of some of them have been studied. Phenotypes A, B, C, D and E have been identified for F4 (K88) fimbriae. Phenotype A is associated with 210 and 240 kDa proteins which bind all three K88 variants ab, ac and ad; Phenotype B of the same proteins binds K88 ab and K88 ac; Phenotype C binds K88 ac and K88 ad; Phenotype D binds K88 ad and Phenotype E none of the three forms. The expression of these receptors is under genetic control. Homozygotes with the genotype SS and heterozygotes Ss are susceptible to attachment and to F4 (K88) ac ab-mediated *E.coli* diarrhoea. Homozygotes with the genotype ss are resistant. A similar system Dd exists for F4 (K88) ad. Attachment sites for F4 (K88) antigen are more common in the anterior small intestine and also in younger pigs. F4 specific glycoprotein receptors of 90 kDa, 61 kDa and 28 kDa in mucus appear to increase with age. Attachment by F5 (K99) and F6 (987P) bearing *E.coli* strains occurs lower down the small intestine, particularly to sialic acid residues in the ileum. Receptors for both determinants have been defined and the expression of the receptors has been shown to be under genetic control. Some E. coli strains colonise the mucosa by means of non-fimbrial factors such as enteroaggregative E. coli (especially EAST1 and AIDA),

iii) producing enterotoxin. Enterotoxigenic *E.coli* (ETEC) closely adherent to the brush border produce enterotoxins which affect cell membrane receptors which contain a ganglioside compound. LT stimulates the production of 3'5' cyclic AMP by adenyl cyclase and this acts on the ion-transport systems within the membrane to cause active secretion of chloride ions into the lumen. These are followed passively by water and sodium ions. The effect of LT toxin is sustained and it also affects tissues outside the gut. STa enterotoxin affects the cyclic guanosine monophosphate (GMP) transport system with a similar net result, but produces a more immediate reaction than LT toxin. EAST1, a 4.1 kDa peptide related to STa appears to be common in F4 infections. STb appears to cause alterations in the apical epithelium of villi and to impair active alanine absorption. It is sensitive to trypsin. Some of the secreted fluid is reabsorbed lower down the intestine but the large intestinal capacity to absorb it is overcome and diarrhoea results. Metabolic acidosis and dehydration occur leading to circulatory collapse and death. Some strains of enterotoxigenic *E.coli* (ETEC) possess the gene (*stx* 2) for SLT/VTIIe but this toxin makes no contribution to enteritis.

iv) multiplication in the small and particularly the large intestine where they invade and destroy the epithelial cells of the mucosa to cause enteritis and subsequent diarrhoea. Systemic spread may occur. Cytotoxins are produced by some of these *E.coli* strains. (Colonisation and Necrotising Factor, CNF). Others attach to the brush border and efface microvilli becoming attached by pedestals. (Attaching and Effacing *E.coli* AEEC). These strains may also destroy epithelial cells. Haemorrhagic lesions may result from enterohaemorrhagic *E.coli* (EHEC)

b) *E.coli* populations cause disease and reach high numbers in the pig intestine when the defence mechanisms (gastric acidity, other bacterial populations and antibody protection) are deficient in some way or when stress or infection with other infectious agents reduces their protective effect.

i) Genetic factors. The resistance of certain strains of pig to F4 (K88) infection because of the phenotype of their brush borders has been noted above. This type of resistance also occurs with F5, F6 and F18 adhesins and similar systems apply for mucus receptors.

ii) Gastric acidity does not reach high levels until 3 or 4 days after birth. This may allow higher than normal numbers of E.coli to enter the small intestine.

iii) Gut flora changes. The intestine of the new born pig is bacteriologically sterile and the first organisms to colonise it multiply rapidly to reach high numbers. Some of these bacteria, e.g. lactobacilli and streptococci, are considered harmless but some strains of E.coli can produce disease at this stage. After colonisation, a balance forms between the members of the normal flora. Colonisation with E.faecium and pig strains of lactobacilli (especially L.sobrius) has been shown to reduce mortality from E.coli diarrhoea but not to prevent colonisation or to prevent the occurrence of diarrhoea.

iv) Non-specific colostral protection. It is becoming clear that fat globules in milk, whey proteins other than immunoglobulins and substances such as lactoferrin act together with maternal leucocytes in the milk to reduce the effect of E.coli disease in a non-specific manner.

v) Specific immune protection. The piglet can absorb colostral antibodies until 36 hours after birth, but until it does so, it is susceptible to septicaemia caused by environmental E.coli. The passive immunity obtained in this way protects against systemic invasion by E.coli strains experienced by the sow and lasts for 6-10 weeks. Passive immunity in the form of IgA, IgG and IgM antibodies directed against E.coli encountered by the sow is present in the milk and the IgA antibodies are adsorbed to the mucosa of the piglet's intestine. Here they prevent the adhesion or penetration of pathogenic E.coli and neutralise LT toxin thus preventing diarrhoea. In addition to anti-adhesive and antitoxic activity, the multiplication rate of E.coli in the lumen is reduced and phagocytosis by neutrophils is increased. Dams with the genotype ss do not form antibody to F4 (K88) and any progeny with the genotype Ss are unprotected against F4 (K88)-bearing pathogens. From 1-2 weeks of age, the piglet intestine is capable of producing antibodies to E.coli and from 2 weeks of age IgM and IgA antibodies are produced in gradually increasing quantities until, by 6 weeks of age, the full IgA response to intestinal antigens is operating. This response is protective against E.coli strains present in the normal intestine and feed but pathogenic strains of E.coli not previously experienced by the sow or the piglet may still colonise the gut and cause disease. However, the acute diarrhoea and septicaemia seen in the neonatal piglet is less common in older pigs because of increasing antibody protection. Diarrhoea may occur in piglets of 3-4 weeks of age at a time when passively-acquired IgG antibody levels in the serum are falling. IgA antibodies in the milk are still present, but their efficiency may be reduced by the presence of solid food in the diet. At this time, the piglet's own immune competence in terms of IgG and IgA antibody production is not yet sufficient to reduce the severity of E.coli infections.

vi) <u>Infection with other agents</u>. Infections with rotavirus, epidemic diarrhoea virus, coccidia, cryptosporidia and bacterial agents other than *E.coli* may also be important predisposing factors and cause syndromes which may be confused with *E.coli* infections or occur with *E.coli* in the field.

vii) <u>Intestinal motility and secretions</u>. The normal flow of food and secretions may exert a "flushing" effect of bacterial populations in the lumen. If interrupted, e.g. by stress or weaning, <u>E.coli</u> numbers may build up sufficiently in the small intestine to cause disease. Frequent small feeds reduce the severity of diarrhoea when compared with 1 or 2 daily feeds.

viii) <u>Environmental and management factors</u>. Changes such as chilling have now been shown to affect the duration of diarrhoea by an indirect effect through cortisol levels on immunity. Starvation, water, deprivation, other forms of stress and change in diet disturb the normal balance and allow pathogenic <u>E.coli</u> strains to multiply in the small intestine and cause disease. Mixing commonly accompanies management changes and exposes non-immune piglets to infection. Dirty accommodation and high protein feeds increase the number of infecting bacteria and make clinical disease more likely.

From this point onwards the syndromes caused by *E.coli* will be considered separately.

Neonatal *E.coli* Septicaemia

Clinical signs

One or more newborn piglets in a litter may become ill within 12 hours of birth and die within 48 hours. Affected piglets stand apart from the rest of the litter with drooping tails, sink into recumbency and die after a period of unconsciousness, sometimes accompanied by convulsions and paddling movements. The body temperature may be high in the earlier stages of the disease but becomes subnormal before loss of consciousness occurs. Mortality from the septicaemic form approaches 100% of the affected piglets. Once body temperature has fallen below 35°C euthanasia should be considered.

Pathological findings

Piglets may be in good bodily condition, sometimes with cyanosis of the extremities. The carcase muscles may appear congested, the spleen may be enlarged and the stomach is filled with curd. When animals have not died immediately, there may be fibrinopurulent polyserositis, polyarthritis and meningitis. Pneumonia may be present. Occasionally the intestine may be distended with pale contents indicating the presence of neonatal diarrhoea.

E.coli can be isolated from liver, spleen and heart blood in cases of septicaemia. The isolates may be identifiable as a pathogenic serotype.

Epidemiology

<u>Neonatal septicaemia</u> results from the infection of non-immune piglets which have not ingested colostrum or which ingest colostrum lacking specific antibody. The organism is present in dirty farrowing accommodation or in the

intestinal flora of the sow. Continuous farrowing, inadequate cleaning and poor environmental temperature control increase the likelihood of infection. A strain new to a farm may precipitate an outbreak. Disease may occur in the progeny of recently-purchased gilts or sows. 0115 F165 *E.coli* may be responsible.

Diagnosis

Piglets with neonatal septicaemia can be distinguished by their good condition from those dying of starvation. Deaths occur only during the first 12-48 hours from this cause. The isolation of *E.coli* from freshly-dead carcases confirms. Other causes of neonatal death should be considered. Strains associated with septicaemia such as 08K87, K88, 0781K80 and 0115 K-F165 may be isolated from heart blood, liver and spleen as well as from gut.

Treatment

Affected piglets may be given parenteral or oral antimicrobial. The prognosis for affected piglets is poor. The remainder of the litter should be treated, also depressed piglets of similar age in adjacent litters. Suitable agents for injection include ampicillin, amoxycillin, streptomycin, gentamycin (where registered), apramycin, spectinomycin, neomycin, oxytetracycline and chlortetracycline, chloramphenicol (not EU), thiamphenicol, cephalosporins, fluoroquinolones such as enrofloxacin and danofloxacin (where registered), baquiloprim and trimethoprim: sulphonamide. Long acting formulations of ampicillin, amoxycillin and oxytetracycline may be used to continue therapy.

Oral dosers may be used for 3-5 days, to treat the apparently unaffected litter with products which are active systemically. These include amoxycillin, ampicillin, trimethoprim sulphonamide, where available. Supportive treatment using electrolyte replacers, correct heating etc., should be given.

Control

Ensure that colostrum has been taken and that temperature is adequate. No specific vaccines are yet available. If supplementary feeding of piglets is necessary, colostral substitutes may be of value.

Neonatal Diarrhoea

Clinical signs

Piglets affected by neonatal enteric colibacillosis show varying degrees of watery diarrhoea before death or recovery. Affected piglets may still suck but often stand with drooping tails and appear shrunken, lose the bloom from their skin and have erect coat hairs. Loss of flesh is apparent, particularly over the hips and backbone. The diarrhoeic faeces may be difficult to see on casual inspection as it is often pale, creamy yellow in colour. Dried crusts of diarrhoeic faeces may be seen on the thighs or perineum and there may also be scalding about the anus. Affected pigs may enter a coma and die or recover without subsequent loss of condition after 3-6 days. Diarrhoeic faeces may be present in creeps and on the bars of slatted floors and may be blood-stained diarrhoea.

Outbreaks of neonatal diarrhoea and septicaemia occur in farrowing houses where successive litters, particularly those of gilts or newly purchased sows, may be affected. In some cases the morbidity may reach 70% of all piglets born. Seventy per cent of piglets affected with diarrhoea in the first few days of life may die. Mortality rates then decrease rapidly until less than 10% mortality occurs in affected pigs over 2 weeks of age. Piglets which are extremely dehydrated and which do not respond to treatment should be killed.

Pathology

The carcase is dehydrated and the liver dark in colour. The stomach usually contains milk curd and may have infarctions of the wall, the small intestine is dilated, flaccid and mildly congested. In freshly-killed or very recently dead animals, the villi may be intact and finger-like in some enterotoxic diarrhoeas and in others some degree of villous atrophy may have occurred. The jejunum is the principal area affected by F4 (K88)+ve strains and the lower jejunum and ileum by F5 (K99)+ve and F6 (987P)+ve strains.

Blood may be present in the large intestinal contents where CNF-producing strains are involved. Both enterocolitis and interstitial pneumonia have been recorded in experimental infections. Microvillous effacement and pedestal formation may be visible in histological sections of the colons of freshly-killed piglets with AEEC.

Strictly enterotoxigenic *E.coli* strains are isolated only from the gut.

Epidemiology

Infection may originate from the sow, from residual contamination in poorly-cleaned pens or by lateral spread from adjacent affected litters. Failure to ingest colostrum and chilling predispose to the condition as does genetic susceptibility to F4 (K88), F5 (K99) or F6 (937P)-bearing organisms. The widespread use of vaccination of sows has reduced the prevalence of F4 (K88) in neonatal diarrhoea and may be responsible for the widespread occurrence of EAST1 *E. coli* in some countries. It may also be more common in gilt litters.

Diagnosis

Watery diarrhoea in neonatal piglets is usually caused by *E. coli*. From 24 hours of age, it may be confused with that caused by T.G.E., epidemic diarrhoea, rotavirus, *Clostridium perfringens* type A or type C, or *Campylobacter coli*. The piglets do not vomit (T.G.E. and epidemic diarrhoea), other pigs on the farm are rarely affected (T.G.E. and epidemic diarrhoea) and there is little gastritis and little villous atrophy (T.G.E., epidemic diarrhoea rotavirus and other viruses). In most cases there is no blood (*C.perfringens* type C, type A), no necrosis of the small intestinal mucosa (Clostridia) and no mucoid small intestinal or colonic contents (*C.coli*). Coccidial and cryptosporidial infections do not occur until the end of this period.

Where blood is present in the intestine, the condition may be distinguished from *C.perfringens* type C disease by the age of onset (earlier) and the pattern of mortality (100% of the affected litter in the clostridial disease), Confirmation depends upon bacteriology.

Laboratory confirmation of neonatal *E.coli* diarrhoeas can be obtained from faecal samples or rectal swabs. The isolation of a pathogenic serotype in profuse or pure culture may suggest *E.coli* diarrhoea but, unless examinations for virus, other bacteria and protozoa are carried out, the identification of *E.coli* as the cause is only presumptive. It is better to send a carcase or a live piglet to the laboratory as T.G.E. and epidemic diarrhoea can then be ruled out and the characteristic post-mortem findings may be seen. Specific antibody or monoclonal antibody to pilus/fimbrial antigens has been used to identify pathogenic serotypes in frozen sections which may also be used for T.G.E. and epidemic diarrhoea diagnosis. The isolation of apparently pure cultures of pathogenic serotypes from the small intestine provides strong confirmatory evidence for the diagnosis of *E.coli* disease. ELISA tests for pilus antigens [F4 (K88), F5 (K99), F6 (987P) and F41] may be used on faeces, intestinal contents or swabs. Isolated colonies may be examined using reverse passive latex agglutination tests for pilus antigens F4, F5, F6 and F41 (Fimbrex, Central Veterinary Laboratory, UK) and for LT and ST enterotoxins. F5 and F6 antigens may only be expressed when cultures are grown on Minca medium.

DNA probes and primers have been used to determine the pathogenic determinants of isolates and they are frequently serotyped using polyclonal sera to common pathogens e.g., Abbottstown. Polymerase chain reaction primers have now been described for most pathogenic determinants of *E.coli* and their use in diagnosis is increasing, often as multiplex PCRs to detect a range of pathogenic determinants.

Treatment

Neonatal diarrhoea and other scours due to *E.coli* in sucking pigs may be treated parenterally using the agents listed for septicaemia and also ceftiofur, but it is preferable to use oral therapy for 3-5 days with them and the following agents: neomycin preparations and furazolidone (not EU), spectinomycin, apramycin, sulfamethopyrazine and enrofloxacin or other fluoroquinolones Electrolyte replacement with glucose:glycine or other preparations should be available or be given if piglets cannot drink. Maintaining adequate environmental temperature is important.

Failure of treatment may be due to antimicrobial resistance. Antimicrobial sensitivity should be determined. If organisms are sensitive and there is response to therapy, reconsider the diagnosis or the treatment schedule.

Control

Farrowing accommodation should be clean, dry and should be disinfected and, if possible, fumigated between farrowings. All-in-all-out husbandry (batch farrowing) should be practised. The sow may be scrubbed on entry to reduce contamination and creep heating should be arranged so as to ensure the piglets an even temperature of 35°C, 95°F for the first week of life. Soft sterilised sawdust bedding will improve comfort. All piglets should take colostrum. If this is not available, colostrum substitutes may be of value. Supplementary feeding should be carried out using proprietary sow milk replacer for best results. Water should be available and electrolyte solutions may be provided if neonatal diarrhoea occurs commonly. Oral medication given as soon as colostrum has been taken may prevent outbreaks in unprotected litters.

The prime method of prevention is by vaccination of the sow prior to farrowing to provide passive immunity in the colostrum.

Killed *E.coli* vaccines given parenterally may induce serum antibody which is passed on to the piglets in the colostrum. Vaccines usually consist of strains carrying fimbrial and enterotoxin antigens or the purified pathogenic determinants themselves. Examples available in the UK include: Colisorb (Intervet), mixed killed cells (including O157 F4ac, K' V17') and containing *E. rhusiopathiae*; Gletvax 6 (Schering Plough), *C.perfringens* type C, F4 (K88) ab, ac, F5 (K99) and F6 (987P); Suvaxyn *E.coli* P4 (Fort Dodge) adjuvanted pili F4 (K88, K99, 987P F41), Neocolipor (Merial) F4, F5, F6 and F41 and alum adjuvat; and Porcilis Porcol 5, Intervet (LT toxoid, K88 ab, K88 ac, K99 and 987P in an oil adjuvant). A primary course requires two doses 4 to 6 weeks apart with boosters every six months. Vaccination within two weeks of farrowing is not advised for most sow vaccines.

A killed oral vaccine containing 7 enteropathogenic serotypes (Intagen Roche was formerly available combined with vaccination of the sow prior to farrowing with a killed *E.coli* vaccine to provide protection. A number of experimental vaccines have been described since then, but none are currently on the market. F4 (K88) plasmid may be eliminated from *E.coli* in the gut of vaccinated pigs directly or by selection in the population. Autogenous vaccines from the farm of origin may be prepared and given dead or live (Kohler type) in some countries (but not in Britain). The live vaccine must be given some time prior to farrowing to avoid mortality and loss of productivity in the litter. Immunity from such vaccines may only last for a single lactation.

Recent experimental studies suggest that the inclusion of F41 antigens improves protection. STb has been shown to be poorly immunogenic.

Passive immunisation using hyperimmune sera to *E.coli* may still be available in some countries and provide some degree of protection. The most common form of passive immunity is provided by colostrum substitutes which are given to neonatal piglets by stomach tube at birth. These may contain porcine or bovine antibodies to *E.coli* (not necessarily to pathogenic determinants) and may be of value in the control of neonatal diarrhoea problems.

The efficacy of all biological methods of control varies and although mortality is reduced and loss of productivity is prevented, protection may not be complete. The failure of ss genotype dams to recognise K88 antigen in vaccines may be partly responsible, also the involvement of serotypes of *E.coli* not included in the vaccines and the uneven intake of colostrum and protective milk in sucking piglets which can reduce protection. Failure of a vaccination programme should involve re-examination of the diagnosis, the methods of administering the vaccine, environmental factors such as temperature and hygiene and the intake of colostrum in neonates. Finally, confirmation of the compatibility of vaccines and the serotypes/pathotypes present on the farm should be assessed, as changes in fimbrial types have occurred in *E.coli* populations following vaccination programmes.

Probiotics are sometimes given to piglets soon after birth but whatever their claimed efficacy in the prevention of neonatal diarrhoea, they do not protect non-immune piglets against experimental challenge.

E.coli diarrhoea between the neonatal period and weaning (3 week scour, milk scour).

Clinical signs

A greyish or whitish diarrhoea may occur in unweaned piglets between 10 and 28 days of age. Affected animals become emaciated and hairy and may remain permanently stunted. Diarrhoea of this type may also occur, sometimes with fever, in piglets of any age fed on milk replacer diets or where creep feed of unsuitable quality is given. This is traditionally attributed to *E.coli* and the organisms may be present but many other agents have been incriminated.

Whole litters are rarely affected, but the larger animals in almost every litter may be affected on some farms. Mortality is usually less than 20%.

Haemorrhagic gastroenteritis may occur from 8 days onwards. Affected piglets die suddenly or after the passage of a brownish diarrhoea.

The faeces of recovering animals becomes progressively firmer but usually remains white. The most common indication for humane slaughter is chronic stunting.

Pathology

Similar to that of neonatal diarrhoea. In most cases pathogenic *E.coli* is isolated from lesions of coccidiosis, rotavirus infection or coronavirus infection, as a secondary invader.

Epidemiology

Primary *E.coli* outbreaks are most likely in this age group in the litters of gilts or when a new serotype is introduced to a herd. In most cases the disease which occurs in successive litters is initiated by coccidia or rotavirus and some infection persists from neonatal diarrhoea.

Diagnosis

The demonstration of features of *E.coli* enteritis described under neonatal diarrhoea and the isolation of pathogenic *E.coli* in pure and profuse culture suggest primary *E.coli* diarrhoea.

The above features may distinguish *E.coli* enteritis from other conditions, but in this age period (from 4 days-weaning), mixed infections are not uncommon. Sudden death, with or without brownish diarrhoea and congested intestines may indicate haemorrhagic enteritis. As coccidiosis, cryptosporidium and *C.perfringens* type C secondary infection can all occur in this age group, bacteriological and histological findings for *E. coli* infection should be present before diagnosis is confirmed.

Treatment

As neonatal diarrhoea, ensuring that electrolyte is present in the pen. Antimicrobials have been included in sterilised peat but no controlled studies of uptake have been carried out.

Control

Sow vaccination may have a residual effect on *E.coli* in pigs of this age and medicated first creep given fresh in small quantities daily may reduce the occurrence of disease. Water medication and electrolyte may also reduce the involvement of *E.coli* in diarrhoea at this age.

Postweaning Enteritis (Post weaning diarrhoea)

Clinical signs

Postweaning diarrhoea occurs within 10 days of weaning, often within 4-5 days of the change of diet. Affected pigs pass greyish, brownish, or watery diarrhoeic faeces with no traces of blood. Haemorrhagic diarrhoea is extremely uncommon. Mucus is rarely present. The diarrhoea is usually transient and resolves within 3-5 days but it may persist, and deaths from dehydration or septicaemia may occur in adverse husbandry conditions. In some cases fever (up to 40.6°C, 105°F) may occur over a period of 4 or 5 days and affected animals may be anorexic and depressed. Chronic post-weaning enteritis may cause permanent stunting in recovered pigs. Faeces may be difficult to see in flat decks or in veranda houses with slatted floors. The feeders in flat decks and the corners of the dunging areas in veranda houses should be examined for signs of diarrhoea in full-slatted accommodation. Where inspection is difficult, affected animals may be identified by their dehydrated appearance, and perineal staining.

20-50% of all weaned pigs may be affected, but mortality from the uncomplicated disease is less than 10% of those affected unless complications occur. Even when diarrhoea is only transient, marked reduction in the rate of daily liveweight gain may occur in the remainder of an affected group.

Chronically stunted or severely dehydrated animals which are unable to rise should be killed.

Pathology

The carcase is usually dehydrated, the eyes sunken and there may be some faint cyanosis of the extremities. The serous surfaces are sticky, the liver is congested and the stomach is full of feed in most cases. The gastric mucosa may be congested (a non-specific change) and the small intestine is dilated and congested with watery, buff-coloured contents which can be seen through the wall. The mucosal epithelium is congested and the villi are intact. Mesenteric lymph nodes are enlarged and pale in colour. The colon and rectum contain fluid faeces or are empty.

Histological examination may be useless due to autolysis, but in freshly-killed piglets, the villi appear intact, are often congested and may sometimes be covered with adherent bacteria. Varying degrees of cell shedding may be seen. In haemorrhagic enteritis associated with attaching and effacing *E.coli*, characteristic palisades of attached organisms may be seen on the brush border with effacement of the microvilli and cup and pedestal formation of the lumenal surface. This type of lesion may be seen in the duodenum as well as further down the tract. Haemorrhage and ulceration may occur in the large intestine in this rare form of the disease.

Pure growths of ß-haemolytic F4 (K88), LT-positive *E.coli* can usually be isolated from the anterior small intestine or F5 (K99)-positive or F6 (987P) E.coli from the posterior small intestine in enteric colibacillosis but not from other organs outside the gut. Isolates may subsequently be identified as known pathogenic serotypes or pathotypes. It is not uncommon for more than one pathotype to be present in affected animals after recovery but only pure cultures are usually present during acute disease.

Epidemiology

The mixing of immune carrier and non-immune piglets at weaning, the loss of maternal immune protection, the provision of high protein feeds ad lib, the change of environment and contact with poorly cleaned pens or drainage from pens containing other affected pigs all contribute to the development of the disease. The purchase of pigs, their mixing and introduction to new diets and cold dirty pens or houses with an existing problem may be contributory factors in outbreaks.

On a national scale, a particular *E.coli* serotype may be associated with outbreaks of clinical disease and may then be succeeded by other serotypes. However, certain serotypes have been isolated consistently from enteric colibacillosis over long periods of time. Examples include 0149 K91 F4 (K88) ac (Abbottstown) which still accounts for many outbreaks in the UK. Recent developments in molecular epidemiology are adding to knowledge of the relationships between infections within farms and in outbreaks

Diagnosis

The clinical findings of a grey-brown watery diarrhoea 3-5 days after weaning are suggestive of *E. coli* post weaning diarrhoea. T.G.E. and epidemic diarrhoea rarely affect the post-weaning age group alone and are rarely associated with fever or mortality. In salmonellosis, high fever, necrotic material in the faeces, discoloured skin and a septicaemic carcase may be seen. The post-mortem appearance in *E.coli* post-weaning enteritis is characteristic. The isolation of pure cultures of pathogenic *E.coli* confirm the diagnosis. *E. coli* isolates may be identified further by antigenic analysis or by multiplex PCR. Spirochaetal diarrhoea has an incubation period of 6-7 days or more, and the slightly mucoid appearance to the faeces and the restriction of lesions to the large intestine distinguishes it from *E.coli*. Spirochaetes are present in large numbers in the faeces. In rotavirus diarrhoeas the agent may be identified and where *C.perfringens* type A or other clostridia are involved large numbers of sporulating *C.perfringens* type A are present and enterotoxin or specific cytotoxins are identifiable by vero cell assay or the Reverse Passive Latex Agglutination test. Cryptosporidial infection is usually chronic and does not affect pigs so acutely.

Treatment

Severely affected pigs may be treated parenterally using the products listed for neonatal septicaemia, but therapy is normally given in feed or water. Water medication is preferable using antimicrobials such as ampicillin, amoxycillin, apramycin, neomycin, tetracyclines, trimethoprim:sulphonamide combinations, spectinomycin, furazolidone (not EU), gentamicin (not UK), fluoroquinolones (where registered) and cephalothin or ceftiofur (where registered). Treatment should be continued for 3-5 days and should be started as soon as clinical signs are noted.

In feed medication at therapeutic levels can also be given either after the outbreak has begun or over the period of risk and should be continued for at least 10 days and preferably for 3-5 weeks. Agents for in-feed medication include chlortetracycline, oxytetracycline, apramycin, neomycin, sulphonamide, trimethoprim: sulphonamide and enrofloxacin (not registered UK). Furazolidone is effective but cannot be used in the EU.

Treatment should be accompanied by correction of environmental temperature, and by disinfection of the pen towards the end of the treatment period and may be supplemented by fluid replacement with glucose: glycine electrolyte (Lectade, Pfizer), or antibiotic containing proprietary electrolyte-replacing solutions. If there is no response to treatment which has previously been effective, re-examine diagnosis and check antimicrobial sensitivity of *E.coli* as antimicrobial resistance can develop readily in this organism.

Toxin antagonists. Experimental studies have been carried out with enterotoxin antagonists and these show some promise but are not yet available.

Egg yolk antibody. Use of egg yolk antibody from hens immunised with *E. coli* F4, F,5, F6 and rotavirus cured diarrhoea within 1 day in experimental studies.

<u>Bacteriophage treatment</u>. Experimental and field studies suggest that phage suspensions specific for enteropathogenic *E.coli* strains can be used in treatment.

Control

Recently-weaned pigs should be maintained at an even temperature for the first week. If kept dry and warm in clean surroundings, postweaning enteritis is less likely to occur. Dusty surroundings and chilling exacerbate morbidity. Affected piglets should be treated promptly and other litters of susceptible age watched.

Dietary factors may reduce the severity or occurrence of post weaning diarrhoea. Avoid change of feed at weaning and reduce quantity of feed slightly. Ensure feed is clean and fresh. The use of totally digestible diets may also reduce diarrhoea at weaning. Creep feed fed before weaning may reduce enteric disease at weaning. Bromelain (a protease) inhibits the receptors for *E. coli* F4, and reduces susceptibility of treated animals to that of the resistant phenotype in controlled experiments. Lactic acid in the diet may reduce gastric pH and reduce the multiplication of *E.coli*. Probiotics containing porcine lactobacilli, toyocerin and *E.faecium* may reduce the severity of disease but do not prevent it in controlled experiments.

Medication at treatment level may be given over the period of risk. Water medication is preferable as it does not require a change of ration.

Antimicrobial growth promoters with an effect on *E.coli* may be incorporated in the feed (creep or weaner ration) over the period of risk and may help prevent the development of the disease. Examples include carbadox and olaquindox (Bayonox, Bayer) where registered (not EU). Treatment may also be given over this period.

Zinc Oxide is incorporated in post weaning rations of 70% UK farms at levels of 3.2kg to give 2600 ppm zinc in the ration for 2 weeks and results in a dramatic reduction in post weaning diarrhoea. Continued incorporation may result in eventual toxicity or in residues. There are concerns over the environmental effects.

Complete protection of the piglet against *E. coli* post-weaning diarrhoea by means of vaccine is still not possible. Vaccination of the sow may have some residual effect if weaning is at 3-4 weeks of age but protection of the piglet at weaning requires vaccination of the piglet. Vaccines used for sows could be used to vaccinate piglets in the first week of life, but none are so registered (UK). Oil adjuvanted vaccines should be avoided unless there is a specific claim for protection. Endotoxin levels in vaccines containing whole cells may be unsuitable for piglets. Live, unattenuated vaccines should not be used. Experimental studies suggest that protection is not complete.

Experimental vaccines consisting of live, attenuated, Aro-ve salmonellae expressing F4 have been used. Pure F4 fimbriae given orally have also been shown to provide some protective immunity.

References

Broes, A., Fairbrother, J.M., La Riviere, S., Jacques, M. and Johnson, W.M. (1988). Virulence properties of enterotoxigenic *E.coli* 08 KX105 strains isolated from diarrhoeic piglets. Infection & Immunity 56, 241-246.
Chandler, D.S., Mynott, T.L. (1998). Bromelain protects piglets from diarrhoea caused by oral challenge with K88 positive enterotoxigenic *E. coli*. Gut 43, 196-202.

Cupere, F. de., Deprez, P., Demeulenaere, D., Muyle, E. (1992). Evaluation of the effect of 3 probiotics on experimental E.coli enterotoxaemia in weaned piglets. J.Vet Med., Series B **39**, 277-284.

Erickson, A.K., Baker, D.R., Bosworth, B.T., Benfield, D.A., Francis, D.H. (1994). Characterisation of porcine intestinal receptors for the K88ac fimbrial adhesin of E. coli as mucin type sialoglycoproteins. Infection and Immunity **62**, 5404-5410.

Fairbrother, J.M., Broes, A., Jacques, M., La Riviere, S. (1989). Pathogenicity of E.coli 0115 K "V165" strains isolated from pigs with diarrhoea. Am.J.Vet.Res. **50**, 1029-1036.

Fairbrother, J.M., Nadean, E., Gyles, C.L. (2005). Escherichia coli in postweaning diarrhoea in pigs: an update on bacterial types, pathogenesis and prevention strategies. Animal Health Reviews **6**, 17-39.

Faubert, C., Drolet, R. (1992). Haemorrhagic gastroenteritis caused by E.coli in piglets. Clinical, pathological and microbiological findings. Canadian Vet. J **33**, 251-256.

Helie, P., Morin, M., Jacques, M., Fairbrother, J.M. (1991). Experimental infection of newborn pigs with an attaching and effacing E.coli O45K "E65" strain. Infection & Immunity **59**, 814-821.

Kelly, D., O'Brien, J.J., McCracken, K.J. (1990). Effect of creep feeding on the incidence, duration and severity of post-weaning diarrhoea. Res.Vet.Sci. **49**, 223-228.

Kortbeek Jacobs, J.M.C., Kooten, P.J.S. van, Donk, J.A. Vander Dyk, J.E., van, Rutten, V.P. (1984). The effect of oral immunisation on the population of lymphocytes migrating to the mammary glands of the sow. Vet.Microbiol. **9**, 287-299.

Kuyogushima, M., Ginsburg, V., Kiwan, H.C. (1989). E.coli K99 binds to N-glycolyl sialoparagloboside and N glycolyl GM3 found in piglet small intestine. Arch.Biochem. **270**, 391-397.

Metcalf, J.W., Krogfelt, K.A., Krivan, H.C., Cohen, P.S., Laux, D.C. (1991). Characterisation and identification of a small intestine mucus receptor for the K88 ab fimbrial adhesin. Infection & Immunity **59**, 91-96.

Mynott, T.L., Luke, R K.J., Chandler, D.J. (1996). Oral administration of protease inhibits enterotoxigenic E. coli receptor activity in small intestine. Gut **38**, 28-32.

Nagy, L.K., Painter, K.R. and Mackenzie, T. (1985). Vaccination with K88, K99 and 987P. Evaluation of procholeragenoid against experimental colibacillosis in piglets of vaccinated dams. Vet Rec. **116**, 123-125.

Penrith, M.L., Henton, M.M., Clay, C.G. (1995). CNF1 toxin-producing strains of E. coli isolated from weaner pigs with necrotic enteritis in South Africa. Vet. Rec. **136**, 493-494.

Rose, R., Moon, H.W. (1985). Elicitation of enteroluminal neutrophils by enterotoxigenic and non-enterotoxigenic strains of E.coli in swine. Infection and Immunity **48**, 818-823.

Smith, H. and Huggins, M.B. (1983). The effectiveness of phages in treating experimental F coli diarrhoea in calves, piglets and lambs. J.Gen.Microbiol. **129**, 2659-2675.

Wray, C., Piercy, D.W.T., Carroll, P.J., Cooley, W.A. (1993). Experimental infection of neonatal pigs with CNF toxin-producing strains of E.coli. Res.vet.Sci. **54**, 290-298.

Oedema disease (Bowel Oedema)

Definition

Oedema disease usually occurs shortly after weaning but may occur in older pigs. Facial oedema, nervous signs and sudden death occur in variable numbers of pigs in a pen. It is caused by enteric infection with E.coli strains which produce a verotoxin which is absorbed to affect the arterial walls

Incidence

Occurs worldwide and on individual farms it may be important, but not common in Britain at present.

Aetiology

The syndrome is caused by infection with *E.coli* strains, carrying the gene *stx* 2 and capable of expressing the toxin designated VTIIe, VT2e, SLT IIe or SLT2e and known as enterotoxaemic *E.coli* (ETEEC). They usually belong to serotypes 0139: K12: H1, 0138 K81 NW, 0141 K85 ab H4 and 0141 K85 a, c H_4, but VT may be present in other strains along with enterotoxins. The major fimbrial type is now designated F18 and exists in two forms, F18ab and F18ac. 86% *E.coli* isolates from cases of oedema disease have been shown to express F18 ab (formerly F107) fimbriae (major subunit protein MW 15.1 kDa).

Pathogenesis

The *E.coli* strains responsible for Oedema Disease multiply throughout the small intestine and adhere to the brush borders of the epithelial cells by means of the F18 fimbriae. Receptors expressed on mature epithelial cells are under genetic control and the organism does not adhere to epithelial cells from pigs phenotypically resistant to Oedema Disease. This resistance has been localised to basepair 307 in the α (1,2) fucosyltransferase 1 (FUT1 (M307)) gene.

E.coli levels reached 4×10^9 per ml in the mid jejunum and the organism clusters on and adheres to the villous epithelium. *E.coli* levels are greatest 2-4 days post-infection and prior to the appearance of clinical signs of oedema disease which appear about 5 days after infection. Toxin is produced and absorbed to a range of tissues including the smooth muscle cells of the media of arterioles to cause hypertension following which angiopathy develops in the submucosal arterioles.

Lesions in the blood vessels begin 2 days post-infection with swelling and vacuolation of endothelial cells followed by sub-endothelial deposition of fibrin, perivascular oedema, microthrombus formation, necrosis of the tunica media and endothelial proliferation. There may also be damage to the submucosal nervous plexuses. These changes in the arterial walls appear to be responsible for the oedema seen in the tissues in this disease and for the nervous signs and central nervous system lesions. The toxin appears to damage cells by inhibition of protein synthesis and both lesions and the syndrome can be reproduced by giving as little as 3ng of pure toxin/kg intravenously although 6ng/kg is required to kill pigs.

Enterotoxin production by VT producing strains of *E.coli* may result in concurrent diarrhoea and catarrhal enteritis has been recorded in some outbreaks of oedema. Recovery from infection may be accompanied by the development of antibody to both F18 fimbriae and to a lesser extent to VT2e.

Clinical signs

The disease usually occurs within 10 days of weaning and affects one or more of the better piglets in the group. Outbreaks often commence with one or more pigs being found dead and others with varying degrees of nervous disturbance may be present. Affected pigs appear dull, may appear blind and may show head pressing. General incoordination and loss of balance occur later and may be noted at feeding time. Affected animals lag behind others and are less able to reach the trough. Lateral recumbency with paddling movements leading to coma and death normally follow within 4-36 hours of the onset of clinical signs. Affected pigs may have oedema of the eyelids, nose and ears and early cases may have a peculiar, squeaky voice. Body temperature may reach 40°C, 104°F, early in the disease but rectal temperature is often normal at the onset of clinical signs. Neither constipation nor diarrhoea is a constant feature, but a short period of diarrhoea may precede the onset of oedema disease proper. Affected pigs may recover completely apart from a check in growth or remain with a head tilt, gait disturbance or paralysis. Oedema disease has (1996) been identified in sows in Switzerland as sporadic cases or short outbreaks with inappetance and progressive locomotor disturbance leading within hours or days to loss of control of the hindlimbs and evetual recumbency. Paralysed animals should be killed humanely, as should those where gait disturbances are sufficiently severe for physical damage to develop.

Pathological findings

Dead animals are usually in good condition with full stomachs. Cyanosis is rarely present and oedema of the eyelids and face may be visible in recently dead animals. The most constant finding is oedema of the wall of the greater curvature of the stomach, where it occurs between the mucosa and the muscle layers. Jelly-like areas of oedema may also be present in the mesocolon, in the larynx and in the kidney capsule. Clear fluid may be present in the body cavities. Ischaemia of the kidney cortex and congestion of the medulla may be noted and all the carcase lymph nodes may be oedematous. Oedema disappears rapidly once the carcase is opened and may disappear after death. It may be absent if enteritis is also present. Histological findings usually confirm the presence of oedema in the stomach wall and in the brain where the perivascular spaces may be very pronounced. In chronic cases encephalomalacia is seen. The underlying lesion is hyaline degeneration and fibrinoid necrosis in arteries and arterioles. Proliferative arteriopathy develops as the lesions age and may be seen in pigs which have not died until several days after the onset of the disease. Histological lesions may be present in sub-clinically affected animals.

Epidemiology

The disease may affect 10-30% of recently weaned pigs with up to 100% mortality in the affected animals, is normally restricted to pigs in this age group but has now been identified in sows. The use of treatment may postpone its onset. The disease does not appear to spread from herd to herd and it was rare for many years in Britain but is now increasing in incidence, particularly in early weaned pigs and in those which receive high protein rations with no feed additives. Recent outbreaks have caused 30% mortality for some weeks and may be associated with changes in the susceptibility of breeding stock. A clear example of the transmission of the disease with breeding stock has recently been documented from Denmark. Oedema Disease is not of public health importance, but *E. coli* O157 H7 producing VT1 may colonise pigs and spread to others (the infecting dose is 6 x10^3), but usually dies out in an individual within 2 months. It does not cause Oedema Disease but may cause diarrhoea. A number of other VT producing *E. coli* serotypes which cause disease in humans have been found in pigs.

Diagnosis

The clinical signs, post-mortem findings and histopathology in recently dead animals are distinctive. When cases of sudden death occur alone, the condition must be distinguished from other causes of such deaths such as mulberry heart disease, Hertztod and anthrax. The absence of high fever and the presence of oedema enable the nervous signs to be differentiated from those of

Teschen-Talfan disease, streptococcal meningitis, salt and organic arsenical poisoning. The high, squeaky voice is of use here. Oedema of the colonic mesentery may be seen in early cases of spirochaetal diarrhoea and swine dysentery and, perhaps, *C. difficile* infection, but the involvement of the colon in those diseases is diagnostic.

The isolation of serotypes of *E.coli* such as 0139 K81, 0139 K12 and 0141 K58 from the small intestine provides additional evidence and the identification of genes for VT2e and F18 is confirmatory. VT2e may be detected in culture supernates, in colonies using DNA probes or by PCR using gene sequences. ELISAs have been developed to detect VT2e in faeces from affected pigs and recombinant VT2e has been used to detect antibody in serum from groups of pigs within 2-3 months of infection.

Treatment

Affected pigs rarely recover, but some courses of treatment are frequently adopted and may be of value to the group. They are:

a)   antibiotic therapy - usually injection or water treatment with a tetracycline, streptomycin, enrofloxacin, ampicillin and other antimicrobials effective against *E.coli*, on the basis that reduction of *E.coli* numbers in the gut may prevent further cases. (For antimicrobials see Postweaning Enteritis above. Antimicrobial sensitivity should be determined).

b)   reduction of blood pressure in clinically affected animals. The value of this has not been fully established and in such animals nursing may be of more value. Melperone 4-6mg/kg may be of value (not registered UK)

c)   reduction of feed intake. Restriction of feed intake or the inclusion of bran or other roughage in the diet may reduce the *E.coli* load in the remainder of the group.

Control

Control may be achieved by management alone. Measures designed to prevent the build up of pathogenic *E.coli* populations in the gut include limiting the feed intake of recently weaned pigs physically or by increasing roughage levels, use of acidifiers, correction of any environmental problems and weaning by removal of the sow. It has been suggested that increasing creep levels before weaning may be of value. Unfortunately, the use of sufficient roughage to inhibit *E.coli* colonisation depresses growth and leaves treated pigs susceptible as colonisation never reaches levels required to induce immunity. Weaning with scrupulous attention to hygiene and environment has been coupled with frequent small feeds of digestible rations after weaning in some UK herds. The amounts of feed are gradually increased.

Treatment levels of antimicrobials effective against colibacillosis may be included in the drinking water or feed (see Postweaning enteritis above) during the period of risk. Growth promoters such as olaquindox and carbadox (where registered) and zinc oxide appear to reduce the incidence.

Experimental studies have shown that serum antibody to VTIIe produced by active vaccination or administered as hyperimmune serum is protective. The inactivated toxin is antigenic but is difficult to detoxify and alteration of the molecule has been found to reduce its toxigenicity but retain antigenicity. Immunisation of pigs with F18 fimbriae is also protective. No vaccine is yet available commercially.

It is not yet possible to select resistant pigs on a commercial scale.

Eradication by depopulation was always an option for infected herds, and has been documented in Denmark by depopulating, leaving empty 4 weeks, removingf contaminated soil and material, cleaning and disinfecting using formalin in buildings and lime in the slurry channels and restocking with clean animals after 3 weeks. Some herds remained uninfected.

References

Alexa, P., Hamoik, J., Salajika, E. (1998). Prevention of oedema disease of weaners by administration of immune serum to verotoxin VT2e. Proc IPVS **15**, (3) 105.

Bertschinger, H.U. and Pohlenz, J. (1983). Bacterial colonisation and morphology of the intestine in porcine E.coli enterotoxaemia (Oedema Disease). Vet.Path. **20**, 99-110.

Bertschinger, H.U. and 7 authors (1990). Adhesive fimbriae produced in vivo by E.coli 0139 K12(B) H1 associated with enterotoxaemia in pigs. Vet.Microbiol. **25**, 267-281.

Bertschinger H.U., Stamm, M., Vogell, P. (1993). Inherited resistance to Oedema Disease. Vet.Micro. **35**, 79-89.

Bosworth, B.T., Samuel, J.E., Moon, H.W., O'Brien, A.D., Gordon, J.M., Whipp, S.C. (1996). Vaccination with genetically modified Shiga-like toxin IIe prevents edema disease in swine. Infect. Immun. **64**, 55-60.

Cornick, N.A., Helgerson, A.C. (2004). Transmission and infectious dose of E. coli O157 H7 in swine. Appl. and Environ. Micro. **70**, 5331-5335.

Imberechts, H., Greve, H de., Lintermans, P. (1992). The pathogenesis of edema disease in pigs. Vet.Microbiol. **31**, 221-233.

Imberechts, H., Nagy, B., Sorg, I., Stamm, M., Wild, P., Wittig, W. (1995). Designations F18ab and F18ac for the related fimbrial types F107, 2134P and 8813 of E. coli isolated from porcine post weaning diarrhoea and from oedema disease. Vet. Micro. **45**, 281-295.

Imberechts, H. and 11 other authors (1992). Characterisation of F107 fimbriae of E.coli 107/86 which causes oedema disease in pigs and nucleotide sequence of the F107 major fimbrial subunit gene. Inf. & Immun. **60**, 1963-1971.

Johansen, M., Baekbo, P., Jorsaal, S.E. (1998). Eradication of oedema disease by depopulation. Proc. IPVS **15**, (3)102.

Jorsaal, S.E., Aarestrup, F.M., Ahrens, P., Johansen, M., Baekbo, P. (1996). Oedema disease in Danish pig herds. Transmission by trade of breeding animals. Proc. IPVS **14**, 265.

MacLeod, D.L., Gyles, C.L., Wilcock, B.P. (1991). Reproduction of Edema Disease of swine with purified Shiga-like toxin II variant. Vet.Path. **28**, 66 73.

Methiyapun, S., Pohlenz, J.F.L., Bertschinger, H.U. (1984). Ultrastructure of the intestinal mucosa in pigs experimentally inoculated with an edema disease-producing strain of E.coli (0139: K12 H1). Vet.Path. **21**, 516-520.

Ngeleka, M., Pritchard, J., Appleyard, G., Middleton, D.M., Fairbrother, J.M. (2003). Isolation and association of E.coli AIDA-1/STb rather than EAST1 pathotype with diarrhoea in piglets and antibiotic sensitivity of isolates. J.Vet.Diag. Invest. **15**, 242-252.

Pearce, J.L., Bettelheim, K.A., Reed, B., Cranwell, P.B., Luke, R.K.J. (1994). Isolation of sorbitol non-fermenting, motile E. coli O157 from scouring piglets. Aust. Vet. J. **71**, 156.

Stamm, M. and Bertschinger, H.U. (1992). Identification of pigs genetically resistant to oedema disease by testing adhesion of E.coli expressing F107 to intestinal epithelial cells. Proc. IPVS. **12**, 242.

Sydler, T., Buergi, E., Bertschinger, H.U., Pospischil, A. (1996). Oedema disease in adult swine. Proc IPVS **14**, 272.

Zuniga, A.J., Yokoyama, H., Albicker-Rippinga, P., Eggenberger, E., Bertschinger, H.U. (1997). Reduced intestinal colonisation with F18 positive enterotoxigenic E.coli in weaned pigs fed chicken egg antibody against the fimbriae. FEMS Immunol. Med. Microbiol. **18**, 153-161.

Salmonellosis

Definition

Salmonellosis caused by *Salmonella enterica* may occur as outbreaks of septicaemia, acute enteritis or chronic enteritis and wasting in weaned pigs, but may also occur in other age groups. Morbidity and mortality may be high but infection may only cause mild enteritis or be inapparent.

Incidence

The incidence of salmonellosis varies from country to country. In Denmark, national serological monitoring detected infection on 23% herds between 1995 and 1998 but national control measures have reduced this to around 4%. Figures for infected farms based on culture appear to be higher. In the UK 23% of slaughter pigs were infected in 2003 and only 133 incidents of clinical disease were recorded (170, 2004). These figures are typical of EU countries. Sweden is an exception with single figure incidents in most years. In contrast, 63% Illinois (US) farms were infected in 1997, although figures from elsewhere in the US were lower. Infections in EU countries are rarely due to *S.enterica* serovar Choleraesuis in contrast to the situation in the mid-West of the US where many outbreaks in recently weaned pigs are due to *S.e.* Choleraesuis. Single outbreaks of *S.e.* Choleraesuis are reported in the UK annually.

Aetiology

Salmonellosis is caused by serotypes of *Salmonella enterica*, a Gram-negative coccobacillus which grows readily on MacConkey and other bile agars and does not ferment lactose (*S enterica* serovar Arizona may do so). They are classified into named serovars by the antigenic factors present on their O or somatic antigens and the antigens on their H or flagellar antigens. Final differentiation within serovars is carried out by phage typing, plasmid profiling, restriction endonuclease analysis and resistance pattern. Recent changes to the nomenclature of this group mean that the only species of pathogenic salmonella is *S.enterica* and all others are serovars. *S. enterica* serovar Typhimurium, Derby, Saintpaul, Infantis, Heidelberg, Typhisuis and Choleraesuis may all ocur in pigs. The most common serovar in the UK in 2004 was Typhimurium (64%) followed by Derby (17%). Typhimurium Definitive (phage) Type (DT) 104, a multiantibiotic resistant strain, was most common, whilst phage type 12 was uncommon although important worldwide.

Pathogenesis

Salmonella infections appear to fall into 3 groups: 1) septicaemia which may precede or follow enteritis; 2) enteritis with some degree of local invasion; and 3) colonisation of the intestine or its contents without further penetration. All may be followed by the persistence of small numbers of organisms in the gut mucosa, mesenteric lymph nodes or tonsils in clinically-normal carrier animals. *S.e.*Choleraesuis is primarily a pig pathogen, capable of infecting pig herds for long periods and is the classic example of a septicaemic organism, while Typhimurium causes enteritis with local invasion but can cause septicaemia.

Infection normally follows ingestion of the organism which then multiplies in the small intestine to reach high numbers (Typhimurium). Infection by the respiratory route has been confirmed recently. Organisms may adhere to the epithelium (Typhimurium) and enter enterocytes, M cells or areas of cell shedding within minutes of exposure to pass through them or multiply within them to cause cell death. The genetic control of this process of adhesion and invasion is currently being studied, but may be associated with the possession of a 50 kbp plasmid (Choleraesuis). Choleraesuis, Infantis and other invasive serovars reach the mesenteric lymph nodes within 3 hours after infection and become distributed systemically to cause septicaemia. Other serovars may not do so, although they can be found in extra-alimentary tissues by this time.

Choleraesuis and some other serovars are carried by macrophages in which they may multiply. Organisms may be released in organs such as the liver to form micro-colonies surrounded by necrosis and macrophages. Those which remain within macrophages cause endothelial damage and microthrombus formation throughout the body. The effects of this are most severe where end arteries occur. Systemic effects of the disease are also related to the sites of multiplication. Enteric lesions are associated with loss of the enterocytes and the resulting catarrhal enteritis. The effects of systemic infection on submucosal blood vessels contributes to enteritis in invasive strains (S.e. Choleraesuis) and enterotoxin production has been reported in Typhimurium infection, but differs in its action from E. coli LT. The inflammatory gastrointestinal lesions may become necrotic. Infection is followed by the development of systemic antibodies from day 7 post-infection, peaking at 28 days post-infection and declining but still demonstrable 80 days post-infection. Cellular immunity also develops and animals are immune to challenge. Seronegative pigs often remain carriers.

Clinical signs

Pigs of all ages can be affected by invasive serovars of S. enterica (such as Choleraesuis) although outbreaks are commonest in pigs aged between weaning and 3 or 4 months. The septicaemic form is commonest among younger pigs. Animals may be found dead (mortality almost 100% in this form) or be depressed, dull with weakness and even nervous signs (tremor, head tilt, nystagmus or opisthotonus). Affected animals often bury themselves in straw and show mauve-red cyanosis of the ears, limbs and the centre of the back. Affected pigs have a temperature of 40.6-41.7°C, 105-107°F and die within 24-48 hours. The acute enteric form also occurs in younger pigs and may follow septicaemia in animals which do not die. Affected animals pass a thin watery, yellowish diarrhoea and may be dull and fevered (40.6-41.7°C, 105-107°F. Pneumonic signs, weakness and nervous signs such as paralysis and tremor may occur. In severely affected cases, skin discolouration is present. Recovered pigs may slough affected ears or tails. In the chronic enteric form affected pigs appear severely emaciated and may have intermittent fever. There is persistent diarrhoea.

Infection with the less invasive serovars such as Typhimurium common in Europe and other developed industries rarely result in death except in sucking or recently-weaned pigs. Diarrhoea is the most prominent clinical sign although fever may occur. The diarrhoea is initially brownish (or creamy in sucking piglets) and rarely contains blood. It may contain necrotic material and sometimes has a characteristic smell.

Chronically affected animals may become stunted and some may develop the rectal stricture syndrome in which the rectum may be occluded. Some recovered pigs may have necrotic ear tips. Euthanasia should be carried out on septicaemic animals which are moribund, those with acute respiratory distress, chronically wasted pigs and on those with complete rectal stricture.

Pathological findings

Septicaemic form. The carcases may be in good condition and may show discolouration of the skin and ears. Few gross lesions may be seen, but multiple haemorrhages, enlarged haemorrhagic lymph nodes and enlarged spleens often occur. Widespread focal necrosis and hyaline capillary thrombosis is seen histologically.

Acute enteric form. Skin discolouration may be present. The gut appears inflamed and the contents may be watery with some necrotic material. There may be infarction or ulceration of the gastric mucosa and the mucosa of both small and large intestines may be inflamed and necrotic in later cases. The mesenteric lymph nodes may be enlarged and haemorrhagic. The lungs may be pneumonic and hepatised, the liver is usually pale and there may be petechiae on the kidneys.

Chronic enteric form. The gut is thickened and the mucosa is usually necrotic. Button ulcers are occasionally seen at the ileocaecolic junction and the mesenteric lymph nodes are usually haemorrhagic. "Typhoid nodules", the result of necrotic foci, may be seen in the liver.

Diarrhoeic form due to less invasive serovars. Varying degrees of inflammation of the small intestinal mucosa, enlargement, ulceration and eventual necrosis of the Peyer's patches and lymphadenitis may be present but the changes are not specific. Necrosis of the Peyer's patches and later of the mucosa of both small and large intestine may follow. Rectal strictures associated with mega-colon may be identified. Salmonellae may be isolated from the parenchymatous organs in septicaemic disease and from the tonsil, mesenteric lymph nodes, gall bladder and intestinal mucosa and contents in the enteric form.

Epidemiology

Choleraesuis infection may be enzootic on some farms and appear only in weaned pigs 12-16 weeks of age. Infection is usually introduced to a herd by the purchase of carrier pigs or animals infected by contact at markets or in transit and by exposure of young, non-immune pigs to infected faeces. Recent studies suggest that tonsillar carriage or survival in the environment may be uncommon on infected farms, although the organism persists in wet faeces for 14 days and in dust for 13 months. The reason for the marked difference in incidence and prevalence of this condition between EU countries and mid-Western states of the US is unknown.

Outbreaks of salmonellosis due to other Salmonella serovars usually result from lateral spread within farms by the faecal oral route along lines of drainage contact, within pens and by faecal contamination of food and water. Diarrhoeic faeces contains 10^9 organisms/gram and the infective dose may be as low as 10^3 organisms. Salmonellae may be recovered from carrier pigs where they persist on the tonsils and are shed in the faeces from the tonsils, gall bladder and intestinal mucosa for up to 22 weeks post-infection. Piglets may be infected from carrier sows. Flies, rodents or birds and carnivores such as cats may represent reservoirs of infection and result in contamination of feed or water within a farm. Salmonellae are also present in slurry and in dust within pig housing but the relative importance of these sources in initiating new infections within a farm will depend upon the husbandry system.

Infection is usually introduced with weaners, store pigs or breeding stock or in infected faeces contaminating transport or clothing. Non-immune sows or weaners introduced to an infected herd develop disease. Contaminated pig feed may represent a source of salmonella infection, although the serovars found in pig disease are rarely isolated from pig feed (1.1% pig extrusions and 2.2% pig meals UK 1997). Protein components, are more often contaminated (3.1-5.6%, UK 1997). The widespread use of pelleted or heat-treated feeds and improvements in feed storage in the UK has reduced this source of infection. Breeding stock were responsible for the introduction of multi-resistant Typhimurium DT104 into Denmark.

Septicaemic or bacteraemic pigs and contamination from the tonsils and faeces of carrier pigs can contaminate meat at slaughter and may give rise to human disease. Experimental studies have shown that Typhimurium can be recovered from 93.5% tonsils, 71% caecums, 55% mandibular lymph nodes and 45% ileocaecocolic lymph nodes at slaughter 20-28 weeks after infection. Comparable figures have been obtained from natural outbreaks. Infantis may persist in many carcase organs. Humans may also be infected from contact with live pigs or contaminated effluents.

Diagnosis

The clinical signs lead to suspicion of salmonellosis. The peracute form may be suspected where there is a history of infection on a farm but must be differentiated from erysipelas (skin lesions) and from classical and African swine fever. Post-mortem laboratory examination may rule out these other conditions but they should always be considered. The isolation of salmonellae from all parts of the carcase, especially spleen, lung, intestine and mesenteric lymph node, may suggest salmonellosis but does not rule out the swine fevers.

The presence of necrotic material in the faeces of diarrhoeic animals may suggest salmonellosis or swine dysentery. Fever is not a feature of the latter and the faeces usually contain mucus as well as fresh blood. The isolation of the organism from faecal samples or swabs in profuse culture confirms the diagnosis. Indirect culture confirms the presence of infection but may merely indicate carriage. At post-mortem examination the presence of small intestinal inflammation, enlarged mesenteric lymph nodes, necrosis of Peyer's patches and typhlocolitis or rectal stricture may suggest salmonellosis.

Isolation of salmonellae from parenchymatous organs is significant in the absence of other pathogens. Selective media used for isolation should contain brilliant green or tetrathionate and not selenite which can inhibit Choleraesuis. Faeces, carcases and meat monitoring by culture usually employs a prescribed method such as ISO 6579. Spleen, liver, lung, mesenteric lymph nodes and small intestine from affected pigs should be submitted for bacteriological diagnosis. The isolation of a few colonies of a S.enterica from faeces, slurry, caecal contents, tonsil or lymph nodes, especially following pre-enrichment and enrichment may not be sufficient to confirm salmonellosis as the cause of disease. Such isolations are, however, of potential public health significance and should trigger investigation and control measures for public health reasons and where infection is reportable. Isolations of salmonellae from pigs in the UK must be reported under the Zoonosis Order 1989. The isolation of large numbers of organisms on direct culture may well be significant. Organisms in faeces may be detected by ELISA. PCR has also been described and may detect 1 organism/25g faeces/meat if preenrichment is carried out.

The presence of past infection may be confirmed by the presence of serum antibody. ELISA tests using 'O' antigens are now widespread and may be carried out on serum and on meat juices. The Danish meat juice/serum ELISA is designed to detect a wide range of serovars using 'O' factors 1,4,5,6,7 and 12 in the LPS antigen and a cut off point which gives specificity. It is a herd test and detects 100% Infantis-exposed pigs and 67% Typhimurium-exposed pigs at slaughter. Many EU countries, including the UK, have introduced a similar test

Treatment

Affected animals may be treated individually by the daily injection of a suitable antibacterial agent. Tetracyclines, streptomycin, apramycin, neomycin, ampicillin, amoxycillin, spectinomycin, trimethoprim:sulphonamide, enrofloxacin, danofloxacin, ceftiofur florfenicol and chloramphenicol (not UK) may all be effective. After initial individual treatment, the affected group should be given a course of treatment by water medication with one of the following drugs : tetracyclines; streptomycin; neomycin; apramycin ampicillin; amoxycillin, trimethoprim: sulphonamide, enrofloxacin, danofloxacin, (nitrofurazone; furazolidone; or chloramphenicol not UK), for 3-5 days or until 2 days after the cessation of clinical signs. Animals may remain carriers after the cessation of treatment. In feed medication may also be given but all inappetant animals must be treated individually. Disinfection should accompany courses of treatment.

Failure to respond to antimicrobial treatment may suggest that the organism responsible is resistant to the antimicrobial used and isolation and antimicrobial sensitivity testing should be carried out to confirm its sensitivity.

Control

Uninfected farms. Isolation, the use of salmonella-free stock, the use of clean, heat-treated feed and water, rodent control and netting against birds may all help prevent the introduction of salmonellosis to a farm.

Infected farms. Clinical disease should be treated and strategic medication in feed or water may be given when disease is expected using the agents listed above at therapeutic levels and should accompanied by disinfection. Reduction in salmonella levels may be achieved through a number of practices but elimination of the organism is unlikely by these means. All-in-all-out housing, coupled with isolation of batches by disinfectant barriers and thorough cleaning and disinfection between batches may reduce the spread. Batches moved off farm to clean accommodation may be reared salmonella free. Rodent, bird and fly control may also help. Slatted floors, low slurry levels and solid pen divisions reduce transmission and the use of feed which has been heat treated and contains an organic acid will reduce infection from this source. The use of organic acids (especially formic acid salts) and probiotics or competitive exclusion products in feed may reduce salmonella challenge but cannot eliminate disease from farms. The use of carbadox or olaquindox in feed (where allowed) may suppress the infection. Simple hygiene such as hand washing and disinfection of boots or implements has been shown to reduce salmonella carriage. In outdoor or straw-based systems many of these practices may not be possible and vaccination may be an option.

Vaccination is possible. A number of live attenuated Choleraesuis and Typhimurium vaccines have been described. Such vaccines, given at least 14 days prior to exposure (introduction to an infected farm or house, or housing) may protect against clinical disease. Effective live vaccines may not be available in all countries but where they are eg for *S.e.*Typhimurium, they have been shown to reduce the clinical and subclinical effects of salmonella infection with the same serovar (diarrhoea and growth depression) and reduce salmonella carriage at slaughter. The effects on serological monitoring (ZAP Salmonella, UK) are not yet clear. Killed vaccines are also protective.

Eradication of the organism is difficult but has been achieved by complete depopulation, or, in a limited number of instances, by treatment of a whole herd, coupled with rigorous cleaning, disinfection and a 3 week empty period. The organism can persist in dust for up to a year, so disinfection is vital. Salmonella – free breeding stock must be available for restocking.

Decisions on control and treatment may be aided by carrying out bacteriological examination of the herd and the farm to determine the distribution of infection.

Clinically-affected animals should not be sent for slaughter, and infected or contaminated carcases can only be used safely if the meat is heat treated. The use of serological monitoring for infected herds and carcase sampling under the EU Food Hygiene Directives (from 1st January 2006) mean that control programmes may be required by the Official Veterinarian for food safety reasons.

References.

Barber, D.A., Bainson, P.B., Isaacson, R., Jones, C.L., Weigel, R.M. (2002). Distribution of Salmonella in swine production ecosystems J.Food Protection 65, 1861-1868.

Davies, R., Wray, C. (1997). Studies of multiresistant S. typhimurium infection in pig herds: preliminary findings. Pig J. 40, 80-88.

Fedorka-Cray, P.J., Whipp, S.C., Isaacson, R.E., Nord, N., Lager, K. (1994). Transmission of S. typhimurium in swine. Vet. Micro. 41, 333-344.

Gray, J.T., Fedorka-Cray, P.J., Stabel, T., Kramer, T.T. (1996). Natural transmission of S. choleraesuis in swine. Appl. and Env. Micro. 62, 141-146.

Kramer, T.T., Roof, M.B., Matheson, R. (1992). Safety and efficacy of an attenuated strain of S.choleraesuis for the vaccination of swine. Am.J.Vet.Res. 53, 444-448.

Kranker, S., Alban, L., Boes, J., Dahl, J. (2003). Longitudinal study of S.enterica serotype Typhimurium infection in 3 Danish farrow to finish swine herds. J.Clin Micro 41, 2282-2283.

Loynachan, A.T., Nugent, J.M., Erdman, M.M., Harris, D.L. (2004). Acute infection of swine by various salmonella serovars J.Food Protect. 67, 1484-1488.

Mousing, F., Thode Jensen, P., Halgaard, C., Bager, F., Feld, N., Nielsen, B., Nielsen, J.P., Bech Nielsen, S. (1997). Nationwide Salmonella enterica surveillance and control in Danish slaughter swine herds. Prev. Vet. Med. 29, 247-261.

Nielsen, B., Baggesen, D., Bager, F., Haugegaard, J., Lind, P. (1995). The serological response to S. serovar Typhimurium and Infantis in experimentally-infected pigs. The time course followed with an indirect anti-LPS ELISA and bacteriological examinations. Vet. Micro. 47, 205-218.

Nielsen, B., Sorensen, L.L., Mogelmose, V., Dahl, J., Wingstrand, A., Johansen, M., Emborg, H.D., Baggesen, D.L. (1998). Eradication of multiresistant S. typhimurium DT104 infections in Danish Swine. Proc. IPVS 15, (2) 80.

Reed, W.M., Olander, H.J., Thacker, H.L. (1985). Studies on the pathogenesis of Salmonella heidelberg infection in weanling pigs. Am.J.Vet.Res. 46, 2300-2310.

Reed, W.M., Olander, H.J., Thacker, H.L. (1986). Studies on the pathogenesis of S.typhimurium and S.choleraesuis. var kunzendorf infection in weanling pigs. Am.J.Vet.Res. 47, 75-83.

Wood, R.L., Pospischil, A., Rose, R. (1989). Distribution of persistent Salmonella typhimurium infection in the internal organs of swine. Am.J.Vet.Res. 50, 1015-1021.

Wood, R.L., Rose, R., Coe, N.E., Ferris, K.E. (1991). Experimental establishment of persistent infection in swine with a zoonotic strain of S.newport. Am.J.Vet.Res. 52, 813-819.

Wray, C., McLaren, I.M., Beedell, Y.E. (1993). Bacterial resistance monitoring of salmonellae isolated from animals. National experience of surveillance schemes in the UK. Vet.Micro. 35, 313-319.

Wray, C., Wray, A. (Eds) (2000). Salmonella in domestic animals (Wallingford, UK, CABI Publishing, 463 pp ISBN 0-85199-261-7

Swine Dysentery

Definition

Swine dysentery is an infectious mucohaemorrhagic colitis of pigs characterised clinically by loss of condition and the passage of diarrhoeic faeces containing varying amounts of mucus, blood and necrotic material. A proportion of untreated affected pigs may die and others remain stunted.

Incidence

Occurs worldwide. Recent figures vary from country to country but in 1993, 11% of herds in the US were considered to be infected. Figures for the UK in 1994 suggested that 4.7% of herds were infected (10.5% breeding herds), but the disease is still the second most commonly diagnosed enteric disease of pigs. The increasing number of herds founded using swine dysentery-free breeding stock, the use of such pigs exclusively in feeding enterprises and separate site weaning and rearing operations have reduced the incidence in Europe and the US to below the historic levels (1982-1984) of 30-40%.

Whole sectors of an industry such as breeding companies and their multiplying herds may be free from the disease.

Aetiology

A large anaerobic spirochaete, *Brachyspira* (formerly *Serpulina* or *Treponema*) *hyodysenteriae* initiates swine dysentery and can be isolated from field cases of the disease. *B.hyodysenteriae* is 6-l0 μm in length, flexible and active when viewed by phase contrast microscopy and stains readily with aniline dyes. The cell contains a protoplasmic cylinder 350 nm in diameter with pointed ends and 7-14 fibrils inserting at each end and surrounded by an envelope. The organism can be grown on horse blood agar in atmospheres containing 5% CO_2 and 95% H_2 and forms colonies 1 mm in diameter surrounded by ß-haemolysis after 48 hours' incubation. ß-haemolysis results from the secretion of a powerful haemolysin, hlyA, stimulated by the presence of ribonucleic acid. The gene for hlyA has been cloned and is distinct from those for tylA, tylB and tylC.

B.hyodysenteriae is strongly ß-haemolytic, indole positive, α-galactosidase negative, hippurate negative and is antigenically distinct from other *Brachyspira spp.* (specific antigens include a 36 kDa protein, 10 kDa envelope protein and a 46 kDa periplasmic flagellar protein). Multilocus enzyme electrophoresis, 16S rRNA sequences, DNA:DNA hybridisation, whole cell DNA probes, restriction enzyme analysis (REA) and, more recently and repeatably, Restriction Fragment Polymorphism (RFLP) can all be used to identify *B. hyodysenteriae*. The species can be sub-divided into 11 serogroups based on lipopolysaccharide antigens and these can be further sub-divided into serovars and REA or electrophoretic types. It is sensitive to drying and acid pH <6.0 and is readily destroyed by heat but can survive in organic matter for days or weeks.

Pathogenesis

Infection with *B.hyodysenteriae* is by the oral route. The organism is protected from stomach acid by mucus in dysenteric faeces and reaches the large intestine. There, invasion of the mucus and crypts of the mucosa occurs within 2 hours of exposure. The organism is attracted to colonic mucin and to sialic acid, L-fucose, L. serine and blood and colonises the mucin by means of its flagellae (gene deletion reduces motility). The bacteria multiply in the crypts, invade goblet cells and epithelial cells and damage or disrupt them. Invasion through epithelial cell junctions may occur. Mature epithelial cells may be damaged by the haemolysin(s) (hlyA, tlyA,B and C) and *tlyA*-negative mutants are of lowered pathogenicity. A cytotoxin and lipopolysaccharide may also be involved in damage to the cells. The organism may be found outside the gut in anaerobic or effusive lesions.

An inflammatory response develops associated with mast cell degranulation and production of interleukin 6. Inflammatory change results in loss of tissue and blood and failure by the colonic epithelium to re-absorb chloride and sodium ions. Diarrhoea containing blood and mucus develops and death by dehydration or ion imbalance results. A phagocytic response occurs within 2-3 days of the onset of clinical disease and serum antibody can be demonstrated within 7-10 days of the onset of clinical signs and persists for up to 19 weeks. Serum antibody may be related to protective immunity and IgG, IgA and IgM antibody in the lumen of the large intestine may reduce the rate of mucosal colonisation. Cellular immunity has also been demonstrated. IgA immunity to envelope antigens has been demonstrated in sow's milk and appears to protect sucking piglets. Healing lesions may persist as local foci of inflammation for 40-50 days after clinical recovery and the intestinal mucosa may remain infected although grossly normal.

Studies of *B.hyodysenteriae* infections in gnotobiotic pigs indicate that the organism can cause the disease alone. Lesions in conventional pigs are colonised by bacteria such as *Campylobacter coli*, *Bacteroides vulgatus* or *B. fragilis*, *Acetivibrio ethanolgignens*, *Fusobacterium necrophorum* and other spirochaetes which may aid in the development of the lesion. Only *B.hyodysenteriae* will initiate the disease. Disease may be exacerbated by the presence of fermentable food residues reaching the caecum and colon.

Clinical signs

The first signs of the disease include twitching of the tail, abdominal discomfort, hollowing of the flanks, slight reddening of the skin and slight inappetence. A transient fever of 40-40.6°C (104-105°F) may occur, but usually disappears at the onset of the diarrhoea which persists throughout the course of the disease. Diarrhoea may be the clinical sign first noted. Blood, mucus and, later, pieces of necrotic material appear in the faeces which are yellowish in colour at first and later become brownish-red, liquid in consistency and foul-smelling. When recovery begins after 7-14 days, motions containing large quantities of mucus are produced.

Affected pigs show a marked and rapid loss of bodily condition and appear thin with sunken eyes, hollow flanks and prominent ribs and backbones. The coat may be rough, the tail limp and the perineum stained with faeces. Affected pigs show a variable reduction in appetite but all continue to drink. The feed conversion rate and daily liveweight gain may be permanently depressed. Permanently stunted pigs may pass khaki liquid faeces. The depression in bodily condition may cause depression of reproductive performance in outbreaks of disease in sows.

Pigs of all ages are affected although the peak incidence is in weaned pigs of 6-12 weeks of age. The disease can be particularly severe in sows at farrowing or mid-lactation. Production depression on an affected farm may result in an extension of the rearing time from birth - 100 kg of up to 30 days and a 15% increase in farm costs. The presence of passive or incomplete active immunity, treatment of inadequate duration or level and the use of some growth promoters may all reduce the severity of the clinical signs.

Animals with chronic disease, low rectal temperatures (<38°C) and chronic khaki diarrhoea should be killed on humane grounds.

Post mortem findings

Pigs which have died from swine dysentery are usually in poor bodily condition, and the carcase may appear pale and faintly cyanotic.

The large intestine is the only organ consistently affected. It is usually flaccid and may appear dark or congested with a shiny surface due to oedema of the serosa. The mesenteric lymph nodes are frequently pale and swollen but are rarely congested. Pale patches 1-2mm in diameter on the serosal surface are inflamed lymphoid diverticula. The contents are fluid, foul smelling and contain varying proportions of mucus, undigested food and necrotic material and are brownish-red in colour. The appearance of the mucosa varies with the age of the lesion. In early cases it is swollen and congested, later becoming covered with blood-streaked mucus and patches of fibrinous diphtheritic material. There is an extensive layer of necrotic material in older lesions and this may become dislodged in patches to expose the bleeding mucosa.

In some cases the liver may appear swollen and friable and the gastric mucosa may appear inflamed. The stomach contents may be fluid or contain fibrous material. Microscopic lesions are confined to the large intestinal mucosa which is inflamed. The mucosal epithelium is displaced and the underlying capillaries are exposed or covered with a layer of cellular debris, fibrin, bacteria and red blood cells. Spirochaetes can be demonstrated in the crypts of the colonic mucosa in the earliest lesions in silver-stained, fluorescent antibody, enzyme-linked antibody treated sections or by in situ hybridisation. Large spirochaetes can be demonstrated in wet smears of the lesions and *B.hyodysenteriae* can be isolated from them in profuse culture.

Epidemiology

Swine dysentery is transmitted to healthy, susceptible pigs by the ingestion of the faeces of affected or carrier animals. The incubation period of the disease in the field varies between 7 and 60 days but is usually 4-14 days in experimentally infected animals. Carriers may remain infected and may be able to transmit the disease for at least 90 days after clinical recovery. Farms on which an outbreak of the disease has occurred remain infected unless depopulation and disinfection or a whole herd treatment have been carried out. At least two electophoretic types (ET) or REA types have been identified on individual farms, and *B. hyodysenteriae* appears to be a recombinant species with an epidemic population structure, most isolates belonging to a few ETs. RFLP evidence suggests that the same RFLP type may remain on one farm for up to 10 years, and it may evolve into new types or acquire resistance.

Pigs of all ages are affected although the peak incidence is in weaned pigs of 6-12 weeks of age. The disease can be particularly severe in sows at farrowing or mid lactation. The disease is usually introduced to farms by the purchase of infected pigs, spreads slowly from pen to pen by means of drainage channels or movement of infected pigs, by pig-to-pig contact or on infected boots and implements.

Morbidity may reach 75% of all pigs on the farm and mortality varies between 5 and 25%. Some immunity results from infection with swine dysentery and recovered pigs rarely suffer relapses upon re-infection. Antibodies to the causal spirochaete have been identified in the sera, colonic secretions and colostrum of recovered animals and may be detected on a herd basis by agglutination and ELISA tests.

B.hyodysenteriae can persist in moist faeces at 5°C for up to 40 days and in faeces diluted 1:10 with tapwater for up to 60 days. It can persist in slurry for at least 6 days and in soil for up to 41 days at -20°C, 18 days at 14°C, 2 days at 22°C and less than 5 hours at 37°C. The organism can be demonstrated for much longer by PCR. Transmission to susceptible pigs from infected soil is difficult. Drying or disinfectants such as formalin, phenols and hypochlorites eliminate the organism from contaminated pens within hours. Recent studies show that oxidising disinfectants such as Virkon S and Farm Fluid S (Antec) act within minutes.

Mice, rats, flies and dogs have been shown to carry the organism experimentally, and dogs, rats, mice and flies have been identified as carriers in the field. *B.hyodysenteriae* isolated from mice on infected farms have been shown to be pathogenic for pigs and the organism can be maintained in mouse populations.

Diagnosis

Swine dysentery is usually diagnosed on the basis of the history of the outbreak, the clinical signs shown by affected pigs and the post-mortem findings. The presence of spirochaetes in Gram-stained air-dried or wet smears of faeces provides additional evidence for swine dysentery. Isolation of the organism may be attempted using spectinomycin blood agar containing 400µg spectinomycin/ml or selective media containing additional antibiotics, but care should be taken in assessing the results as weakly-haemolytic spirochaetes may also be isolated. Haemolysis and isolation rates can be improved by slicing the agar or punching holes in it. A direct fluorescent antibody test using acetone-fixed faeces smears has been used. The fluorescent antiserum is prepared in rabbits and absorbed with non-*B. hyodysenteriae* spirochaetes in order to enhance specificity. Spirochaetal isolates may be confirmed as *B.hyodysenteriae* by growth inhibition tests using specific antisera or by slide agglutination tests using similar sera. Enzyme analysis using the API ZYM system is useful as *B.hyodysenteriae* isolates lack alpha-galactosidase. They are indole-positive. Multilocus enzyme electrophoresis is able to distinguish between *B.hyodysenteriae* and other spirochaetes and increasing use is made of monoclonal antibodies to specific proteins in fluorescent antibody, agglutination and ELISA tests for *B.hyodysenteriae* isolates. DNA probes and polymerase chain reaction primers using DNA sequences from 16 S rRNA genes have been described. Specific tests are rarely commercially available and a combination of characters may have to be used.

Isolates may be serotyped. Serological tests such as microtitre agglutination tests and ELISA tests can be used on a herd basis to identify infected herds. Current studies suggest that neither is 100% sensitive and specific, and that neither can identify individual infected animals. The main problem is that these tests may detect antibody to common antigens present in non-*B.hyodysenteriae* spirochaetes and statistical interpretation may be required. Herd infection can also be detected using an ELISA for faecal antigen which can detect 10^2 organisms/ml of faeces or slurry in spite of drug treatment or prolonged storage which makes isolation impossible. Herd monitoring can be carried out using rectal faeces swabs or samples from recently weaned pigs, for culture or immunofluorescence, serum ELISA, faecal ELISA and by culturing 10 sites in the colonic mucosa of slaughter pigs. The polymerase chain reaction may be useful and primers capable of identifying 10 ng of DNA in faeces have been described. Pre-incubation with selective broths may increase sensitivity.

The presence of fresh blood and mucus in the diarrhoea differentiate this condition from most other enteric conditions. Salmonellosis is often associated with fever, post-weaning *E.coli*, Salmonella, and spirochaetal colitis and diarrhoeas rarely contain thick mucus or frank blood. T.G.E. and epidemic diarrhoea occur in explosive outbreaks rather than spreading slowly from pen to pen. Faecal blood in gastric ulceration and proliferative haemorrhagic enteropathy is altered and blackish. At post-mortem examination the restriction of lesions to the large intestine rules out all but spirochaetal diarrhoea (a milder disease) or *Trichuris suis* infection.

Swine dysentery may occur with other diseases and then be atypical. In this situation and following incomplete drug treatment, laboratory examination is required for confirmation of the presence of *B. hyodysenteriae*. Experimental animal infection may be necessary for this.

Treatment

Treatment is best administered in the drinking water, but individual severely-affected animals should be treated by injection. This is particularly important if feed medication is to be used. The treatments given below may not all be available in any one country for regulatory reasons.

Tiamulin is extremely effective when given by injection at 10 mg/kg, in the drinking water at 60 ppm for 5 days (Tiamutin, Leo, Novartis) to give 8.8 mg/kg body weight, and in the feed at 120 ppm for 14-21 days. Resistance to tiamulin is rare in the field, but MICs of 4.0 mg/L have been identified in isolates from UK, Hungary, Poland and Germany and are associated with clinical resistance. Tiamulin should not be given in conjunction with monensin, salinomycin or narasin where these are still used..

Valnemulin (Econor, Novartis) is a pleuromutilin resembling tiamulin but more active, available in feed in the EU for treatment for 7-28 days at 75ppm (3-4mg/kg bodyweight per day) and for prevention at 25 ppm (1-1.5 mg/kg bodyweight) for 7-28 days. It is also incompatible with ionophores.

Lincomycin may be used as a feed additive (110 g/ton, 21 days), by injection at 10 mg/kg in the drinking water at 44 ppm and in combination with spectinomycin (Lincospectin, Pharmacia Upjohn) in the drinking water or feed. The water soluble product is not registered for use in pigs in the UK. Resistance to lincomycin occurs at an MIC of around 33mg/L.

Macrolides may be given by intramuscular injection (tylosin Tylan, at 15 mg/kg) in the drinking water (tylosin at 200 ppm for 7-10 days) or in the feed (tylosin at 100 ppm for 21 days). Resistance to tylosin is widespread amongst *B.hyodysenteriae* isolates in Britain and elsewhere but where organisms are sensitive it is effective. Aivlosin has been shown to be effective when tylosin resistance is present.

Organic arsenicals such as sodium arsanilate in the drinking water (175 ppm, 6 days), arsanilic acid (500g/tonne, 21 days), sodium amino arsonate and monosodium 3-nitro 4-phenyl arsonate were formerly used.

Nitroimidazole drugs are also extremely effective but are not registered in the EU or US. Dimetridazole should be given at 260 ppm in the drinking water for 5-7 days and in the feed at 500 ppm for 7-14 days. Ronidazole may be given for 3-5 days in the drinking water at 60 ppm and at 120 ppm in the feed. Strains resistant to dimetridazole were identified.

All animals in drainage contact should be treated at the same time and disinfection of pens or a move to clean pens after treatment will give best results.

Control

a)   Medication

The disease may be prevented using medication at therapeutic levels just after weaning and mixing. Groups of treated pigs should enter cleaned, dried and disinfected accommodation and may be maintained in isolation until slaughter. Treatment into all-in-all-out systems is very effective and can maintain a rearing or finishing herd free from the disease even when infected breeding stock are present.

Continuous low level medication can be used for a period at any time during the rearing and finishing period. Tiamulin can be given at 30-40g/tonne, valnemulin at 25g/tonne, lincomycin at 44g/tonne, [carbadox in feed at 50 ppm to 35 kg only, or dimetridazole at 200g/tonne and ronidazole at 60g/tonne, not EU]. Interruption of feed intake resulting from intercurrent disease or management changes may result in the appearance of clinical or sub-clinical disease which should be treated promptly. Failure to respond to treatment may be due to the development of resistance or to the presence of other enteric pathogens such as salmonella.

b)   Management

General hygiene reduces the spread of the disease within a unit. The use of all-in-all-out husbandry, coupled with proper cleaning, disinfection and drying helps reduce the spread. Spread from house to house can be reduced by disinfecting pathways and by using disinfectant foot dips and separate implements.   Slatted floors, solid partitions between pens, control of flies and rodents and lowering of slurry levels all reduce the spread of the disease.

The use of multiple site rearing may reduce the incidence of disease and, coupled with treatment at movement (Medicated Early Weaning see Enzootic Pneumonia), "Isowean" or introduction to a clean drainage unit/house may reduce the number of disease outbreaks dramatically.

Prompt treatment of clinical disease also reduces spread. Dietary manipulation by the inclusion of non-starch polysaccharides can reduce the severity of disease in some circumstances.

c)   Vaccination

No vaccines are currently (2006) registered for use in the UK. Killed whole cell vaccines made from one or more serotypes and enriched with envelope proteins have been used in the field. They appear to reduce the prevalence of disease, to improve performance and reduce the number of treatments required. They do not appear to prevent disease completely or to prevent infection. Experimental vaccines composed of digests of *B.hyodysenteriae*, subunits such as envelopes and flagellal proteins, live naturally-attenuated and transposon mutants of the tly gene have all been shown to produce some protection.

d)   Eradication

Eradication has been carried out in a number of ways:

Depopulation and restocking

The sale or slaughter of the stock is followed by scrupulous cleaning, manure disposal, disinfection, an empty period to allow drying (best in summer) and rodent and fly control. The clean unit is then restocked with swine dysentery-free pigs (usually originally hysterectomy derived) from a breeding company and maintained in isolation except for the purchase of disease-free breeding stock. Such herds remain disease-free indefinitely. Depopulation may take place as a single event or pigs may be moved to other holdings to reduce the unprofitable time. Similarly, clean breeding stock may be maintained on a clean unit to occupy the cleaned and disinfected unit immediately it is safe to restock.

Treatment of the whole herd, accompanied by disinfection and rodent control. A number of antimicrobials, (tylosin, dimetridazole, ronidazole, lincocin, tiamulin and valnemulin have been shown to eliminate *B.hyodysenteriae*. Treatment at the recommended rate (extended to double the usual period for safety) of the whole herd with a product to which sensitivity has been established, followed by cleaning, disinfection and the isolation of all farrowing sows and their litters until both have undergone full periods of treatment eliminates the disease. Partial depopulation helps the cleaning process and allows for the increase in growth rate which follows successful eradication. Breeding stock should be bought from clean herds.

e)   Partial eradication accompanied by control

Where hygiene and management are good, the breeding stock may be treated and the organism eliminated. Treated pigs are isolated from the contaminated remnant of the herd by a disinfectant barrier along drainage lines which is moved forward ahead of the clean piglets being born. Sufficient space for cleaning must be cleared by partial depopulation of the feeding herd and clinical disease should be suppressed by prompt treatment or continuous medication.

Such schemes are often cost effective, the cost being recouped within 6 months and may reduce finishing periods by 7-21 days. Isolation and treatment of all incoming animals should be practised.

Isolation of the herd and the purchase of clean breeding stock are essential for continued success.

f)   Medicated Early Weaning and 'Isowean'

The use of medicated early weaning (see Enzootic Pneumonia) and the movements of pigs at intervals in the 'Isowean' system may allow the maintenance of swine dysentery-free finishing enterprises. These may be used as sources for swine dysentery-free breeding stock although hysterectomy-derived stock is safer.

g)   Monitoring for freedom from swine dysentery

A number of programmes have been devised to monitor the success of eradication campaigns and the continued freedom from infection of breeding companies. Herds to be monitored should not use treatments which can suppress swine dysentery or growth promoters (where in use) such as carbadox and olaquindox and salinomycin which can affect its appearance. Farm staff should monitor freedom from clinical signs of swine dysentery and report for investigation any outbreaks of other

163

diarrhoeas. A quarterly veterinary inspection which includes inspection of slatted pens and rectal faecal examination confirms these procedures. A regular programme of monitoring any dead pigs post-mortem helps pick up early or mild intestinal lesions.

This programme can be augmented by serology (where available) using blood samples from slaughtered pigs or those aged more than 10-12 weeks. Inspection of colons at slaughter may be carried out. Culture of colonic lesions from slaughtered pigs or those which have died may be carried out on a regular basis. Diarrhoeic faeces or rectal samples taken at quarterly inspections can be examined for *B.hyodysenteriae*. Animals with post-weaning diarrhoea, those recently mixed and young gilts at service are most likely to yield evidence of infection in a sub-clinically-infected herd. Monitoring may be by faecal ELISA, PCR, or culture but the laboratory carrying out the examination must be capable of distinguishing between *B.hyodysenteriae* and other spirochaetes, as they may not be eliminated by the treatments described.

References

Alexander, T.J.L., Taylor, D.J.. (1969). The clinical signs, diagnosis and control of swine dysentery. Vet. Rec. **85**, 59-63.

Argenzio, R.A., Whipp, S.C. and Glock, R.D. (1980). Pathophysiology of swine dysentery: Colonic transport and permeability studies. J.Infectious Dis. **142**, 676-684.

Egan, I.T., Harris, D.L. and Joens, L.A.(1983). Comparison of the microtitration agglutination test and the ELISA for the detection of herds affected with swine dysentery. Am.J.Vet.Res. **44**, 1323-1328.

Elder, R.O., Duhamel, G.E., Schafer, R.W., Mathiesen, M.R., Ramanathan, M. (1994) Rapid detection of S. hyodysenteriae in diagnostic specimens by polymerase chain reaction. J. Clin Micro. **32**, 1497-1502.

Glock, R.D. (1984). Eliminating swine dysentery from selected herds. Modern Vet.Practice. **65**, 611-614.

Glock, R.D. and Harris, D.L. (1972). Swine dysentery II. Characterisation of lesions in pigs inoculated with *Treponema hyodysenteriae* in pure and mixed culture. Vet.Med. Small Anim.Clin. **67**, 65-68.

Hampson, D.J. (1997). Rapid identification of porcine *Serpulina sp.* Vet Rec **140**, 51.

Hampson, D.J., Mhoma, J.R.L., Combs, B., Buddle, J.R. (1984). Proposed revision to the serological typing system for *T.hyodysenteriae*. Epidemiology and Infection **102**, 75-84.

Harris, D.L., Glock, R.D., Christensen, C.R. and Kinyon, J.M. (1972). Swine dysentery I. Inoculation of pigs with *Treponema hyodysenteriae* (new species) and reproduction of the disease. Vet.Med. S.A.C. **67**, 61-68.

Hsu, TsungDa, Hutto, D.L., Minion, F.C., Zuerner, R.L., Wannemuehler, M.J. (2001). Cloning of a β haemolytic gene of *Brachyspira (Serpulina) hyodysenteriae* and its expression in *E. coli*. Inf. and Immun. **69**, 706-711.

Joens, L.A. and Marquez, R.B. (1986). Molecular characterisation of proteins from porcine spirochaetes. Infection and Immunity **54**, 893-896.

Kramomtong, I., Neramitmansook, W., Whipp, S.C., Joens, L.A., Limawongpranee, S. (1996). Comparison of ELISA and selective culture in the diagnosis of swine dysentery in Thailand. Vet. Rec. **138**, 332-333.

Lymbery, A.J., Hampson, D.J., Hopkins, R.M., Combs, B., Mhoma, J.R.L. (1990). Multilocus enzyme electrophoresis for identification and typing of *T.hyodysenteriae* and related spirochaetes. Vet.Microbiology. **22**, 89-99.

Lysons, R.J., Kent, M.A., Bland, A., Sellwood, R., Robinson, W.F., First, A. (1991). A cytolytic haemolysin from *T.hyodysenteriae*: a probable virulence determinant in swine dysentery. J.Med.Micro. **34**, 97-102.

Olson, L.D. (1996). Enhanced isolation of S. hyodysenteriae by using sliced agar media. J.Clin. Micro. **34**, 2937-2941.

Pluske, J.R., Pethick, D.W., Durmic, Z., Mullan, B.P., Hampson, D.J. (1996). The incidence of swine dysentery in pigs can be reduced by feeding diets that limit the amount of fermentable substrate entering the large intestine. J. Nutrition **126**, 2920-2933.

Rees, A.S., Lysons, R.J., Stokes, C.R., Bourne, F.J. (1989). Antibody production in the pig colon during infection with *T.hyodysenteriae*. Res.Vet.Sci. **47**, 263-269.

Schmall, L.M., Argenzio, R.A. and Whipp, S.C. (1983). Pathophysiologic features of swine dysentery: cyclonucleotide independent production of diarrhoea. Am.J.Vet.Res. **44**, 1309-1316.

Siba, P.M., Pethick, D.W. and Hampson, D.J. (1996). Pigs experimentally infected with S. hyodysenteriae can be protected from developing swine dysentery by feeding them a highly digestible diet. Epidemiology and Infection **116**, 207-216.

Taylor, D.J., Alexander, T.J.L. (1971). The production of dysentery in swine by feeding cultures containing a spirochaete. Brit.Vet.J. **127**, 58-61.

Taylor, D.J., Lysons, R.J., Bew, J., Stevenson, R. and Lemcke, R.M. (1985). Survival of *Treponema hyodysenteriae* in samples of dysenteric pig faeces sent by post and stored at room temperature. Vet.Rec. **116**, 48-49.

Trott, D.J., Oxberry, S.L., Hampson, D.J. (1997). Evidence for S. hyodysenteriae being recombinant with an epidemic population structure. Microbiology (Reading) **143**, 3357-3365.

Windsor, R.S. and Simmons, J.R. (1981). Investigation into the spread of swine dysentery in 25 herds in East Anglia and assessment of its economic significance in 5 herds. Vet.Rec . **109**, 482-484.

Wood, E.N. and Lysons, R.J. (1988). The financial benefits from the eradication of swine dysentery.). Vet.Rec. **122**, 277-279.

Spirochaetal Diarrhoea
(Porcine Intestinal Spirochaetosis, Porcine Colonic Spirochaetosis)

Definition

A syndrome in which infection with spirochaetes other than *B. hyodysenteriae* results in diarrhoea, sporadic dysentery and depression of weight gain in young weaned pigs.

Incidence

Increasingly recognised and apparently widespread. Seen in France, Sweden, Poland, Germany, Britain, Italy, China, Korea, Australia, U.S. and Canada. Clinical disease seen in minimal disease pigs, following withdrawal of antibiotics and where non-immune pigs are mixed with carriers. It is particularly common where no growth promoters are used.

Aetiology

A number of strains or species of weakly ß-haemolytic spirochaetes have been isolated from the faeces or colonic mucosa of pigs using the media and conditions used for *B. hyodysenteriae*. Extensive studies by electron microscopy, antigenic analysis, biochemical profiles, restriction endonuclease analysis, multilocus enzyme electrophoresis and sequence analysis of 16S rRNA has identified four species, *Serpulina. innocens*, only rarely associated with disease, *S. murdochi*, a non-pathogen, *B. intermedia*, a cause of diarrhoea and colitis and *B. pilosicoli*, the most common pathogen and the major cause of the syndrome described here. All of these are distinct from *B.hyodysenteriae* on ultrastructural, gene sequence, biochemical or antigenic grounds.

B. pilosicoli is 6-l0μm in length, 0.25μm in diameter and with 4-7 fibrils in the axial filament. It is weakly β haemolytic, generally indole negative and β glucuronidase negative, D-ribose positive and generally hippurate positive. A specific antigen of 80kDa appears to be present in the cell envelope. Restriction endonuclease analysis (REA) and multiple locus enzyme electrophoresis indicate that a number of REA and ETs exist and RFLP has been useful in subdividing the species, but serotyping has not yet been carried out.

Pathogenesis

Pathogenicity has not been studied exhaustively but infection is oral. Colonisation of the colonic mucosa and consequent failure of colonic absorption appear to be more important than epithelial invasion in this condition. Organisms appear to produce colonic failure by colonising densely the lumenal border of mature epithelial cells. Spirochaetal cells are arranged end on and may be invaginated into the epithelial cell membrane displacing the brush border. Large micro colonies of the organisms develop in the crypts. Spirochaetal colonisation is associated with mild inflammation and is followed by plasma cell accumulation in the lamina propria. In some circumstances spirochaetes may invade damaged mucosa and they have been recorded in anaerobic areas and effusions elsewhere in the body.

Recovery and resistance appear to occur as for swine dysentery. Serum antibody is difficult to demonstrate. In addition to primary infections, the organism colonises lesions of the colon in cases of proliferative haemorrhagic enteropathy, *Trichuris suis* infection, swine dysentery and other enteric diseases.

Clinical signs

Clinical signs are seen most commonly in young, weaned animals, mostly from 20-40 kg, but may occur in non-immune animals of any age. The incubation period varies from 5-20 days, animals have a slight fever (40°C, 105°F) appear "tucked up" and may be off their feed. Recovery occurs within 7-10 days and mortality is rare (less than 1%). A marked reduction in the rate of daily liveweight gain may occur and recovered animals may appear hairy. In some units older animals may also be affected and chronic diarrhoea may occur.

Pathology

The large intestinal serosa may be oedematous and the colon contents fluid. The mucosa is thickened and hyperaemic, with excess clear mucus or local bleeding points and some diphtheritic material. In recovering animals, islands of necrotic material may be seen on the mucosa. The mucosa is oedematous with dilated crypts which may be filled with silver-stained organisms. *B. pilosicoli* may be isolated from the mucosa or colon contents or demonstrated as a false brush border on the cells of the mucosal epithelium using silver stains or fluorescent antibody, and, in complicated infections, is present in pre-existing lesions caused by other pathogens.

Epidemiology

B. pilosicoli appears to survive to a much greater extent in the environment than *B. hyodysenteriae* in swine dysentery., surviving for longer in the soil and in slurry lagoons. In particular, its presence in mice, dogs and some bird species makes its elimination by cleaning and disinfection more difficult. Studies of ETs and RFLP suggest that many types exist. The *B. pilosicoli* isolated from dogs, birds, rodents and man contain clones which cross species boundaries. Some are found in common in pig and man, although most human isolates have different RFLP from porcine isolates. Human strains and some rodent strains can cause disease in pigs. Infection in species other than the pig may account for *B. pilosicoli* infections in newly-established hysterectomy-derived nucleus herds.

Diagnosis

Spirochaetal diarrhoea should be suspected when chronic, non-fatal diarrhoea with little or no blood and some clear mucus occurs in recently weaned pigs in herds free from swine dysentery or following withdrawal of a growth promoter. The post-mortem findings are suggestive, and the isolation of weakly β haemolytic spirochaetes from faeces or colonic contents on spectinomycin blood agar contributes to the diagnosis. The identification of the isolate as *B. pilosicoli* confirms the presence of the disease. The techniques available include biochemical characters (indole, enzyme analysis using API ZYM and hippurate), growth inhibition, multilocus enzyme electrophoresis, immunofluorescence and immunoperoxidase using specific monoclonal or polyclonal antibody and the polymerase chain reaction (PCR), capable of detecting 10^4 cells in faeces. *B. intermedia* is also a primary cause of spirochaetal diarrhoea, but *S. innocens* and *S. murdochi* are likely to be incidental to the development of disease. Other agents such as salmonella, *Trichuris suis* or *Lawsonia intracellularis* may be present. It is important to confirm the identity of spirochaetes isolated from mild colitis in herds where swine dysentery is thought to have been eradicated or to be absent.

Treatment and control

Similar to that used for swine dysentery, ie. tiamulin, valnemulin, lincomycin, or aivlosin (and dimetridazole where srtill possible). Tylosin and other macrolides are more often effective and olaquindox is more effective against spirochaetal diarrhoea than against swine dysentery. All animals in drainage contact should be treated and treatment should be followed by cleaning and disinfection. The organism can then be eliminated from the faeces of a group. Control of rodents and other vector species is particularly important during management for this disease. The organism or the disease can be eliminated from a herd by medicated early weaning.

There is no vaccine, as experimental studies have been unsuccessful.

References

Binek, M. and Szynkiewicz, Z.M. (1984). Physiological properties and classification of strains of *Treponema spp.* isolated from pigs in Poland. Comparative Immunology, Microbiology and Infectious Diseases 7, 141-148.

Felstrom, C., Petterson, B., Thomson, J., Gunnarsson, A., Persson, M., Johansson, K.E. (1997). Identification of *Serpulina sp.* associated with porcine colitis by biochemical analysis and PCR. J. Clin. Micro. 35, 462-467.

Lee, J.I., Hampson, D.J., Lymbery, A.J., Harders, S.T. (1993). The porcine intestinal spirochaetes: identification of new genetic groups. Vet.Micro. 34, 273-285.

Lymbery. A.J., Hampson, D.J., Hopkins, M., Combs, B. and Mhoma, J.R.L. (1990). Multilocus enzyme electrophoresis for identification and typing of *T.hyodysenteriae* and related spirochaetes. Vet.Micro. 22, 89-99.

Neef, N.A., Lysons, R.J., Trott, D.J., Hampson, D.J., Jones, P.W., Morgan, J.H. (1994). Pathogenicity of porcine intestinal spirochaetes in gnotobiotic pigs. Infection and Immunity, 62, 2395-2403.

Park, N.Y., Chung, C.Y., McLaren, A.J., Atyeo, R.F. and Hampson, D.J. (1994). Polymerase chain reaction for identification of spirochaetes associated with intestinal spirochaetosis. Proc.IPVS. **13**, 192.

Stanton, T.B., Fourme-Amazouz, E., Postic, D., Trott, D.J., Grimont, P.A.D., Baranton, G., Hampson, D.J., Saint Girons, I. (1997). Recognition of two new species of intestinal spirochaetes: *Serpulina intermedia sp. nov.* and *Serpulina murdochi, sp. nov.* Int. J. Syst. Bact. **47**, 1007-1012.

Taylor, D.J., Simmons , J.R. and Laird, H.M. (1980). Production of diarrhoea and dysentery in pigs by feeding pure cultures of a spirochaete differing from *Treponema hyodysenteriae.* Vet. Rec. **106**, 324-332.

Tenaya, I.W.M., Penhale, W.J., Hampson, D.J. (1998). Preparation of diagnostic polyclonal and monoclonal antibody against outer envelope proteins *of S. pilosicoli.* J. Med. Micro. **47**, 317-324.

Thomson, J.R., Smith, W.J., Murray, B.P. (1998). Investigations into field cases of porcine colitis with particular reference to infection with *S. pilosicoli.* Vet Rec **142**, 235-239.

Trott, D.J., Constantine, C.L., Oxberry, S.L., Hampson, D.J. (1998). Population structure and molecular epidemiology of S. pilosicoli in Australian piggeries. Proc. IPVS **15**, 3,128.

Trott, D.J., Stanton, T.B., Jensen, N.S., Duhamel, G.E., Johnson, J.L., Hampson, D.J. (1996). *Serpulina pilosicoli sp. nov.,* the agent of porcine intestinal spirochaetosis. Int. J. Syst. Bact. **46**, 206-215.

Campylobacter enteritis

Definition

Campylobacters cause a mucoid creamy diarrhoea which may contain blood in piglets 3 days - 3 weeks of age. They may also cause enteritis in non-immune weaned pigs, and contribute to inflammatory conditions of the ileum and large intestine. Mucus in the faeces in other enteric conditions may indicate their presence

Incidence

The organisms are ubiquitous worldwide but clinical signs are rarely ascribed to the infection. 100% pigs may be infected with *C.coli* but not all may be infected with the other species (*C. jejuni* 4.6% Japan, 5% Denmark, 20-30% in other studies).

Aetiology and Pathogenesis

C.coli is a microaerophilic curved Gram-negative rod forming sprawling watery colonies of blood agar after 48 hours. It is catalase-positive, grows at 43^oC but not at 25^oC and does not produce H_2S on T.S.I. medium and is hippurate negative. Following infection, multiplication occurs in the small intestine, particularly the ileum where the organism is closely associated with the mucosa. A brief bacteraemic phase may occur but the organism does not appear to penetrate the epithelium in any numbers. Recent studies suggest that the organism may produce a cytotoxin which could cause the inflammatory changes seen. Colonisation of the large intestine occurs. Clinical signs begin after an incubation period of 1-3 days after infection.

Other campylobacters are also present in the porcine intestine. *C.hyointestinalis* subsp. *hyointestinalis* or subsp. *lawsonii*, *C.jejuni*, *C.mucosalis*, *C. hyoilei*, *C.lari* and *C.lanienae* have all been identified and may reach high numbers and be associated with enteritis, particularly in weaned pigs.

Clinical signs

Affected piglets may have a mild fever (to 40.6°C, 105°F) which may be maintained for 2-3 days. A watery or creamy diarrhoea containing mucus with occasional streaks of blood is present. These clinical signs may continue for some days. In weaned pigs *C.coli* infection may be associated with chronic mucoid diarrhoea in which no blood is seen. In both forms of the disease loss of condition occurs but mortality is rare.

Infection may not cause clinical signs in immune pigs but experimental infection of hysterectomy-derived, colostrum-deprived or gnotobiotic pigs with *C.coli, C.jejuni, C.hyointestinalis* or *C. sputorum* may produce diarrhoea after 1-4 days.

Pathological findings

In neonatal pigs gross changes are slight and are confined to the small intestine which is slightly inflamed with thickening of the ileum, especially of the terminal portion. The mesenteric lymph nodes are prominent. The ileal mucosa is mildly inflamed and mucoid contents may be present at this site or in the caecum. The mucosa of the large intestine is usually mildly inflamed or normal. Stunting of the ileal villi may be seen. Histological changes are slight, the most prominent being massive enlargement of the lymphoid tissue in the terminal ileum. Crypt abscesses may be present. The ileal thickening results from the lymphoid hyperplasia and not from any proliferation of the mucosal epithelium. In weaned pigs, thickening of the small intestine, particularly of the terminal portion, may be prominent. Large intestinal changes resembling chronic mild swine dysentery may be seen. *C.coli* or other campylobacters, including *C. jejuni*, may be isolated on selective medium from the small intestine in large numbers, and curved Gram-negative rods are present in smears made from the mucosal surface.

Epidemiology

Pigs in most farms are infected with *C.coli* and some farms have high prevalences of *C. jejuni*. Infection takes place by the faecal/oral route in piglets from maternal faeces, contaminated water or horizontal transmission. Maternal immunity normally prevents clinical disease but does not prevent colonisation. Infected animals remain carriers for long periods and pass 10^3-10^4 organisms/g faeces for months. Carriage is in the gall bladder, ileal mucosa and large intestinal mucosa.

Introduction of a campylobacter species to which immunity is absent can result in outbreaks of diarrhoea. *C.jejuni*, or *C.lari* from other species of animal origin or from water may cause disease.

Contamination of pigmeat with campylobacters may lead to human infection. *C.coli* infection is relatively rarely identified in man in the UK, but 6% pig livers were contaminated with campylobacters in one UK survey and *C. jejuni* has been identified on pigmeat or in livers in a number of countries.

Diagnosis

C.coli or *C. jejuni* infections should be suspected when a mucoid diarrhoea containing blood stained mucus occurs in piglets with little mortality and some loss of condition. To confirm, the organism must be present in profuse culture in the ileum and other causes of diarrhoea, such as rotavirus, epidemic diarrhoea, *Clostridium perfringens, E.coli,* coccidia and cryptosporidia should be eliminated to reach a diagnosis of primary *C.coli* infection. *C. jejuni* can be isolated from some watery, mucoid diarrhoeas of weaned pigs. Histological lesions of proliferative enteropathy (P.E.) should be absent. Colonic lesions should be distinguished from PE., spirochaetal diarrhoea and swine dysentery.

Isolation has recently been supplemented by DNA probes and PCR for *C.jejuni*, *C.sputorum* and *C.hyointestinalis*.

Treatment

Oral treatment with neomycin, other amino-glycosides, tetracyclines, macrolides and fluoroquinolones may all eliminate or markedly reduce Campylobacter infection. Treatment, is however, rarely carried out.

Control

Control has rarely, if ever, been attempted in the pig. Low level antimicrobial treatment would be the most appropriate method, coupled with hygiene and chlorination of water supplies. It is possible to maintain pig units founded from primary hysterectomy derived stock free from infection by strict isolation

References

Mafu, A.A., Higgins, R., Nadeau, M., Cousseau, G. (1989). The incidence of salmonella, campylobacter and *Yersinia enterocolitica* in swine carcases and slaughterhouse environment. J.Food Production 52, 642-645.

Mansfield, L.S., Gauthier, D.T., Abner, S.R., Jones, K.M., Wilder, S.R., Urban, J.F. (2003). Enhancement of disease and pathology by synergy of Trichuris suis and Campylobacter jejuni in the colon of immunologically-naïve swine. Am. J. Trop. Med and Hygiene, 68, 70-80.

Moore, J.E., Madden, R.W. (1998). Occurrence of thermophilic Campylobacter spp. in porcine liver in Northern Ireland. J. Food Protection 61, 409-413.

Olubunmi, P.A. and Taylor, D.J. (1982). Production of enteritis in pigs by the oral inoculation of *Campylobacter coli*. Vet.Rec. 111, 197-202.

Taylor D.J. and Olubunmi, P.A. (1981). A re-examination of the role of *C.fetus* subsp *coli* in enteric disease of the pig. Vet.Rec. 109, 112-115.

Vitovci, J., Kondela, B., Sterba, J., Tomancova, I., Matyas, Z., Vladiz, P. (1989). The gnotobiotic piglet as a model for the pathogenesis of *C.jejuni* infection. Zbl.fur Bakt. 271, 91-103.

Weijtens, M.J.B.M., Plas, J. van der, Bijker, P.G.H., Urlings, H.A.P., Koster, D., Logtestijn, J.G.van, Huis in t'Velds, J.H.J. (1997). The transmission of campylobacter in piggeries: an epidemiological study. J. Appl. Microbiol. 83, 693-698.

Weijtens, M.J.B.M., Urlings, H.A.P., Plas, J. van der, (2000). Establishing a campylobacter-free pig population through a top down approach. Letters in Appl. Microbiol. 30, 479-.

Helicobacter spp

Helicobacters have been isolated from the stomachs of pigs (*H. heilmannii*, (also called *Gastrospirillum suis*) and from faeces (*H. pametensis*). *H. heilmannii* has been found in large numbers in the mucosa of pigs with gastric ulceration and has been shown to infect gnotobiotic pigs in experiments. Its significance in the pig is unknown although it is likely to be involved in gastritis and causes inflammation and lymphoid accumulations in experimental infections, but has not caused gastro oesophageal ulceration. Other, as yet unnamed species may do so. *H. pylori* readily infects pigs in experimental studies but has not been isolated from pigs. Porcine species may give rise to human infections.

References

Eaton, K.A., Morgan, D.R., Krakowka, S. (1989). *Campylobacter pylori* virulence factors in gnotobiotic pigs. Inf. and Immun. **57**, 1119-125.

Krakowka, S., Eaton, K.A., Rings, D.M., Argenzio, R.A. (1998). Production of gastro-oesophageal erosions and ulcers in gnotobiotic swine monoinfected with fermentative commensal bacteria and fed high carbohydrate diet. Vet. Path.**35**, 274-282.

Krakowka, S., Rings, D.M., Ellis, J.A. (2005). Experimental induction of bacterial gastritis and gastric ulcer disease in gnotobiotic swine inoculated with porcine *Helicobacter*-like species. Am. J. Vet. Res. **66**, 945-942.

Yeoman, N.D., Holt, S.D. (1996). *Helicobacter heilmannii* (formerly *Gastrospirillum*) association with pig and human gastric pathology. Gastroenterology **111**, 244-247.

Arcobacters

These campylobacter-like organisms (*A. cryoaerophila*, *A.skirrowii* and *A. butzleri*), which grow at 25°C have been isolated from the vagina, uterus and aborted foetuses in cases of infertility and abortion. They have also been isolated from enteritis. They can be identified by PCR and relationships can be established by RFLP. Experimental infection of HDCD piglets has resulted in isolation from all parts of the piglet *(A. butzleri)* or from the gut alone (*A. cryaerophilus*).

They can infect man and cause enteritis and have been found in pigmeat.

References

Hume, M.E., Harvey, R.B., Stanker, L.H., Drolesky, R.E., Poole, T.L., Zhang HongBin (2001). Genotypic variation among arcobacter isolates from a farrow-to-fininsh swine facility. J.Food Protect. **64**, 645-651.

On, S.L.W., Jensen, T.K., Bille-Hansen, V., Jorsal, S.E., Vandamme, P. (2002). Prevalence and diversity of Arcobacter spp. Isolated from the internal organs of spontaneous porcine abortions in Denmark. Vet.Micro **85**, 159-167.

Wesley, I.N., Baetz, A.L., Larson, D.J. (1996). Infection of caesarian-derived, colostrum deprived, day old piglets with *A. butzleri*, *A. cryaerophilus* and *A. skirrowii*. Inf and Immunity, **64**, 2295-2299.

Proliferative Enteropathy

Definition

An infectious bacterial condition in which proliferative changes occur in the epithelium of the small and large intestinal mucosa. The condition underlies necrotic enteritis, regional ileitis and proliferative haemorrhagic enteropathy. Affected pigs appear pale, may be stunted and may die suddenly with clotted blood in the lumen of the small intestine.

Incidence

The disease has been described in Canada, USA., Taiwan, Korea, Japan, Brazil, Mexico, Australia and Europe, including Britain, and is particularly noticeable in herds which were originally hysterectomy-derived. Recent surveys using clinical, pathological or PCR evidence suggest that 56% (Australia), 50% (Japan), 35% (Brazil and Mexico), 31% (UK), 30% (Denmark) of herds are affected/infected but much higher prevalences may be found in slaughter pigs e.g 87% Poland.

Aetiology

Proliferative enteropathy is caused by the obligate intracellular bacterium *Lawsonia intracellularis*. The organism is related to *Desulfovibrio desulfuricans* using 16S rDNA (91% homology) but not to any enteric pathogen. It is a Gram-negative curved rod I.5 μm in length with tapered ends which multiplies by septation within cells. At present it is cultured in a rat enterocyte cell line 1EC-18 in the cells of which it forms micro colonies after 7-14 days. The organism can be sub-cultured in this cell line and can survive outside the cells for up to 2 weeks at 5°C but not multiply. Pure cultures of the organism harvested from these cell cultures have been given to conventional and gnotobiotic pigs and reproduce the lesions of the disease within 21 days. Monoclonal antibodies and DNA probes confirm that this organism is present in the lesion and the association between organism and lesion has been confirmed statistically with an odds ratio of ≥ 14 and an estimated attributable fraction of $\geq 92\%$.

Pathogenesis

Infection is oral and the organism enters epithelial cells of the crypts of the small intestine. The bacteria lie adjacent to the apices of the epithelial cells and enter by endocytic vacuole formation. The vacuoles may fuse with lysosomes but the organisms survive and enter the cytoplasm in which they become more electron lucent and divide by septation. They are located near mitochondria and rough endoplasmic reticulum. Numbers increase until micro colonies of >50 organisms are present within a cell. Infected cells survive parasitism with only minor changes to mitochondrial structure but eventually rupture apparently by apoptosis to extrude the organisms. Those shed to the exterior are electron dense and may enter other cells or pass out in the faeces.

These developments in the intestinal epithelial cells are responsible for the microscopic and gross changes seen in the pig gut. The earliest changes occur as hyperplasia of the glandular epithelium of the terminal small intestine. Goblet cells disappear, the epithelial cells become elongated with many mitoses and the crypts elongate and branch. They may be filled with polymorphs. Capillaries dilate and then rupture at the apex of the villi. Blood loss into the lumen occurs leading to anaemia and hypoalbuminaemia. These changes can take place in germ-free gnotobiotic pigs but colonisation with *Bacteroides vulgatus* and pathogenic *E.coli* increase their severity.

The incubation period is dependent on the inoculum and can be as short as 4 days with high numbers of organisms in infected in infected tissue inocula. The changes in the mucosal epithelium are first visible 8-10 days after experimental infection with small numbers of organisms, reach their maximum extent after 21 days and then may regress, become necrotic (necrotic enteritis, sometimes caused by salmonellosis or nicotinic acid deficiency) or continue to proliferate to give rise to a benign adenomatosis. Mucosal proliferation and erosion may result in changes in the terminal ileum, the muscular coats of which become hyperplastic to give regional ileitis or hosepipe gut. The presence of infection and lesions in the large intestine may lead to failure of colonic absorption.

L. intracellularis is first shed in the faeces 13 days after infection (but sooner with high inocula) and shedding may reach 10^8/g and continue for up to 10 -12 weeks. Serum IgG antibody can be demonstrated by indirect immunofluorescence or ELISA from 21-28 days post infection onwards. Antibody can be demonstrated from 2 weeks post shedding of the organism as determined by PCR) and may persist for more than 3 months. During this period the organisms may be demonstrated in the apical cytoplasm of affected cells or by PCR in the faeces. Haemorrhage in proliferative haemorrhagic enteropathy occurs at the same time as destruction of the organisms and other mucosal changes and may be immune mediated. Maternal antibody can be demonstrated for up to 5 weeks of age but does not protect against colonisation.

Clinical signs

The clinical disease is most commonly seen in recently-weaned pigs and lasts for about 6 weeks. It has an incubation period of 3-6 weeks and can occur in animals of any age from 3-4 weeks to adults. The first signs are failure to gain weight or loss of weight and capricious appetite. Affected pigs appear pale, may vomit, are anaemic (P.C.V. as low as 20%) and may have blackened faeces due to melaena. Some animals pass loose granular faeces which spread on concrete like portions of wet cement especially where other infections are present (see intestinal spirochaetosis and campylobacter enteritis). After 4-6 weeks they may recover completely. Some pigs die suddenly with proliferative haemorrhagic enteropathy (PHE). These usually appear pale with a low body temperature (37.8°C,100°F), 1-2 hours prior to death and may be of any age from 6-10 weeks upwards. Breeding stock may die when the disease first enters a herd (from proliferative haemorrhagic enteropathy) or if clean stock are introduced to an infected herd. Some animals remain stunted. Morbidity may reach 12% and mortality 6% in such cases. Affected pigs may appear thin, pale and may have mild diarrhoea.

The presence of the disease in breeding herds may lead to a decrease in production of up to 8%, partially due to abortion which follows 6 days after clinical signs develop in pregnant sows. There are two indications for humane slaughter: when animals are suffering from severe blood loss, hypothermia, and are unable to rise, and severely stunted pigs with chronic disease.

Pathological findings

Pigs which die from the disease are pale with a thickened small intestine which may appear dark or pale, swollen, reticulated and flaccid from the serosal surface. The lesions of proliferative enteropathy occur in the ileum and upper third of the spiral colon. The wall of the gut may be thickened and flaccid. The surface of the mucosa may be thrown into folds reminiscent of those seen in Johne's disease of cattle and the tips of the rugae may show bleeding points. Plaques of thickened mucosa resembling that of the affected small intestine may be seen in the large intestine and polyps may also be present. This underlying lesion may disappear or develop to give the following changes:

In necrotic enteritis the lining of the intestine may be covered in yellow or greyish masses of friable necrotic material closely adherent to the surface.

In regional ileitis ("hosepipe gut") the wall of the lower small intestine is smooth and rigid, particularly in the terminal region of the ileum. Upon section, the muscle layers are thickened and the lining is ulcerated or covered in granulation tissue.

In proliferative haemorrhagic enteropathy the lesions are largely restricted to the small intestine. The lower third is distended and filled with clotted blood mixed with food. Bleeding points can only be seen using a dissecting microscope and are very localised. The mucosa is often highly folded. The contents of the large intestine are blackish and tarry. The carcase is pale and the blood watery.

In histological sections, the affected mucosa is thicker than normal and contains branched crypts packed with dividing cells. There is a marked absence of goblet cells. Affected tissue may lie next to normal tissue, particularly at the edge of a polyp. In silver-stained sections the apical cytoplasm of the cells lining the crypts may be seen to contain large numbers of bacteria which may be identified as *L.intracellularis* with specific fluorescent antibody or using DNA probes.

Other bacteria such as campylobacters may be present in lesions in both small and large intestine. Their presence may affect the pathological findings.

Epidemiology

L. intracellularis can be detected in faeces by the polymerase chain reaction (PCR), although antimicrobial treatment and growth promoters may reduce levels of detection and the degree of shedding. One infection profile obtained from a herd with enzootic infection using PCR demonstrated infection in 1.9% piglets 0-24 days old, 22.9% animals 10-24 days post weaning, 12.9% growers and finishers, 3.4% slaughter pigs, 0.9% gilts and in no boars or sows to give an overall prevalence of infection of 6.8%. Many infection profiles suggest that higher infection rates are common and some show peak shedding periods at 10-12 weeks or even later where antimicrobial treatments have been given. The organism survives outside cells for up to 2 weeks at 5°C, and field evidence suggests that emptying, cleaning and resting of buildings for two weeks reduces environmental infection. It may survive in rodents and other small mammals as it is possible to infect hamsters experimentally and similar organisms have been identified in rats, rabbits and ferrets but not in mice. Infection profiles obtained by PCR on faeces are mirrored by serum antibody demonstrated by indirect immunofluorescence and ELISA, but begin 2 weeks after shedding is first demonstrated.

Transmission of the disease from herd to herd is in carrier pigs (both growers and breeding stock), but the role of vectors is not clear. The development of disease within an affected farm is affected by immunity and clinical signs rarely occur in piglets and recovered animals remain immune. Disease is most obvious when non-immune animals are introduced to an infected herd, when the disease is introduced to a non-immune herd and when courses of treatment or the use of growth promoters such as tylosin, salinomycin and virginiamycin delay infection until near slaughter.

Diagnosis

Based on the clinical signs of failure to thrive, the occurrence of pale pigs and the presence of altered blood in the faeces in proliferative haemorrhagic enteropathy. This occult blood may be detected using biochemical methods. The point at which the disease develops may be determined clinically by sequential weighing. Loose faeces or diarrhoea commonly occur, but faecal consistency is not a reliable guide to the presence of the disease. The presence of the infection in faeces can be confirmed by PCR the specific 319bp product using 16S rDNA sequences.

The disease may be identified by post-mortem examination of pigs which die on farm or be found at the slaughter house. The gross lesions of ileal thickening, mucosal lesions and presence of blood in the lumen are suggestive and can be confirmed as P.E. by demonstrating the organism in smears of intestinal lesions stained by Koster's method (red bacilli). The identification of organisms in the apical cytoplasm of the epithelial cells of affected gut by histopathology by silver staining (presumptive only), by the use of specific antibody in immunofluorescence or immunoperoxidase or by the use of DNA probes or PCR confirms the presence of the disease. Indirect fluorescent antibody testing of serum can demonstrate infection in 90% pigs infected for 28 days and it, or ELISA serology, are generally equivalent to PCR in herd testing.

Treatment

Individual clinically-affected pigs may be treated with injectable long-acting tetracycline. Water medication of affected groups with tetracycline at 400ppm for 4 days usually results in a clinical cure. Chlortetracycline at 400ppm in feed for two weeks will have the same effect and tiamulin (150ppm) valnemulin 75 ppm, lincomycin (110ppm), aivlosin (42.5 ppm) or tylosin (100ppm) have also been shown to be effective when given for the appropriate period. In some cases, the use of these drugs postpones the onset of the disease when elimination of organisms occurs without the development of protective immunity. A regime in which tetracycline treatment (or other effective antimicrobial) in feed at 300 or 600 ppm (treatment level) for two weeks (or 400 ppm for 4 days in water) is followed by no treatment and then by another course of treatment after 18 days (less than the common incubation period) has been suggested on the basis that organisms are eliminated and re-infection in the majority of pigs is prevented by immunity following the initial exposure. When spirochaetosis, salmonellosis or other bacterial disease is present, the treatment should be modified accordingly.

Control

The introduction of genetic material into nucleus herds free from the disease should be by hysterectomy, AI or embryo transfer to prevent the possible introduction of infection with carrier pigs. Within a herd the disease may be suppressed by continuous low level medication using one of the products named above or by carrying out a treatment regime intended to stimulate natural immunity. The use of tylosin, spiramycin, virginiamycin or salinomycin as growth promoters (not EU) may reduce the extent of infection and the severity of any clinical disease. Any form of treatment may leave a variable proportion of the animals non-immune and susceptible to disease. Epidemiological evidence suggests that the disease is more common where weaned pigs are kept on slatted floors. Quaternary ammonium, iodine and Virkon S (Dupont) disinfectants have been shown to be effective against the agent.

Vaccination with an attenuated strain of L. intracellularis is now widely available and can reduce clinical disease and improve performance. Vaccine is given orally from 3 weeks of age or in clean drinking water. Care must be taken not to inactivate the vaccine by antimicrobial treatment. Protection lasts for 17 weeks.

References

Boesen, H.T., Jensen, T.K., Moeller, K., Nielsen, L.H., Jungersen, G. (2005). Evaluation of a novel ELISA for serological diagnosis of porcine proliferative enteropathy. Vet. Micro. 109, 105-112.

Kroll, J., Roof, M.B., McOrist, S. (2004). Evaluation of protective immunity in pigs following oral administration of an avirulent live vaccine of Lawsonia intracellularis. Am. J. Vet. Res. 65, 559-565.

McOrist, S., Gebhart, C., Boid, R., Barns, S.M. (1995). Characterisation of Lawsonia intracellularis gen. nov. sp. nov., the obligately intracellular bacterium of porcine proliferative enteropathy. Int J. Syst. Bacteriol. 45, 820-825.

McOrist, S., Gebhart, C.J. and Lawson, G.H.K. (1994b). Polymerase chain reaction for diagnosis of porcine proliferative enteropathy. Vet. Micro. 41, 205-212.

McOrist, S., Lawson, G.H.K. (1989). Reproduction of proliferative enteritis in gnotobiotic pigs. Res.vet.Sci. 46, 27-33.

McOrist, S. Roberts, L., Jasni, S., Rowland, A.C., Lawson, G.H.K., Gebhart, C.J., Bosworth, B. (1996). Developed and resolving lesions in porcine proliferative enteropathy. Possible pathogenetic mechanism. J.Comp. Path. **115**, 35-45.
McOrist, S., Shearn, M.F.H., Morgan, J. (1999). Control of porcine proliferative enteropathy by oral administration of chlortetracycline. Vet. Rec. **144**, 48-49.
McOrist, S., Smith, S.H., Green, L.G. (1997). Estimate of direct financial losses due to porcine proliferative enteropathy. Vet. Rec. **140**, 579-581.
McOrist, S., Smith, S.H., Klein, T. (1999). Monitored control programme for proliferative enteropathy on British pig farms. Vet. Rec. **144**, 202-204.
Moller, K., Jensen, T.K., Jorsal, S.E. (1998). Detection of L. intracellularis in endemically infected pig herds. Proc IPVS **15**, (2) 63.
Rowland, A.C. and Lawson, G. (1974). Intestinal adenomatosis in the pig : Immunofluorescence and electron microscopic studies. Res.vet.Sci. **17**, 323-330.
Rowland, A.C. and Lawson, G.H.K. (1975). Porcine intestinal adenomatosis : A possible relationship with necrotic enteritis, regional ileitis and proliferative haemorrhagic enteropathy. Vet.Rec. **97**, 178 180.
Smith, S.H., McOrist, S. (1997). Development of a persiistent intestinal infection and excretion of L. intracellularis by piglets. Res. vet. Sci. **62**, 6-10.
Stege, H., Jensen, T.K., Moeller, K., Vestergaard, K., Baekbo, P., Jorsal, S.E. (2004). Infection dynamics of L.intracellularis in pig herds. Vet. Micro. **104**, 197-206.

Yersinias in porcine enteritis and human health

Definition

Yersinias (principally *Y.enterocolitica*) are capable of causing enteritis and typhlocolitis in weaned pigs and contaminating carcases to cause human food poisoning.

Incidence

Worldwide, tonsillar carriage of *Y.enterocolitica* appears to vary but is often 60% of pigs at slaughter. In some US surveys, >90% lots slaughtered contain infected pigs.

Aetiology

Yersinia are Gram-negative coccobacilli which form 1-2 mm colonies on blood agar after 48 hours at 37°C but which also grow at temperatures as low as 4°C. They are divided into biotypes and also serotypes based on O groups.
Clinical disease in pigs is principally associated with *Y.enterocolitica* and *Y.pseudotuberculosis* and human food poisoning with *Y.enterocolitica* of biotype 4, serotype O3 although biotype 2:09, and biotype 1:08 also occur. *Y. enterocolitica* from human food poisoning is capable of expressing virulence determinants such as a 220 kDa outer membrane protein and an enterotoxin both of which are present in pig isolates.

Pathogenesis

Oral infection with *Y. enterocolitica* can lead to infection of the tonsils and multiplication in the ileum and large intestine. Faecal shedding occurs between 5 and 21 days post infection and continues for up to 10 weeks. Systemic spread may occur within 3 hours of infection but is uncommonly recorded. 10^4 organisms appear necessary to produce colonisation and shedding. A serological response occurs from day 19 post infection and lasts for at least 10 weeks. *Y.pseudotuberculosis* is more commonly associated with septicaemic spread and the development of micro abscesses in liver, spleen, mesenteric lymph nodes and gut as well as the enteric lesions. Infection may localise on the tonsil and the anal ring.

Clinical signs

Y.enterocolitica is associated with mild fever (40°C, 104°F), diarrhoea which may be watery and dark in colour and with blood-stained mucus on solid faeces. It has also been recovered from lesions in cases of rectal stricture. Diarrhoea may last only 4-5 days and most infections are inapparent *Y.pseudotuberculosis* is associated with dullness, inappetence, oedema and blood-stained diarrhoea and has been isolated from rectal strictures. Poor feed conversion has been reported.

In man *Y.enterocolitica* is associated with enteritis and appendicitis. Pigs normally recover spontaneously and rarely require humane slaughter.

Pathology

No gross or microscopic findings are associated with tonsillar carriage. *Y.enterocolitica* may give rise to a catarrhal enterocolitis in which micro colonies of the organism may be seen surrounded by neutrophils. Similar findings with button ulcers of the colon, micro-abscesses in the gut wall, mesenteric lymph nodes, liver and more obvious inflammatory lesions are found in *Y.pseudotuberculosis* infection.

The organisms may be isolated from tonsil, systemic lesions and gastrointestinal tract in affected pigs.

Epidemiology

Both species may be carried by pigs for long periods of time on tonsils and *Y.enterocolitica* may be detectable in faeces for up to 30 weeks after recovery from clinical disease. Herd studies have confirmed that faecal shedding occurs first in weaners (30%), increases in growers (50%), reaches a peak in finishers (75%) and declines in gilts (20%) and is absent in sows and sucking pigs. Serum antibody is absent in sucking pigs and weaners, occurs in growers (30%), finishers 80%, gilts (90%) and sows (100%). The organism may survive in the environment and is capable of infecting other species such as rats, mice, flies and man. It has been identified in water in some farms and has been recovered from feed. The same organism is generally found in the pig farm environment and the pigs.

In slaughter houses infection from tonsils, tongues and gut contents may contaminate carcases directly or indirectly by way of equipment. Workers may be exposed. O:3 from pigs appears to be identical with that isolated from human enteritis as Restriction Endonuclease Analysis types and restriction fragment polymorphism gel electrophoresis (PFGE) were identical in one study.

Diagnosis

Y. enterocolitica infection is usually suspected following post-mortem examination or bacteriology rather than from the clinical signs. Isolation from faeces may require enrichment in phosphate buffered saline at 4°C or specific enrichment broths followed by culture on selective and indicator media. Both organisms may be isolated directly from parenchymatous organs and may be demonstrated in tissue by DNA probes. Y. enterocolitica may be detected by PCR in faeces at 5-10 cfu/ml and 1pg DNA using primers based on ail,yst and virF genes. Enrichment increases the sensitivity of PCR.

Antibody to Y. *enterocolitica* can be detected using ELISAs with lipopolysaccharide antigen and is a useful herd test. Antibody to serotype O:9 may interfere with testing for *Brucella suis*.

Treatment

Y.enterocolitica enteritis may respond to treatment with tetracyclines, synthetic penicillins, furazolidone (not EU) and enrofloxacin in water or feed.

Control

Low levels of the above antimicrobials may suppress infection in pigs at risk but control of rodents, hygiene (especially with all in, all out husbandry) and prompt treatment of outbreaks reduces the incidence. The control of rodents and flies is important.

Vaccination using autogenous vaccines has been described.

Transmission to man may be controlled by hygiene amongst abattoir workers and by care during evisceration, removal of tongues and tonsils and by cleaning of machinery, flooring and prevention of splashing.

References

Barcellos D.E.S.N. de and Castro, A.F.P. de, (1981). Isolation of *Y.pseudotuberculosis* from diarrhoeas in pigs. Br.Vet.J. **137**, 95-96.

Fukushima, H. Wakamura, R., Ito, Y. and Saito, K. (1984). Ecological studies of *Y.enterocolitica*. II Experimental infection with *Y.enterocolitica* in pigs. Vet.Micro. **9**, 375-389.

Harnett, N., Liu, Y.P., Krishnan, C. (1996). Detection of pathogenic *Y. enterocolitica* using the multiplex PCR. Epidemiology and Infection **117**, 59-67.

Harper, P.A.W., Homitzky, M.A.Z., Rayward, D.G. (1990). Enterocolitis in pigs associated with *Y.pseudotuberculosis* infection. Aust.vet.J. **67**, 418-419.

Neef, N.A., Lysons, R.J. (1994). Pathogenicity of a strain of *Y.pseudo tuber-culosis* isolated from a pig with porcine colitis syndrome. Vet.Rec. **135**, 58-63.

Nielsen, B., Heisel, C., Wingstrand, A. (1996). Timecourse of the serological response to *Y. enterocolitica* O:3 in experimentally-infected pigs. Vet. Micro. **48**, 293-303.

Thibodeau, V., Frost, E.H., Chenier, S., Quessy, S. (1999). Presence of *Yersinia enterocolitica* in tissues of orally-inoculated pigs and the tissues and faeces of pigs at slaughter. Can. J.Vet Res.**63**, 96-100.

Thibodeau, V., Frost, E.H., Quessy, S. (2001). Development of an ELISA procedure to detect swine carriers of pathogenic *Yersinia enterocolitica*. Vet Micro.**82**, 249-259.

Wingstrand, A., Nielsen, B. (1996). Cross-sectional investigation of pig herds for *Y. enterocolitica* O:3. Proc. IPVS **14**, 320.

MYCOPLASMA INFECTIONS

A number of species of Mycoplasmas and some related organisms have been isolated from pigs, but only three species have been repeatedly associated with clinical syndromes in the field. They are: *M.hyopneumoniae* the causal agent of enzootic pneumonia, *M.hyorhinis* which causes polyserositis and arthritis in younger pigs, and *M.hyosynoviae* which causes arthritis in pigs of over 35 kg. liveweight.

Other mycoplasmas isolated from pigs include the following species: *M.flocculare* (from the respiratory tract), oral cavity; *M.hyoarthrinosa* (from joint lesions); *M.hyogenitalium* (from the uterus of a sow), *M.sualvi* and *M.hyopharyngis* from intestinal and vaginal samples. Other mycoplasmas may be isolated occasionally and include *M.salivarium*, *M.gallisepticum*, *M.iners*, *M.bovigenitalium*, *M.buccale*, *M.mycoides* and *M.arginini*. Acholeplasmas do not require sterols for growth and *A.laidlawii*, *A.granularum*, *A.axanthum*, *A.oculi* and others have been isolated from the upper respiratory tract, joints and conjunctivitis but have primarily been isolated (*A.laidlawii*) from faeces. The renamed *Eperythrozoon suis* (*M.haemosuis*) has been covered earlier.

Ureaplasmas have been isolated from the genital tracts of sows and from boar semen.

Anaerobic mycoplasmas unique to the pig have been demonstrated in large intestinal contents and the large intestinal mucosa.

Enzootic Pneumonia

Definition

Enzootic pneumonia is a contagious pulmonary disease of the pig caused by *Mycoplasma hyopneumoniae* and characterised clinically by coughing, unthriftiness and very low mortality. Clinical signs may be more severe when a non-immune herd is affected.

Incidence

The disease is found throughout the world and is an important cause of economic loss. Herds free from enzootic pneumonia have been established and maintained in many countries. Infected herds are more common than those with clinical signs or lesions at slaughter as management, treatment, vaccination and, recently, eradication (Switzerland and Finland) have all affected the incidence.

Aetiology

The cause of enzootic pneumonia is *M.hyopneumoniae* which is 200-500 nm in size, and may be seen in Giemsa-stained smears as a delicate pleomorphic organism in the form of cocci, rings, signet rings, bipolar and triangular shapes. The cell surface bears fimbriae which are more numerous in vivo that *in vitro*. The genome has been sequenced. The organism can be grown only on complex media containing porcine serum and little if any penicillin (it is inhibitory) in aerobic and microaerophilic conditions (5-10% carbon dioxide) and can form colonies after 2-10 days on solid media. It requires cholesterol for growth and ferments glucose but not arginine or urea. Growth inhibition studies on solid media suggested antigenic differences between strains and isolates of *M.hyopneumoniae* and the existence of different strains has been confirmed by restriction endonuclease analysis and PFGE. *M.hyopneumoniae* is antigenically related to *M.flocculare* and *M.hyorhinis* in the same subcluster of *M.fermentans*. A number of antigens are specific to *M.hyopneumoniae*. They include a 36 kDa lactate dehydrogenase protein, 40, 43, 64, 74 and 97 kDa antigens which can be used to distinguish *M.hyopneumoniae* from *M.flocculare* and *M.hyorhinis* both of which may occur in the lesions of enzootic pneumonia. *M.hyopneumoniae* is inactivated within 48 hours of drying on cloth or hair but may persist for up to 17 days in rain water at 2-7°C. It is sensitive *in vitro* to penicillin G (important for isolation) and to tiamulin, valnemulin, tylosin, lincomycin, other macrolides such as spiramycin, fluorinated quinolones such as enrofloxacin, ciprofloxacin and danofloxacin and to a lesser extent to tetracyclines including doxycycline.

Pathogenesis

Infection with *M.hyopneumoniae* takes place by the inhalation of infected aerosols produced by infected pigs or by direct contact, and the mycoplasma becomes established in the respiratory tract where it localises on the ciliated cells of the tracheal, bronchial and bronchiolar epithelium. Attachment appears to depend upon a 97kDa protein located in a fuzzy layer of the mycoplasma surface which binds to a series of lipids on the apex of the cilia. It persists in these sites for a period of weeks or months and initiates the sequence of pathological changes described below. These changes appear to be due to the presence of the organism on the surface of the epithelium where it often lies between the cilia and the apical cytoplasm of the cells. Cilia on infected cells are clumped by mycoplasma and are then shed. The apical cytoplasm of the denuded cells then bulges and the cells degenerate. A cytotoxic effect associated with the cell membrane has been demonstrated. The cytotoxin appears to be a heat-sensitive antigenic protein inactivated at 100°C for 15 minutes. Penetration of the organism into the tissues does not usually occur. Recent studies in gnotobiotic and SPF pigs show that systemic spread is possible following intravenous inoculation and may result in arthritis. Differences in the virulence of *M. hyopneumoniae* isolates have been demonstrated experimentally.

Infection of the ciliated epithelium of the respiratory tract appears to prevent normal clearance of secretory products from the tract. The lesions have been considered to result from the pooling of such material in the lobes of the lung. The earliest lesions appear 3 days after experimental infection as small dark red areas in anterior lung lobes. These areas enlarge after seven days and coalesce by 13 days post infection to give consolidation of the anterior lobes of the lung. The mediastinal and bronchial lymph nodes become greatly enlarged.

Three weeks after infection, the consolidated areas lose their reddish colour and become greyish pink, gradually fading to grey by the 8th week post infection and disappearing by 80-100 days after infection. At their maximum extent they occupy a mean of 5.7% of consolidated lung volume (28 days p.i.) in uncomplicated infection. Histological changes first appear 3 days after infection with inflammation associated with congestion of the capillaries of the alveolar septa, and the accumulation of neutrophil polymorphs in the airways and lamina propria of bronchioles. Five days post infection lymphocytes and macrophages appear, and by the 7th day, lymphoid accumulation about the bronchi and bronchioles becomes marked and the alveoli contain many large mononuclear cells, polymorphs, lymphocytes and IgA and IgG plasma cells. There is hyperplasia of the bronchiolar epithelium, and proliferation of type 2 pneumocytes. Later changes include proliferation of the lymphoid tissue to cause occlusion of some bronchioles. Hypertrophy of the bronchial glands occurs and mucus and a mononuclear cell exudate are found in the airways. This results in the only measurable effects on respiratory function - a decrease in the respiratory:expiratory resistance ratio from 1.08 (normal) to 0.6, reduced oxygen consumption and hyper-ventilation. Affected animals eventually recover and the lesions regress after about 12 weeks, so that older sows (2-4 litters) may be free from infection, although, in one study, freedom was not found until 8-11 litters.

IgA antibody develops in the tracheal mucosa and may be demonstrated in secretions from 30 days p.i. followed by IgG. Alveolar washes contain IgG from 45 days p.i. and levels peak at 80 days p.i. Serum antibody develops 8-46 days p.i., and may peak at 70-80 days p.i., persisting for at least a year. Antibody is passed by immune sows to their piglets in the colostrum and may be demonstrated in piglet serum for at least four weeks and up to 9 weeks after birth. It protects against infection.

Secondary infection with *M.hyorhinis* and *Pasteurella multocida* is common and in the case of *P.multocida* may affect the extent of the lesions and the severity and duration of clinical signs. Other organisms such as *Haemophilus parasuis* and *Actinobacillus pleuropneumoniae* may also invade the lesions. Influenza virus, circovirus and PRRS infections often occur at the same time. The combination with PRRS is particularly severe.

Clinical signs

Two distinct clinical syndromes occur in enzootic pneumonia, a rare, acute form associated with the reintroduction of the disease into a S.P.F. herd, and the common, chronic type found in herds where the disease is enzootic. In many S.P.F. herds, however, reinfection with *M.hyopneumoniae* has resulted in clinical signs and has had no effect on daily liveweight gain or feed efficiency.

Acute Form

Pigs of all ages may be affected and may show anorexia, pyrexia of 40.6-41.7°C, 105-107°F and respiratory distress accompanied by coughing. Some adults and up to 50% of piglets may die, often before coughing is apparent. Boars may not work and there may be delayed weaning to service intervals and other reproductive disturbances.

Chronic Form

In most cases few clinical signs of infection are apparent. Young pigs of 3-10 weeks of age become infected and within 10-16 days develop clinical signs. These begin with transient diarrhoea and a dry cough, although sneezing may be observed in sucking pigs. A low fever may occur. Later the clinical signs consist of a barking cough, particularly in finishing pigs. Coughing is most obvious when the animals are disturbed first thing in the morning. Coughing spreads gradually to most members of the group (over a period of 3-14 weeks) and lasts for about 50 days. Signs of respiratory embarrassment are rare unless secondary infection occurs. Secondary infection can lead to outbreaks of pneumonia and coughing which is particularly severe in 2-4 month old pigs and has been reported particularly in the US at 18-20 weeks.

An important clinical sign is the gradual development of uneven size amongst animals of the same weaning weight because of unequal infection in a litter. This leads to delay in marketing a batch and to husbandry problems. Uncomplicated infection depresses growth rate by as much as 15.9% from 5 to 85 kg with worsening of feed conversion ratios by as much as 13.8%. Effects are often less dramatic than this with an average reduction in feed efficiency of 0.2. Adverse environmental factors such as dusty atmospheres, chilling or high humidity or ammonia levels may exacerbate these effects on growth. The production effects appear to be proportional to the volume of lung affected and both are more severe when other infections are present.

Animals with severe respiratory distress sufficient to cause prostration, failure to suck (if piglets), and subnormal rectal temperatures and congestion of the extremities should be killed humanely.

Pathological findings

Evidence of enzootic pneumonia is usually found incidentally at slaughter or after death from other causes, e.g. complicated pneumonia. Lesions are found bilaterally in the apical, cardiac and intermediate lobes and in the anterior parts of the diaphragmatic lobes and are fawn/pink or plum-coloured and clearly demarcated from the normal lung tissue. The bronchial and mediastinal lymph nodes are enlarged. Lung lesion scores can be constructed to give quantitative results from lung maps.

Histological examination normally shows marked peribronchial and peribronchiolar lympho-reticular hyperplasia. There is proliferation of cells on the alveolar walls and many type 2 pneumocytes and macrophages occur in the lumen of the alveoli. Plasma cells also occur in the alveolar lumen. In older lesions, alveolar collapse may occur.

Mycoplasmas are present in Giemsa-stained impression smears made from the lesions but they are difficult to identify as *M.hyopneumoniae* by their morphology. Isolation of the organism is not feasible in many cases, as *M.hyorhinis* often grows more profusely and masks *M.hyopneumoniae* colonies. If isolation attempts are made, presumptive *M.hyopneumoniae* colonies may be identified by a fluorescent antibody method or the growth inhibition test. The methods described by Friis (1975) or Friis *et al.* (1991) are most widely used for isolation. PCR techniques are increasingly widely used to confirm the presence of the organism. *M.hyopneumoniae* may also be identified in lung tissue using immunofluorescence on smears or on frozen sections. Organisms can be seen as a yellow-green granular layer on the surface of the bronchial and bronchiolar epithelium. Immunoperoxidase techniques can demonstrate organisms in fixed sections as can labelled DNA probes.

Epidemiology

Enzootic pneumonia is normally transmitted to susceptible pigs by direct contact with infected animals or by their inclusion in the same air-space. Young pigs normally become infected from carrier sows soon after birth or when introduced into an airspace containing infected animals. Maternal immunity may protect piglets from infection and the infection of a group may be uneven, taking several weeks under some circumstances and sometimes leaving members of the group uninfected for 16-20 weeks. The organism becomes progressively less easy to isolate from 85 days post-infection but can be demonstrated by PCR for up to 185 days post infection. Many gilts of 8 months of age may be free from infection and by the second or third parity infection is rare. PCR sampling of nasal swabs suggests that infection may remain in some sows until parity 8.

The widespread use of serological testing has confirmed that spread of infection within a unit depends upon the husbandry system and that clinical signs and slaughterhouse monitoring of lungs do not reflect the onset or prevalence of infection very well. Differences in the onset of infection of 3-4 weeks may occur in different houses on the same unit. Infection is transmitted most rapidly within common airspaces in continuous stocking systems with open pen divisions, where animals are in direct contact (28 days), 7 times less frequently where solid partitions exist (42 days) and least frequently in all-in-all-out systems and outdoor systems. It may die out in small (<25 sow) herds. Aerosol spread can occur (to 150m) but occurs less frequently when buildings are even 10 m apart.

Spread between buildings on clothing and implements is also possible, but the organism does not appear to persist in human respiratory passages or to occur in reservoir hosts such as rats and mice.

Infection is usually introduced to uninfected farms by the purchase of carrier pigs but aerosol transmission between units may occur up to 3.2 km (2 miles). Sources of aerosol infection include infected farms (especially units with more than 500 animals and where forced ventilation leads to plumes of infected air) and the transport of infected pigs past the farm. Transmission of infection between farms by man, other animals or fomites appears to be rare.

Diagnosis

Enzootic pneumonia is normally diagnosed on the basis of findings in a herd rather than in an individual animal. The most useful criteria are:

1. The presence of a chronic pneumonia in the herd, particularly in fattening pigs, resulting in uneven growth rate and poor feed conversion efficiency but with no mortality.

2. Clinical signs in the 2-4 month old age range - a dry non-productive cough without fever or respiratory distress.

3. Post-mortem findings of a sharply demarcated, "cuffing" type of pneumonia in the anterior lung lobes. The histological findings are not specific, but help to confirm the diagnosis.

4. Confirmation by laboratory tests is essential for diagnosis, especially in monitoring schemes. Infection can be confirmed by:

Culture from freshly collected lung tissue with and without lesions from apical and cardiac lobes. Access to a competent laboratory is required and the methods of Friis *etal*. (1991) may be most appropriate.

Immunofluorescence uses the same material as culture for smears or frozen sections and specific monoclonal or absorbed polyclonal antisera.

Polymerase chain reaction (PCR) using swabs from all three stem bronchi of both lungs and primers from the 16S rRNA gene. Nasal swabs may be examined using nested PCR and real-time PCR (ReTiPCR) has been described..
Antigen ELISA using specific monoclonal antibody can be used on the same swab samples.

All three of these methods are equivalent to culture at 14 and 28 days post-infection but, with the exception of PCR, their sensitivity declines to 60-90% by day 57 p.i. and 11-40% by day 85 p.i.

DNA probes have been described but may only be 60% as efficient as immunofluorescence.

Immunoperoxidase may be used on fixed sections.

Antibody may be detected in serum using a number of tests. Most repeatable and specific results have been obtained with ELISAs using the 36 kDa engineered lactate dehydrogenase enzyme or other recombinant proteins as antigen. Monoclonal blocking ELISAs and Tween 20 ELISAs are also available.

All of these three serological tests (and others using fractions extracted from *M.hyopneumoniae*) are specific for that organism and do not cross-react with *M.flocculare*, *M.hyorhinis* or *M.hyosynoviae* in use. Antibody levels are first detectable at 10 days post-infection and remain detectable for at least 80 days post infection.

Other agents commonly complicate enzootic pneumonia. *M.hyorhinis* and *P.multocida* are common invaders, the latter frequently being present in the more severe and prolonged cases of enzootic pneumonia with the most extensive lesions. PRRS and circovirus may also be present. Enzootic pneumonia can be differentiated from Haemophilus infection, pleuropneumonia and swine influenza by the lack of fever except, possibly, in non-immune herds, and from parasitic infection such as Ascaris and Metastrongylus infections by the post-mortem findings. The lesions of enzootic pneumonia are distinctive but may need to be differentiated from those caused by Chlamydia. Acute disease in SPF herds should be differentiated from swine influenza.

Treatment

Infection with mycoplasmas is difficult to eliminate entirely, but the clinical manifestations of enzootic pneumonia can be reduced by treatment with a number of antimicrobials. Water medication with tetracyclines will prevent infection with mycoplasmas and treatment with tylosin (100pm in feed) may also reduce infection. Tiamulin, (Tiamutin, Novartis) 10-15 mg/kg reduces and may eliminate lesions from infected pigs when given in the water, and in the feed, but may not eliminate the mycoplasma. Treatment may have to be continued for 5-10 days. Best results have been obtained by tiamulin treatment using injectable drug at 15 mg/kg for three successive days. It may also be used with chlortetracycline. Valnemulin (Econor, Novartis) has been shown to be effective when given in feed for 3 weeks at 200 ppm (10-12 mg/kg bodyweight per day). Aivlosin (42.5 ppm in feed) and tulathromycin (Draxxin, Pfizer, 2.5 mg/kg parenterally) and tilmicosin (pulmotil, Elanco 200-400ppm in feed) may be used. Lincomycin and spectinomycin:lincomycin combinations may also be of value. Fluorinated quinolones such as enrofloxacin (Baytril, Bayer, 2.5mg/kg, injectable and water soluble forms), marbofloxacin, (Marbocyl ,Vetoquinol) 2 mg/kg) and danofloxacin (Advocin, Pfizer, 1.25mg/kg) can also be used. The lung lesions of enzootic pneumonia take some time to regress after treatment and are not completely eliminated by treatment although significant production improvement can be expected.

Control

a) Husbandry methods to mitigate the effect

1. All-in, all-out policy for buildings or units. Each house should be emptied at the same time, fumigated and re-filled.
There are clear advantages in this practice and productivity is higher and general disease levels are lower. The effects are particularly marked if all-in, all-out husbandry is applied to whole sites. When combined with treatment of a batch upon entry, this practice may reduce economic effects considerably.

Isowean[TM] (PIC) is a system in which piglets are weaned at less than 3 weeks, moved to a clean site and reared for four weeks. They are then moved to clean grower sites and the rearing site cleaned ready for a new batch. After 4-6 weeks in grower sites, pigs move to clean finisher sites. This application of the all-in, all-out principle may be accompanied by treatment at entry and has reduced disease losses dramatically. The minimum age of weaning of 4 weeks in the EU reduces the effect of this procedure.

2. Low stocking densities for housed pigs. Each pig is allowed individual accommodation and forced ventilation is used. Expensive, but when applied to groups with good ventilation, enzootic pneumonia may be reduced. Studies have shown that ammonia does not predispose to *M.hyopneumoniae* infection but exacerbates complicated lesions. Periodic use of organic acid aerosols may reduce the severity of disease.

3. Pigs in extensive systems rarely develop enzootic pneumonia, but finishing pigs by this method is generally uneconomic. Infection may persist in animals reared outdoors.

b) Vaccination

A number of vaccines have been produced and evaluated. Most are parenteral and consist of killed organisms or extracts of them, combined with aluminium hydroxide or proprietary adjuvants. Aerosols, oral vaccination, intraperitoneal vaccination with oil-adjuvanted killed organisms, intradermal vaccination, subunit vaccines, vaccines using Salmonella vectors, and DNA vaccines and live attenuated vaccines have all been described. Six vaccines are now commercially available in UK (2006) Suvaxyn M-hyo (Fort Dodge); Stellamune and Stellamune Once (Pfizer), Hyoresp (Merial) M+PAC (Schering Plough) Ingelvac M hyo (Boehringer) have been tested in a number of countries. In controlled trials they reduce the number and extent of lesions by 50% and improve daily liveweight gain, feed conversion and days to slaughter to a variable extent which is usually economic. Numbers of treatments are also reduced. Responses are most satisfactory when pigs are vaccinated at 3 and 5 weeks as opposed to 1 and 3 weeks. Colostral antibody may reduce the response, and, where infection occurs late, 10 week vaccination may be useful. Single injections have been used.

c) Treatment

1. Continuous medication

Low levels of medication may be given continuously/for 4 week periods e.g., tiamulin at 40 ppm in feed to prevent the development of clinical signs and lesions.

2. Pulse medication

Treatment may be given at therapeutic levels to all pigs in a building or in the finishing portion of the herd. Treatment usually lasts for two days in each week, allowing for withdrawal periods for units sending pigs for slaughter weekly.

3. Strategic medication

Treatment may be given at therapeutic level to all pigs entering an airspace. This is particularly effective when coupled with all-in, all-out husbandry.

Any of the products listed above could be used but combinations such as tiamulin and chlortetracycline may be more effective on some units where enzootic pneumonia is complicated.

d) Serum/infection profiling

The availability of ELISAs for serum antibody testing has allowed antibody profiles to be constructed for herds and individual houses within a herd. PCR (especially ReTiPCR) on nasal swabs can also be used The time of infection can be determined directly (PCR) or indirectly (10 days prior to initial antibody detection) and allows vaccination or treatment measures to be applied precisely.

e) Eradication

Enzootic pneumonia may be eradicated in four main ways:

1. Hysterectomy and isolation

Piglets removed by hysterectomy and reared apart from the dam in isolation are free from enzootic pneumonia and many other infective conditions. Complete repopulation of herds by this means is rarely a practicable proposition on the average farm, but has been used to provide enzootic pneumonia (and other disease) free stock for repopulation. The nucleus herds of large hybrid organisations are mostly enzootic pneumonia-free, are maintained in strict isolation and are given new blood lines only by hysterectomy. Isolation should include at least 3.2 km separation from the nearest infected unit under U.K. conditions for it to be effective for long periods. Isolated units should be sited away from main roads and visiting personnel and transport should be closely controlled.

In the U.K. many herds of this type are monitored for infection by means of quarterly or six-monthly clinical inspections, the recording of incidents of respiratory disease and the examination of lungs from pigs at slaughter by culture, histopathology or PCR with further investigation of any circumstance which suggests enzootic pneumonia or infection with M.hyopneumoniae. A regular programme of serological monitoring is now possible. Monitoring of finishing pigs should be supplemented by sampling of sows and their colostrum for serum antibody or PCR of nasal swabs. In some circumstances new blood may be introduced by A.I. or embryo transfer which pose little risk of infection.

Breakdown rates of 4-10% p.a. have been recorded in such schemes in the U.K., Switzerland, Denmark and the U.S.A.

2. Slaughter and re-stocking

Enzootic pneumonia-free stock is available in Britain and other countries, on a commercial basis. Farms should be cleared of all pigs, cleaned, disinfected and fumigated, left free from pigs for four weeks and then repopulated with disease-free animals. The sources of these animals are usually the nucleus or multiplying herds of commercial hybrid organisations, many of which are free from the disease.

186

3. Treatment and isolation as means of eradication

Medicated early weaning: Tiamulin and valnemulin have been used in two ways for the eradication of enzootic pneumonia from pig herds. In the Medicated Early Weaning technique, farrowing sows are treated with tiamulin and their litters snatched or weaned at 5 days and reared artificially. For the first 10 days of life, oral therapy with tiamulin at 10 mg/kg is given. Mortality can be high, but the organism is apparently eliminated in most cases.

The piglets produced can be reared in isolation and tested for the development of antibody before introduction to a clean herd.

Whole herd treatment after partial depopulation. Breeding stock can be treated with tiamulin in the feed (at 200 ppm) or in drinking water to give 10 mg/kg daily for 10 days following removal of weaned, growing or finishing pigs. Provided no untreated pigs are present on the farm, pigs may remain free from enzootic pneumonia for years. The absence of infection can be confirmed by serological and clinical monitoring of the new finishing herd. Successful eradication has been reported using valnemulin and lincomycin, but results have been less clear with enrofloxacin

4. Segregation and isolation

This method is laborious. The progeny of older sows (more than 2 and possibly more than 8 parities) are often free from infection and can be reared in isolation. They may be protected from disease by colostral immunity and remain carriers. Exhaustive serological or PCR testing and slaughter monitoring of these pigs may be required to confirm that an enzootic pneumonia-free herd has been produced.

Piglets reared and later finished on successive all-in, all-out isolated sites (Isowean) may also be free from infection, but careful monitoring is needed before they could be introduced to nucleus or multiplying herds.

References

Alexander, T.J.L., Thornton, K., Boon, G., Lysons, R.J. and Gush, A.F. (1980). Medicated early weaning to obtain pigs free from pathogens endemic in the herd of origin. Vet.Rec. 106, 114-119.
Barford, K., Sorensen, V., Feld, N.C. (1994). Evaluation of a monoclonal blocking ELISA detecting antibodies on a single pig level. Proc.IPVS 13, 189.
Blanchard, B., Vena M.M., Cavalier, A., Lannic, J. le., Gouranton, J., Kobisch, M. (1992). Electron microscopical observations of the respiratory tract of SPF piglets inoculated with M.hyopneumoniae. Vet.Micro. 30, 329-341.
Calsamiglia, M., Pijoan, J., Bosch, G.J. (1999). Profiling M.hyopneumoniae in farms using serology and a nested PCR technique. Swine Health and Production 7, 263-268.
Doster A.R. and Lin, B.C. (1988). Indirect immunoperoxidase used to identify M.hyopneumoniae in porcine lung. Am.J.vet.Res. 49, 1719-1721.
Fano, E., Pijoan, C., Dee, S (2005). Dynamics and persistence of M.hyopneumoniae infection in pigs. Can. J.Vet.Res. 69, 223-228.
Feenstra, A.A., Sorensen, V., Friis, N.F., Jensen, N.E. and Bille Hansen, V. (1994). Experimental M.hyopneumoniae infection in pigs. Proc.IPVS 13, 187.
Friis N.F. (1975). Some recommendations concerning primary isolation of M.suipneumoniae and M.flocculare. Nord.Vet.Med. 27, 337-339.

187

Geary, S.J. and Walczak, E.M. (1983). Isolation of a cytopathic factor from *M.hyopneumoniae*. Infection and Immunity, **41**, 132-136.
Goodwin, R.F.W. and Whittlestone, P. (1967). The detection of enzootic pneumonia in pig herds 1. Eight years' general experience with a pilot control scheme. Vet Rec. **81**, 643-647.
Haldimann, A., Nicolet, J., Frey, J. (1993). DNA sequence determination and biochemical analysis of the immunogenic protein P36, the lactate dehydrogenase (LDH) of *M.hyopneumoniae*. J.Gen.Microbiol. **139**, 317-323.
Hannan, P.C.T., Windsor, H.M., Ripley, P.H. (1997). In vitro susceptibilities of recent field isolates of *M. hyopneumoniae* and *M. hyosynoviae* to valnemulin (Econor), tiamulin and enrofloxacin and the in vitro development of resistance to certain antimicrobials in *M. hyopneumoniae*. Res. vet. Sci. **63**, 157-160.
Sorensen, V., Ahrens, P., Barfod, K., Feenstra, A.A., Feld, N.C., Friis, N.F., Bille-Hansen, V., Jensen, N.E., Pedersen, M.W.,(1997). *Mycoplasma hyopneumoniae* infection in pigs: duration of the disease and evaluation of four diagnostic assays. Vet. Micro. **54**, 23-34.
Sorensen, V., Barfod, K., Feenstra, A.A. and Feld, N.C. (1994). The humoral immune response to *M.hyopneumoniae* infection in pigs in relation to clinical signs and pathological lesions. Proc.IPVS **13**, 190.
Stark, K.D.C., Keller, H., Eggenburger, E. (1992). Risk factors for the reinfection of pig breeding herds with enzootic pneumonia. Vet.Rec. **131**, 532-535.
Stark, K.D.C., Nicolet, J., Frey, J. (1998). Detection of *M. hyopneumoniae* by air sampling with a nested PCR assay. Applied and Environmental Microbiology, **64**, 543-548.
Stemke, G.W. (1997). Gene amplification (PCR) to detect and differentiate mycoplasmas in porcine mycoplasmal pneumonia. Letters In Applied Micro. **25**, 327-330.
Strasser, M., Frey, J., Besteti, G., Kobisch, M., Nicolet, J. (1991). Cloning and expression of a species-specific early immunogenic 36 kDa protein of *M.hyopneumoniae* and *E.coli*. Inf. and Imm. **59**, 1217-1222.
Vicca, J., Stakenborg, T., Maes, D., Butaye, P., Peeters, J., Kruif, A de, Haesebrouck, F.(2003). Evaluation of the virulence of M. hyopneumoniae field isolates. Vet. Micro. **97**, 177-190.
Vraa-Andersen, L., Christensen, G., Kuiper, R. (1994). Vaccine efficacy with Suvaxyn *M.hyo* in Denmark. Proc.IPVS. **13**, 192
Zhang, Q., Young, T.F., Ross, R.F. (1995). Identification and characterisation of a *Mycoplasma hyopneumoniae* adhesin. Inf.and Immun. **63**, 1013-1019.
Zimmerman, W., Weiskopf, S. (1996). The use of lincomycin in an enzootic pneumonia eradication programme in pig herds. Proc. IPVS **14**, 235

Infection with *Mycoplasma hyorhinis*

Definition

M.hyorhinis causes polyserositis and arthritis in pigs of 3-10 weeks of age and some strains have been shown to cause pneumonia and otitis media.

Incidence

The clinical syndrome is rarely identified but is probably widespread in Britain as *M.hyorhinis* is a common inhabitant of the nasal cavity of pigs and can be isolated from up to 60% of pigs. It is commonly present in the lesions of enzootic pneumonia (40-60%) It is usually absent from hysterectomy-derived herds maintained in isolation.

Aetiology

M.hyorhinis forms colonies on the same media used for *M.hyopneumoniae* within 1-2 days. However, *M.hyorhinis* cannot always be grown on conventional mycoplasma media and may need to be cultured on media containing cells such as BHK-21 or lysates of them or on mink S and L cells in which a characteristic cytopathic effect is produced. *M.hyorhinis* produces phosphatase and reduces tetrazolium unlike either of the other two common porcine mycoplasmas. Slight antigenic differences between isolates have been identified.

Some of these have been shown to be due to a variable surface lipoprotein Vlp, three forms of which exist, able to produce 10^4 antigenic variations. The genes for these proteins have been cloned.

Pathogenesis

M.hyorhinis enters the body by the respiratory route, colonising the respiratory tract (including the Eustachian tube tract and the middle ear) and is often present in lesions of enzootic pneumonia. It causes a septicaemia and settles out on serous surfaces and in the joints where it causes inflammation. Complement-fixing and metabolic inhibition antibodies are produced.

Clinical signs

An incubation period of 3-10 days is followed by subclinical infection or a slight fever, less than 40.6°C, 105°F, which is present for 4-5 days. Affected pigs are often 3-10 weeks of age and show a reduction in appetite and a marked reduction in growth rate, a hairy coat. Many stretch or breathe in an unusual fashion when disturbed. Arthritis and swelling of the joints may occur, and many pigs remain affected for up to 6 months. Recovery begins 4 weeks after infection. Up to 25% of the pigs may be affected in an outbreak.

Infection commonly complicates enzootic pneumonia without any apparent exacerbation of the condition and pasteurellosis where it may exacerbate clinical signs. It has been isolated repeatedly from otitis media.

Affected animals rarely require humane destruction but it might be indicated following fibrous pericarditis or prolonged lameness unresponsive to antimicrobial treatment.

Pathological findings

At post-mortem examination, affected pigs are seen to be thin, with fibrinous pericarditis, pleurisy and peritonitis. In later cases, adhesions may be present between the organs in the affected cavity. Joint lesions occur, particularly in the tarsus, stifle, carpus and shoulder. Affected joints contain large amounts of serofibrinous or serosanguineous synovia, and villous hypertrophy of the synovial membranes and erosion of the articular cartilages is often present. The villous hypertrophy is associated with accumulations of plasma cells and lymphocytes.

Inflammatory changes in the respiratory tract include a subacute catarrhal bronchopneumonia which resolves spontaneously and Eustachian tube inflammation. Organisms adhere to the cilia.

Antibody develops following infection.

Epidemiology

Infection spreads between pigs by aerosol or direct contact and between farms principally by infected carrier pigs.

Diagnosis

Distinguished from Glasser's disease, streptococcal meningitis and arthritis and *A.pleuropneumoniae* infection by the absence of fever and low mortality, and from *M.hyosynoviae* by the age affected. Post-mortem findings, bacteriology and immunofluorescence on frozen sections of respiratory tract will confirm. *M. hyorhinis* may be accompanied by *M. hyosynoviae* and *M. hyopneumoniae* in pericardial lesions.

Control and treatment

The use of hyperimmune gamma globulin has been described for both treatment and prevention of *M.hyorhinis* infection but it is rarely available and not in UK. Antimicrobials suitable for use in enzootic pneumonia may be of value and eradication using the methods used for enzootic pneumonia may also be effective. There are no formal accounts of its eradication.

References

Buttenschon, J., Friis, N.F., Aalbaek, B., Jensen, T.K., Iburg, T., Mousing, J. (1997). Microbiology and pathology of fibrinous pericarditis in Danish slaughter pigs. J.Vet. Med. Series A, **44**, 271-280.

Friis, N.F., Feenstra, A.A. (1994). *Mycoplasma hyorhinis* in the aetiology of serositis amongst piglets. Acta Vet Scand **35**, 93-98.

Kazama, S., Yagihashi, T., Morita, T., Awakura, T., Shimada, A., Umemura, T. (1994). Isolation of *Mycoplasma hyorhinis* and *M.arginini* from the ears of pigs with otitis media. Res.Vet.Sci. **56**, 108-110.

Levy, J.A., Sumner, P.E. and Hooser, L.E. (1982). Rapid tissue culture method for detection of *Mycoplasma hyorhinis*. J.General Microbiology **128**, 2817-2820.

Monta, T., Fukuda, H., Awakura, T., Shimada, A., Umemura, T., Kazama, S., Yagihashi, T. (1995). Demonstration of *Mycoplasma hyorhinis* as a possible primary pathogen for otitis media. Vet. Path. **32**, 107-111.

M.hyosynoviae Infection

Definition

M.hyosynoviae causes an arthritis in pigs weighing between 35 kg and 115 kg and is a frequent cause of lameness in recently purchased breeding stock.

Incidence

It was reported to be responsible for 23% of cases of arthritis in fattening pigs over 35 kg liveweight in Iowa . It has been identified in Britain and Denmark by clinical signs, and confirmed by serology and isolation and is now common in pigs from some suppliers.

Aetiology

M.hyosynoviae differs from the other two major pig mycoplasmas by fermenting arginine but not glucose or urea. It is best isolated in anaerobic conditions when it can outgrow *M.hyorhinis*. It may survive drying for up to 4 weeks but is more sensitive *in vitro* to tiamulin than other mycoplasmas.

Pathogenesis

It is commonly found on the tonsils of healthy carrier sows and occurs in the pharyngeal region in 7-8 week old pigs. Infection is by the oronasal route and has taken place in many herds by 10-12 weeks of age. Colonisation of the tonsils usually occurs. Septicaemia may develop 2-4 days after intranasal inoculation and the organism settles out in the joints to a variable extent to produce the characteristic clinical and pathological findings within 4-49 days. It may also occur in the lungs. Early changes in the joints include isolation from 4 days post inoculation, with associated changes in the synovial villi from mild oedema and hyperaemia (day 4) to gradual enlargement of the villi, cell detachment, neutrophil invasion and protein exudation into the synovial fluid by Day 10. Mycoplasmas can be seen at the bases of the villi and between the synovial cells. After 2-3 weeks, the synovial membranes are infiltrated with macrophages and lymphocytes and by 7 weeks, fibrosis has begun.

Clinical signs

Few clinical signs are apparent in most infections. No fever is noted, and the only apparent effect is alteration in the gait of the affected pigs. More severe disease may occur as acute lameness in one or more limbs, progressing from a single affected joint to complete inability to stand within 24 hours. In these animals, there may be a rise in rectal temperature (to 40°C for 1-2 days after exposure), pronounced lameness after bending tests, severe pain on movement and screaming when pushed by penmates. As affected animals cannot compete for food and water, death may result from cannibalism. Affected animals usually weigh more than 35 kg. Bursitis and soft, fluctuating swellings of the joints may develop but external signs may not be apparent. Affected pigs limp, shift weight from one leg to another or may be unable to rise, often adopting a dog-sitting position. In Britain, non-immune gilts or boars introduced into infected herds are chiefly affected with sudden lameness 7-21 days after introduction, and clinical signs may occur 22-24 days after mixing large finishers.

Humane slaughter may be indicated when chronically-affected animals are unable to rise. These acute signs may last for 3-10 days and then decrease, so treatment should be attempted before euthanasia.

Pathological findings

The synovial fluid from affected joints is clear, yellowish-brown in colour and may contain flakes of fibrin and the articular surface is usually normal. Swelling and hyperaemia is seen in the synovial membrane of affected large limb joints. Fibrosis develops in chronic cases. Polyserositis is absent. *M.hyosynoviae* can be isolated from affected joints, lymph nodes and mucous membrane secretions during the acute stage of the disease and from tonsils and pharynx in carriers. Mycoplasma -associated bursitis may be found on the lateroplantar aspect of the tarsus and on the laterodistal aspect of the elbow.

Diagnosis

Acute lameness in older fattening pigs or recently introduced breeding stock with no fever or evidence of polyserositis is suggestive. The withdrawal of joint fluid from tarsal, elbow or knee joint (after sedation) may aid diagnosis. In

M. hyosynoviae infection the fluid is clear, yellowish-brown in colour and may contain flakes of fibrin. In streptococcal arthritis, fluid is haemorrhagic and turbid with many neutrophils and in osteochondrosis, clear and yellowish. Isolation and identification of the organism confirms. Selective media (Friis 1991) may be required to suppress *M.hyorhinis*. The organism may be recovered from blood for 7-11 days from 1-4 days post exposure, from joints from 5-21 days until at least day 64 , tonsil from days 6-61, lymph nodes from 6-15 days and spleen from 6-15 days. ELISA demonstration of circulating antibody may also be used, but maternal antibody commonly persists until 8-10 weeks and active antibody only appears from 8-16 weeks. Erysipelas and osteochondrosis should be eliminated before reaching a diagnosis.

Treatment and control.

Treatment of animals with early clinical signs with tiamulin at 15 mg/kg by injection on 2-3 successive days has been found useful. Isolation of the organism from the joints of such treated animals is difficult. Tylosin, lincomycin or other antimicrobials active against mycoplasmas may also be used for a similar period. Animals in contact should be treated. Where the introduction of breeding stock to infected herds results in lameness (usually after 14-21 days), a course of treatment such as lincomycin in drinking water should be given at least 2-3 days before the expected appearance of the clinical signs and the treatment repeated 10 days later.

References

Burch, D.G.S. and Goodwin, R.F.W. (1984). Use of tiamulin on a herd of pigs seriously affected with *M.hyosynoviae* arthritis. Vet.Rec. **115**, 594-595.
Friis, N.F., Ahrens P., Larsen, H. (1991). *M.hyosynoviae* isolation from the upper respiratory tract and tonsils of pigs. Acta Vet.Scand. **32**, 425-429.
Hagedorn-Olsen, T., Basse, A., Jensen, T.K. Nielsen, N.C. (1999). Gross and histological findings in synovial membranes of pigs with experimentally-induced *M. hyosynoviae* arthritis. Acta Path. Microbiol.Immunol.Scand. **107**, 201-210
Hagedorn-Olsen, T., Nielsen, N.C. Friis, N.F.,(1999). Induction of arthritis with M. hyosynoviae in pigs: clinical response and re-isolation of the organism from the body fluids and organs J.Vet.Med, Series A. **46**, 317-325.
Hagedorn-Olsen, T., Friis, N.F., Nielsen, N.C. (1998). *M. hyosynoviae* infection profiles in three pig herds. Proc IPVS **15**, (2) 203.

M.arthritidis infection

M.arthritidis, a rodent mycoplasma, has been isolated from joints in an outbreak of conjunctivitis, severe polyarthritis and infertility in a boar stud.

Reference

Binder, A., Aumuller, R., Likitsecharote, B., Kirchhoff, H. (1990). Isolation of *M.arthritidis* from the joint fluid of boars. J.Vet.Med. Series B. **37**, 611-614.

Bordetella bronchiseptica infections

Definition

B.bronchiseptica colonises the ciliated epithelium of the upper respiratory tract early in life to cause rhinitis characterised by sneezing, mild turbinate atrophy and some reduction in the rate of daily liveweight gain. *B.bronchiseptica* also colonises the lower respiratory tract to cause a persistent purulent bronchitis and a pneumonia which may persist in the absence of nasal changes to cause depression of the daily rate of liveweight gain.

Incidence

Infection with *B.bronchiseptica* was present in 91% of pig herds in one survey in southern England and the infection is present in all pig rearing countries, often at a similar prevalence. One study from Italy found it in 75/76 farms

Aetiology

B.bronchiseptica is a small (0.5 x 0.8-l.0 μm) Gram-negative aerobic bacillus and is motile. It produces ß-haemolytic 1-2 mm grey colonies on some nutrient blood agars but on richer media is non-haemolytic. On MacConkey agar it produces non-lactose fermenting colonies in 48 hours.

B.bronchiseptica exists in 4 colony phases, I to Vir-. Phase 1 colonies contain fully virulent organisms. The pathogenic determinants produced include fimbriae, the mannose-resistant haemagglutinin, (filamentous hamagglutinin, FHA) and the 68 kDa outer membrane protein pertactin all involved in adhesion. A number of toxic factors are also produced; the haemolysin is an adenyl cyclase; a cytotoxin has been described, an osteocytic toxin and the Dermonecrotoxin (DNT) of 14 kDa has been cloned. Phase II, III organisms may not express all these characters and may be isolated from pigs. All variants, including Vir- may be derived from Phase I organisms *in vitro*. but reversion to Phase I can only take place *in vivo*. There are antigenic and also genetic differences between isolates based on restriction endonuclease analysis (REA) of genes for determinants such as fimbria (*fim*) and flagellae (*fla*)

The organism survives drying and in water for 3 weeks, is sensitive to disinfectants and to antibiotics such as trimethoprim:sulphonamide, ampicillin, macrolides and fluorinated quinolones such as enrofloxacin.

Pathogenesis

Phase I *B.bronchiseptica* infect pigs by aerosol or contact and colonise the ciliated epithelium of the nasal cavity.

It is not clear whether infection of the lower respiratory tract occurs directly or as a result of inhalation or postnasal drip from the infected nasal cavity. The organism attaches to the cilia, microvilli and epithelial cell surfaces by means of surface structures which appear as a fuzzy or stringy structure visible in electron-micrographs and proliferates to reach high numbers ($4x10^{10}$). When levels exceed $3x10^5$, the cilia are lost in the region of greatest bacterial growth and a neutrophil reaction occurs. Pertactin is required for this colonisation. Toxic substances which include adenyl cyclase and DNT diffuse into the tissue and cause changes in osteoblasts of the bones of the nasal cavity within 7 days of infection. Osteoid fibres are reduced and turbinate atrophy has occurred within 14-21 days. In other parts of the body, bony changes and changes in cartilages have been seen but it is not clear whether these are directly attributable to the toxin or to indirect effects of altered nutrition and chronic inflammation. Turbinate atrophy usually resolves in uncomplicated infections by the time of slaughter and within 70 days in experimental infections in gnotobiotic pigs.

In the lower respiratory tract, a bronchopneumonia may develop early in the disease process. It affects the cranial and middle lobes of the lung in particular but may occur as discrete patches in other lobes. The pneumonic areas may contain the bacteria but these are usually restricted to the bronchi where they cause a mucopurulent exudate. The organisms persist in the trachea, bronchi and bronchioles for at least 2-3 months after infection. Lung lesions often resolve by collapse and scarring.

IgM antibody can be detected to the FHA from 1 week post infection and IgA antibody in 2 weeks. IgG antibody is obvious in serum 4-5 weeks after infection. Immunity to infection may develop and is passed on to the offspring as passive immunity, but its presence delays the antibody response. Neither type of immunity appears to eliminate infection and passive immunity can be overwhelmed by heavy challenge. Immunity does appear, however, to reduce the bony changes and restrict lower respiratory tract infection to the bronchioles, bronchi and trachea.   Infection with other bacteria such as *P.multocida*, *Mycoplasma hyorhinis*, *Haemophilus parasuis* can occur in the nose and *Haemophilus parasuis* and mycoplasmas commonly occur in the bronchitis or bronchopneumonia.

Clinical signs

Outbreaks of sneezing occur in baby pigs from 1 week of age and this may be paroxysmal with snorting and sometimes epistaxis. Tear staining is often seen and mucopurulent exudate may be seen on the nostrils, hanging from them or on the pen floor. Occasionally signs of twisting of the snout may develop in uncomplicated infections but this and other persistent changes of atrophic rhinitis such as brachygnathia superior (shortening of the upper jaw) and complete turbinate atrophy are more common in Progressive Atrophic Rhinitis. There may be coughing in the pneumonic form which may begin within 3-4 days of infection and be accompanied by mild fever (to 40°C, 104°F), anorexia and loss of condition and increased respiratory rates. Mortality can occur at this stage in uncomplicated infections and may reach 30%.

Uncomplicated infections with *B.bronchiseptica* have been shown to cause reductions in the rate of daily liveweight gain of 16-19% when compared with minimal disease controls and from 26-30% in conventional pigs.   In complicated infections (eg with PRRSV) these figures could be exceeded in non-immune pigs but in immune pigs may be reduced as would be the severity of the clinical signs. In the progeny of immune sows they may be restricted to sneezing amongst piglets.

Humane destruction may be indicated in young pigs with severe pneumonia and loss of condition or in wasted sucking piglets. It need not be considered unless treatment has proved ineffective.

Pathology

The pathology of uncomplicated *B.bronchiseptica* infection is that of a catarrhal rhinitis accompanied by some failure of the conchal bones and ethmoturbinates to develop and/or some distortion of the nasal septum. The nasal mucosa may be covered in exudate, inflamed and in the later stages may be metaplastic. In all cases, a purulent bronchitis can be demonstrated and in cases of bronchopneumonia, areas of consolidation and reddening may be seen in the cranial and middle lung lobes or as red, pneumonic areas elsewhere. These lesions frequently heal by collapse and fibrosis and leave fissures in the lung which survive until slaughter. The bronchitis can be demonstrated in the absence of gross lung lesions.

Histological changes include a catarrhal rhinitis with loss of the epithelium and heavy infiltration with inflammatory cells. In chronic cases metaplasia and loss of the goblet cells occurs. Fibrous tissue occurs in the submucosal tissues and there is a decrease in the numbers of osteoblasts. In the lower respiratory tract a catarrhal exudate is present in the bronchi and in pneumonic lesions there is congestion, intra-alveolar haemorrhage and accumulation of neutrophils. The healing lesion contains macrophages and fibroblasts. Bacteria may be seen adhering to surviving ciliated epithelium.

B.bronchiseptica can be isolated from the nasal cavity, trachea, bronchi and bronchial lymph nodes in early cases, but only from the ethmoturbinate and sometimes from the bronchi in chronic cases or carriers. Other organisms, e.g. P.multocida may also be isolated.

Epidemiology

B.bronchiseptica infection is usually introduced to a herd by the purchase of infected carrier pigs from an infected herd. These pigs may be clinically normal. On rare occasions the organism may be introduced on clothing or hair on which the organism may be in dust or dried nasal secretions. A number of animal species such as dogs, rodents and man can carry the organism in their respiratory tracts. These organisms can cause disease in pigs but are less likely to colonise the nose in the numbers required for disease than porcine strains. Restriction endonuclease studies and ribotyping confirm that only a few B.bronchiseptica strains occur in pigs and differ from those in other species.

Spread within a farm is by aerosol and by direct and indirect contact. It is enhanced by poor ventilation, by the presence of large numbers of pigs within an airspace and by the weight of infection. In immune herds airborne organisms are most common from 14 days of age in farrowing accommodation and throughout the rearing period.

Evidence from nasal inoculation studies in gnotobiotic pigs suggests that 3×10^5 organisms may be required to cause infection to become established. The development of pneumonia, atrophy of the turbinate changes and distortion of the nasal septum depend upon a number of factors. The most important of these is probably the state of immunity of the pig when infected. Maternal immunity is passed to the piglet and protects against gross changes but not against the establishment of infection. The piglets of non-immune mothers or those with a poor immune status (usually gilts) may develop severe disease. In herds which are rapidly expanding or in which sow turnover is high, clinical disease can be widespread. Infection of susceptible pigs occurs in weaner pools in fattening units, particularly when pigs from different sources are mixed, and the subclinical form of the disease occurs.

Diagnosis

The clinical signs of severe sneezing and tear staining in piglets suggest that B.bronchiseptica infection is present. When it is present alone, growth depression in non-immune pigs and some transient changes in the bones of the nasal cavity may be seen. Tear staining is common and pneumonic changes such as coughing, dyspnoea and some mortality may also occur.

When outbreaks of sneezing occur in piglets or older weaned animals, isolation of *B.bronchiseptica* from nasal swabs (cotton tip, not alginate) may be of use in confirmation. Selective medium containing penicillin, furaltadone, gentamycin and bromthymol blue may be used as may cephalothin media. Isolation may be made on simple blood agar or MacConkey medium at post mortem examination by culturing the turbinates, the sinus epithelium or the tracheal or bronchial epithelium. 48 hours incubation is necessary. Chromosomal DNA probes have been found to improve the sensitivity of detection.

Sneezing should be differentiated from that of inclusion body rhinitis (earlier in non-immune herds and not responsive to antimicrobial therapy) and the pneumonic form from other causes of pneumonia such as enzootic pneumonia, pleuropneumonia and pasteurellosis. If Progressive Atrophic Rhinitis is present, the presence of *B.bronchiseptica* infection in the herd may be assumed in most cases. Agglutination and ELISA tests for serum antibody may be carried out using the 68K outer membrane protein or whole Type 1 organisms as antigen, but antibody to the pathogenetic determinant DNT is rare.

Treatment

B.bronchiseptica may be sensitive *in vitro* to a number of antimicrobials. These include tetracyclines, ampicillin, erythromycin, cloxacillin, enrofloxacin, streptomycin, sulphonamides such as sulphadimidine, and trimethoprim: sulphonamide. Parenteral treatment with any of these agents may be given to severely affected pigs and this should be followed by oral dosing with the same drug if in piglets or water medication in older pigs if possible. Treatment should be continued for at least 10 days and preferably for 2 weeks.

Control

Prophylactic medication

(a) In the feed. Clinical signs can be suppressed by the medication of the feed with trimethoprim:sulphonamides (30 mg/kg daily), tetracycline, sulphonamides such as sulphadimidine. These products may be used to medicate the feed especially in recently weaned pigs. All pigs in the same airspace should be medicated.

(b) By strategic therapy. Parenteral treatment with trimethoprim: sulphonamide given at 3 days, 10 days and 3 weeks of age may prevent clinical signs of the disease and reduce the shedding of *B.bronchiseptica*. Long acting tetracyclines may also produce a similar effect.

Vaccination

(a) Killed vaccines. Formalin-killed, alum-adjuvanted vaccines have been produced and are combined with *P.multocida* toxoid to control Progressive Atrophic Rhinitis (Porcilis AR-T, Intervet). They are used to immunise sows 6 and 2 weeks prior to farrowing and protect piglets from Bordetella bronchopneumonia and rhinitis by means of passive antibody transfer. Active immunity can be stimulated by vaccination of piglets at 7 and 28 days of age. Reduction in clinical signs occurs on a herd basis and the rate of carriage of the organism is reduced. Recent studies have shown that purified adhesive antigens may protect against colonisation.

(b) <u>Live vaccines.</u> An attenuated live vaccine given by nasal instillation establishes in the respiratory tract and is claimed to reduce the incidence of gross lesions. The vaccine strain may not colonise upon first administration because of maternal immunity and may be eliminated accidentally by treatment.

Modern developments with other *Bordetella sp.* have not yet been applied to either killed or live *B.bronchiseptica* vaccines for pigs which remain traditional in nature whether produced alone or in combination with *P.multocida*.

Eradication

The medicated early-weaning technique in which sows are medicated with trimethoprim:sulphonamide prior to farrowing and the piglets dosed orally for 10 days, being weaned at 5 days, has been shown to eliminate *B.bronchiseptica* infection. Similar results have been achieved by medication of the drinking water with the drug at levels of 7 and 35 ppm of trimethoprim:sulphadiazine mixture for 28 days. The use of this treatment coupled with all in, all out husbandry can free finishing herds from the infection and control the disease in a breeding herd.

Husbandry measures

The use of an all-in, all-out housing policy and the provision of good ventilation will reduce the severity of the disease by reducing the weight of infection. On a herd basis, the purchase of animals from herds known to be free from infection, or the treatment of incoming animals may reduce the chance of introducing the disease to any uninfected herd. The use of more old sows as mothers may also reduce the incidence of clinical disease.

References.

Brockmeier, S.L., Register, K.B., Magyar, T., Lax, A.J., Pullinger, G.D., Kunkle, R.A. (2002). Role of the dermonecrotic toxin of *Bordetella bronchiseptica* in the pathogenesis of respiratory disease in swine. Inf and Imm 70, 481-490.

Cameron, R.D.A., Giles, C.J. and Smith, I.M. (1980). The prevalence of *Bordetella bronchiseptica* and turbinate (conchal) atrophy in English pig herds in 1978-1979. Vet.Rec. 107, 146-149.

Collings, L.A., Rutter, J.M. (1985). Virulence of *Bordetella bronchiseptica* infection in the porcine respiratory tract. J.Med.Microbiol. 19, 247-255.

Jong, M.F. de., (1987). Prevention of Atrophic Rhinitis in piglets by means of intranasal administration of live non-AR pathogenic *Bordetella bronchiseptica* vaccine. Vet.Quarterly 9, 123-133.

Jong, M.F. de., Borst, G.H.A. (1985). Selective medium for the isolation of *P.multocida* and *B.bronchiseptica*. Vet.Rec. 116, 167.

Kono, Y., Suzuki, S., Mukai, T., Okazaki, K., Honda, E., Yamashiro, T. (1994). Detection of specific systemic and local IgG and IgA antibodies of pigs after infection with *B. bronchiseptica* by ELISA. J.Vet.Med. Sci. 56, 249-253.

Magyar, T., Chanter, N., Lax, A.J., Rutter, J.M., Hall, G.A. (1988). The pathogenesis of turbinate atrophy in pigs caused by *B.bronchiseptica*. Vet.Micro. 18, 135-146.

Oyant, L.H.S., Bourges, D., Chevaleyne, C., Raze, D., Locht, C., Salmon, H. (2005). Role of *Bordetella bronchiseptica* adenyl cyclase in nasal colonisation and in development of local and systemic immune responses in piglets. Vet. Res. 36, 63-77.

Pullinger, G.D., Adams, T.E., Mullan, P.B., Garrod, T.I., Lax, A.J. (1996). Cloning, expression and molecular characterisation of the dermonecrotic toxin gene of *Bordetella spp.* Inf. and Immun. 64, 4163-4171.

Register, K., Ackermann, M.R., Dyer, D.W. (1995). Non-radioactive colony lift hybridisation assay for detection of *B. bronchiseptica* in swine. J. Clin. Microbiol. **33**, 2675-2678.

Register, K., Boisvert, A., Ackermann, M.R. (1997). Use of ribotyping to distinguish *B. bronchiseptica* isolates. Int. J. Syst. Bact. **47**, 678-683.

Rutter, J.M., Collings, J.A. (1983). The virulence of *Bordetella bronchiseptica* in atrophic rhinitis of pigs. In Atrophic Rhinitis of pigs. Eds. Pedersen, K.B. & Nielsen, N.C. Luxembourg CEE. 77-83.

Silveira, D., Edington, N., Smith, I.M. (1982). Ultrastructural changes in the nasal turbinate bones of pigs in early infection with *Bordetella bronchiseptica*. Res. in Vet.Sci . **33**, 37-42 .

Smith, I.M., and Baskerville, A.J. (1979). A selective medium facilitating the isolation and recognition of *Bordetella bronchiseptica* in pigs. Res.vet. Sci. **27**, 187.

Smith, I.M., Giles, C.J., Baskerville, A.J. (1982). The immunisation of pigs against experimental infection with *Bordetella bronchiseptica*. Vet.Rec. **110**, 488-494.

Underdahl, N.R., Socha, .E. and Doctor, A.R. (1982), Long-term effect of *Bordetella bronchiseptica* infection in neonatal pigs. Am J.Vet.Res. **43**, 622-625.

Progressive Atrophic Rhinitis

Definition

Infection of non-immune piglets with toxigenic *P.multocida* results in severe sneezing, later followed by atrophy of the turbinate bones and distortion of the nasal septum, sometimes accompanied by shortening and twisting of the upper jaw. Depression of the rate of weight gain may occur.

Incidence

Progressive Atrophic Rhinitis has been reported in most intensive pig-rearing countries. Severe atrophy may be found in occasional pigs in Britain. In the United States the condition varies in reported incidence from place to place but appears to be present in at least 10% of herds and more in some areas. The incidence may range from 5% to 40% in other European countries. The recent widespread use of effective vaccines has reduced the numbers of affected pigs without reducing the number of affected herds. Eradication programmes have reduced the incidence of infection in countries such as The Netherlands.

Aetiology

Progressive Atrophic Rhinitis is caused by infection with toxigenic *P.multocida* usually of type D but occasionally of type A.

P.multocida is a Gram-negative coccobacillus 0.3-1.0 μm in diameter and 1.0-2.0 μm in length which shows bipolar staining in tissue smears. It forms grey non-haemolytic watery colonies 3-5 mm in diameter on blood agar and does not grow consistently on MacConkey Agar. Capsules are formed and types A, B and D are recorded in pigs. Strains capable of causing Progressive Atrophic Rhinitis secrete the heat and trypsin labile polypeptide toxin *P.multocida* dermonecrotoxin (DNT) of molecular weight 143,000 Da coded for by the Pm *tox A* gene which may be associated with a prophage. The gene has been cloned and toxin may be produced in *E.coli* whole or in part. Toxigenic *P.multocida* strains form colonies which are indistinguishable from those of non-toxigenic strains and which behave like other *P.multocida* strains. They only occasionally produce fimbriae and are susceptible to drying and a wide range of disinfectants and antimicrobials such as penicillins, tetracyclines, cephalosporins e.g. ceftiofur and fluorinated quinolones. Antimicrobial resistance may occur and can be transferrable.

Pathogenesis

Long lasting atrophy of the conchae can result from the intramuscular or intraperitoneal injection of as little as 250 ng/kg of toxin or the instillation of pure toxin into the nasal passages three times at 27 days of age. The changes produced are seen in the natural disease and include degeneration and necrosis of osteoblasts, accelerated osteoclastic osteolysis and initial stimulation of osteoclast activity to result in the replacement of the bony core of the concha by fibrous tissue. Injection of pure toxin can lead not only to atrophic rhinitis but also to growth retardation and, at high doses, to liver damage, icterus and mortality. In natural disease the changes described above are accompanied by those associated with phase I *B.bronchiseptica* which colonises non-immune pigs and appears to allow toxigenic *P.multocida* of type D and sometimes type A to reach the levels necessary for the production of clinical disease. Infection may occur as early as 3-4 days of age when *B.bronchiseptica* adheres to the cilia of the nasal epithelium. Continued levels of ammonia of 20ppm can trigger this process in neonatal piglets. Some isolates of serotypes 3 and 12 *P.multocida* type D have also been shown to be adherent by means of fimbria-like structures, but most workers agree that adhesion to ciliated epithelium is poor in this species.

The changes in the turbinate mucosa in atrophic rhinitis itself include loss of cilia, hyperplasia and metaplasia of epithelial cells, neutrophil infiltration and the secretion of mucus. Toxigenic *P.multocida* colonises this mucus layer apparently adhering to a low molecular weight (<25 kDa) substance in the mucus and reaching high numbers (10^4-10^7/ml) and producing the toxin which can be absorbed from the nasal mucosa. Toxigenic *P.multocida* may persist in moderate numbers for long periods in the tonsil. Numbers in the nose are reduced in the presence of antibody to toxin but infection is not prevented.

The toxin has been shown to produce a number of effects. It appears to enter cells by endocytosis and affects the uptake of porcine growth hormone. Individual fibroblasts may proliferate and osteoclast precursors are stimulated to develop calcitonin receptors and become osteoclasts. It has systemic effects, and at low levels (0.1 μg) affects levels of hepatic glycogen. At high levels (2.8 or 5.6 μg) hepatocellular degeneration occurs accompanied by icterus, ataxia, blindness and death after five days. Gastric ulceration, polioencephalomalacia, effects on ureters and necrosis of the liver were all seen in addition to turbinate atrophy. It inhibits endochondral bone formation by reducing physeal area and chondrocyte proliferation and thus affects skeletal growth.

Within the nasal mucosa the osteoblastic formation of bone is affected with an increase in the number of osteoclasts and later, a fall in their numbers. Disruption of osteoid synthesis is accompanied by a fibrous hyperplasia and eventually the bony core of the turbinate decreases in size. Secondary atrophy of the mucosa occurs and the whole turbinate may disappear within two weeks especially if the changes occur at the period of maximum growth between 2 and 4 weeks. They are more severe in the ventral conchae.

Sneezing may result from local irritation, the action of toxins and infection with secondary agents such as *Mycoplasma hyorhinis* to cause bleeding from the nose and blockage of the airways for short periods of time. Some degree of resolution may occur before slaughter but this is unlikely in severely affected animals from which the infections have not been eradicated. The severity of conchal changes may be associated to some extent with breed and growth rate.

The absence of turbinates may be reflected in an increased incidence of lower respiratory tract disease but it is not clear whether the absence of conchae *per se* is the cause through reduction in the filtering and warming capacity of the nasal chamber or whether lower respiratory tract disease associated with the two causal agents is directly responsible. Toxigenic *P.multocida* type D appears to colonise the lung only poorly but can cause pneumonia.

Clinical signs

Outbreaks of sneezing occur in baby pigs aged between 1 and 8 weeks of age and are accompanied by blockage of the lachrymal ducts, tear staining or even epistaxis. As the disease progresses, signs of deviation or shortening of the upper jaw may appear with corrugation of the skin of the snout and under shooting of the lower jaw. Signs of pneumonia or stunting may also be noted. In some animals or affected farms, sneezing may be transitory and little outward effect may be seen although turbinate atrophy may be found at slaughter. This form is most common where infection does not occur until after weaning and or where immunity is present.

Severely affected animals may have difficulty in eating and the nasal changes may be seen in pigs of all ages in affected pigs. Rates of daily liveweight gain may be depressed and there may be some mortality amongst piglets. The nasal changes may affect the value of weaners produced for sale. Economic effects on growth rate associated with the bony changes have been estimated at 0.5%, (growth depression of 25-40g/day) or nil, depending upon the study.

Humane slaughter is indicated in young piglets with severe nose bleeding and loss of condition which cannot feed. Infection can normally be reduced by treatment.

Pathological findings

Pigs may be in poor condition with grossly twisted snouts and tear staining. There may be pronounced corrugation of the skin of the snout and nasal discharge may be present.

Atrophy of the turbinates, distortion of the nasal septum and shortening or deflection of the snout are the most prominent findings. The nasal changes are most easily seen in snout cross-sections at the first premolar (level with the corner of the mouth).

The changes may be graded 1-5 in order of severity:-

Grade 1 = slight deviation from normal.
Grade 2 = slight atrophy.
Grade 3 = more severe atrophy.
Grade 4 = loss of at least 1 turbinate.
Grade 5 = loss of all turbinates.

Alternative grading systems include taking prints of the snout or photographing the cavity and recording the Total Perimeter Ratio (TPR normal pigs 1.3-1.5, abnormal 0.4-0.1) and the Turbinate Area Ratio (TAR, normal pigs 0.38-0.4, abnormal 0.16-0.17).

'Swastika' forms or spurs of bone growth out of line with the smooth curve of normal conchae may indicate resolution of pre-existing lesions. The degree of shortening of the upper jaw may also be measured between the upper and lower incisors as an indication of the severity of the changes. A purulent rhinitis may be present and the mucosa may be pale if affected animals are examined early in the disease. The mucosa is normally denuded of its epithelium and heavily infiltrated with inflammatory cells and a catarrhal exudate may be present at the surface. In chronic cases, metaplasia of the epithelium with loss of goblet cells occurs.

B.bronchiseptica and toxigenic *P.multocida* type D may be demonstrated in early cases although in older animals they may be difficult to isolate.

Epidemiology

Infection is transmitted between pigs by aerosol or contact. In aerosols 69% of organisms survive for at least 5 minutes in 79% relative humidity at 37°C and survival is better at lower ambient temperatures. The organism can be recovered from clean water for up to 14 days, slurry for 6 days and from lung washings for 4 days. It may be demonstrated in up to 44% slaughter pigs, 57% young sows but may still be demonstrable in 17% of 3-year old sows.

Transmission between farms is principally by the movement of infected pigs but aerosol transmission and transmission on clothing may be possible over short distances. Toxigenic *P.multocida* from man has been shown to cause disease in pigs but contact with infected rabbits did not. Other species such as sheep and cows also carry toxigenic organisms.

Atrophic rhinitis occurs most frequently in herds in which the toxigenic Pasteurella is present with the almost ubiquitous *B.bronchiseptica* and where the system of management is such that piglets born to non-immune mothers (or colostrum-deprived piglets) are exposed to heavy infection early in life. In herds composed of gilts obtained from a number of sources and farrowed continuously, the disease is likely to be severe. In herds which are closed and have a substantial number of older sows, early infection is less severe as are the nasal changes. Changes may also be severe on such farms when piglets of varying immune status are weaned early and kept in large groups.

Gross changes may develop in weaners purchased by fattening units but this is unusual. Within an affected unit the syndrome may rise and fall in prevalence because of changes in housing, prophylaxis, treatment and composition of the sow population. Low temperature and ammonia concentrations of 10-25 ppm have been associated with exacerbation and increased ventilation with reduction in severity. Infection can be introduced by animals which do not have clinical conchal atrophy or other nasal or facial changes. The introduction of new strains of *P.multocida* to herds with immunity to their existing strain may trigger new outbreaks. Restriction endonuclease analysis and ribotyping suggest that up to 4 REA types or ribotypes may occur in a single herd and that the majority of infections are due to a single type at any one time. A single epidemic strain appears to be important in Denmark.

Diagnosis

1.   Clinical Diagnosis

Progressive Atrophic Rhinitis may be suspected when outbreaks of paroxysmal sneezing occur in piglets and when the changes in the snout appear with age. Measurements of malocclusion of the upper and lower incisors may provide an early indication of severe disease as may biopsy of the nasal mucosa. Turbinate atrophy may also be detected in life by endoscopy, X-ray examination or computer tomography. Atrophy of the conchae and displacement of the nasal septum may be demonstrable.

2.   Pathological Diagnosis

Progressive Atrophic Rhinitis is often suspected first at post mortem or slaughter on transverse section of the snout at the level of the first premolar tooth. Recent studies suggest that additional sections anterior to this may also detect the changes in the tips of the turbinates. The changes can be graded according to the schemes described above. Within the nasal cavity evidence of active rhinitis may also be present and staining with phloxine-alcian blue may demonstrate metaplastic epithelium in longitudinal snout sections. The severity of the problem in a herd can be assessed by a computerised atrophic rhinitis monitoring scheme (A.R.M.S.) based on scores obtained at slaughter but this is only of retrospective value and can only detect changes which have taken place 4-5 months previously. Regular clinical examination and post-mortem examination of piglets found dead is probably a more effective measure of the active disease situation.
In young pigs the condition should be differentiated from cleft lip (cheiloschisis), absence of lower jaw (agnathia) and craniofacial asymmetry (all present before birth), paranasal abscess or bullnose (bacterial infection from tooth-clipping or fighting in unweaned pigs) which occur in individual animals only. In pigs 1-6 months of age, osteodystrophia fibrosa of nutritional of unknown or hormonal origin may occur but spongy bone is present; brachygnathia superior or short snouts may occur especially in Large Whites and Middle White Pigs (a breed character) and mandibular malalignment may occur especially in adults due to bone remodelling and protrusion of lower jaw which develops in association with the vice of bar biting (seen where sow stalls are used).

3.   Demonstration of toxigenic *P.multocida*

This confirms clinical or pathological identification of Progressive Atrophic Rhinitis. The organism is isolated from nasal washings, cotton-tipped swabs from the posterior nares, tonsillar swabs or from the cut surface of crypts of the tonsils at slaughter.
P.multocida can be isolated directly on blood agar, but contamination is common and selective media containing clindamycin 75 mg, gentamycin 75 mg, vancomycin 4 mg and amphotericin 5 mg/L may be of value. Colonies may be identified at 24 and 48 hours or growth harvested at 24 hours for identification. Toxin is usually detected using commercially available ELISAs or occasionally by neutralisation assay on cell cultures. The gene for the toxin may be detected by PCR using oligonucleotide primers. PCR may be used on suspensions of nasal material as well as on early culture material and chromosomal DNA probes may be used to detect both *P. multocida* and *B. bronchseptica* on primary cultures.

4.   Demonstration of immunity

Intradermal injection of toxin produces lesions in non-immune pigs but no lesions in immune pigs. Neutralising antibody may be detected in serum in cell culture assays but antibody to the toxin is difficult to demonstrate by ELISAs in natural infections. It is readily detectable following vaccination.

Treatment

Acute disease in sucking piglets may be treated with trimethoprim sulphonamide, ampicillin, amoxicillin, tetracyclines, ceftiofur or enrofloxacin given by injection or oral doser as appropriate. A single dose may be sufficient for clinical cure or a short course may be required. Animals should be supported with additional food and electrolyte if they cannot suck. Where the B.bronchiseptica component is important, trimethoprim sulphonamide may be the drug of choice.

Disease in weaned pigs can be treated by injection or by water medication using the antimicrobials listed above with the addition of tylosin and penicillin (by injection). Feed medication is considered below under 'Control'.

Control

a) Antimicrobials

Progressive Atrophic Rhinitis may be controlled by the strategic medication of young pigs at 3 days, 10 days and 21 days of age using the antimicrobials listed above, but primarily trimethoprim sulphonamide. Weaned pigs at risk may be treated continuously with antimicrobial in feed or water at therapeutic levels. Feed medication can be given at this stage using the agents listed above. Medication of groups of animals entering an airspace in an all-in, all-out system is the most efficient method.

The development of antimicrobial resistance may make re-assessment of antimicrobial control necessary from time to time and it should be regarded as short-term or appropriate only to systems such as finishers where vaccinated stock cannot be obtained.

b) Vaccination

Killed vaccines containing P.multocida toxoid alone, or with killed B.bronchiseptica antigens, are given to sows 5 and 2 weeks prior to farrowing and protect the piglets with passive immunity to the toxin. Protection may last up to 8 weeks and prevents the bony changes and improves growth rates. Improvements of up to 120g/day have been recorded. Protection depends upon the ingestion of colostrum but does not prevent infection. Piglets may be vaccinated at 7 days and 21 days to provide active immunity, but confirm that the vaccine is safe for them.

c) All-in, all-out systems

Progressive Atrophic Rhinitis and infection may be prevented by a combination of vaccination and isolated farrowing coupled with all-in, all-out rearing with or without medication of animals at entry. The isowean system may also be used.

d) Eradication

Infection has been eradicated consistently by depopulation and restocking with uninfected pigs from clean herds produced by hysterectomy, medicated early weaning (using trimethoprim sulphonamide) or testing and confirmation of freedom.

Testing sows for infection, slaughter of continued carriers coupled with treatment of sows into clean accommodation and batch farrowing and rearing has been shown to eradicate the organism from lightly affected herds (~20% infected sows). Eradication is faster and more reliable if all sows are vaccinated before test and removal begins, and if clean breeding stock are purchased.

e) Monitoring for infection

Primarily by culture of nasal swabs followed by ELISA or PCR for toxigenic *P.multocida*. Additional monitoring by clinical, and particularly post-mortem examination.

References

Chanter, N., Goodwin, R.F.W., Rutter, J.M. (1989). Comparison of methods for the sampling and isolation of toxigenic *P.multocida* from the nasal cavity of the pig. Res.Vet.Sci. **47**, 355-358.

Chanter, N., Magyar, T., Rutter, J.M. (1989). Interaction between *B.bronchiseptica* and toxigenic *P.multocida*, in atrophic rhinitis of pigs. Res.Vet.Sci. **47**, 48-53.

Diemen, P.M.van, Schrama, J.W., Hel, W. van der, Verstegen, M.W.A., Noordhuizen, J.P.T.M. (1995). Effects of atrophic rhinitis and climatic environment on the performance of pigs. Livestock Product. Sci., **43**, 287 294.

Donnio, P.Y., Avril, J.L., Andre, P.M., Vaucel, J. (1991). Dermonecrotoxic toxin production by strains of *P.multocida* isolated from man. J.Med.Micro. **34**, 333-337.

Foged, N.T., Nielsen, J.P., Jorsal, S.E. (1989). Protection against Progressive Atrophic Rhinitis by vaccination with *P.multocida* toxin purified by monoclonal antibody. Vet.Rec. **125**, 7-11.

Fussing, V., Nielsen, J.P., Bisgaard, M., Moyling, A (1999). Development of a typing system for epidemiological studies of porcine toxin-producing *P. multocida subsp. multocida* in Denmark. Vet. Micro. **65**, 61-74.

Gelger, J.O. and 7 others (1992). Elimination of atrophic rhinitis using Isowean 3 site production. Proc. IPVS **12**, 166.

Jolie, R., Thacker, B. (1990). Comparison of atrophic rhinitis morphometric measurements and macroscopic grades of nasal cross sections on computerised tomography scans of pigs. Proc. IPVS **11**, 53.

Jong, M.F. de., Nielsen, J.P. (1990). Definition of Progressive Atrophic Rhinitis. Vet.Rec. **126**, 93.

Kamp, E.M., Bokken, G.C.A.M., Vermuelen, T.M.M., Jong, M.F. de, Buys, H.E.C.m., Reek, F.H., Smits, M.A. (1996). A specific and sensitive PCR assay suitable for large-scale detection of toxigenic *P. multocida* in nasal and tonsillar swab specimens of pigs. J. Vet Diagnostic Invest. **8**, 304-309.

Register, K.B., Lee, R.M., Thomson, C. (1998). Two colour hybridisation assay for simultaneous detection of *B. bronchiseptica* and toxigenic *P. multocida* from swine. J. Clin. Microbiol. **36**, 3342-3346.

Robertson, J.F., Wilson, D., Smith, W.J. (1990). Atrophic rhinitis, influence of the aerial environment. Animal Production **50**, 173-182.

Rutter, J.M. (1989). Atrophic Rhinitis. In Practice **11**, 74-80.

Shryock, T.R., Losonsky, J.M., Smith, W.C., Gatlin, C.L., Francisco, C.J., Kuriashkin, I.V., Clarkson, R.B., Jordan, W.H. (1998). Computed axial tomography of the porcine nasal cavity and a morphometric comparison of the nasal turbinates with other visualisation techniques. Can. J. Vet. Res. **62**, 287 292.

To, H., Someno, S., Nagai, S. (2005). Development of a genetically modified non-toxigenic *Pasteurella multocida* toxin as a candidate for use in vaccines against progressive atrophic rhinitis in pigs. Am.J.Vet.Res. **66**, 113-118.

Voets, M.T., Klaasen, C.H.L., Charlier, P., Wiseman, A., Descamps, J. (1992).   Evaluation of an AR vaccine under controlled conditions. Vet.Rec. **130**, 549-553.

Wallgren, P. and 5 others (1994). Age distribution of pigs carrying *P.multocida* in herds affected with rhinitis. Proc. IPVS **13**, 122.

Pneumonic Pasteurellosis

Definition

Pneumonic pasteurellosis results from the colonisation of existing lung lesions with *P.multocida* to increase their severity and give rise to fever, respiratory distress and death in some cases. Growth may be depressed in chronically-affected animals.

Aetiology

P.multocida subsp. *multocida* of capsular type A, serotype 3 is most commonly isolated from lesions. It forms large, mucoid colonies 3-5 mm on blood agar, is rarely toxigenic and some isolates produce fimbriae. Toxigenic strains of type A and, occasionally of type D, have also been recovered from lesions. Organisms such as *P. multocida subsp. gallicida* have also been isolated from conditions resembling haemorrhagic septicaemia.

Pathogenesis

P.multocida pneumonia is difficult to reproduce experimentally. Pure cultures have only rarely been successful in producing pneumonic lesions when given alone by the intranasal or aerosol routes. Pneumonia can be produced repeatably when pure cultures of non-toxigenic type A strains are given by intra-bronchial inoculation, following lung damage caused by large volumes of saline, lipopolysaccharide, *A.pleuropneumoniae* toxin and infection with *Mycoplasma hyopneumoniae* in enzootic pneumonia. The mechanism by which pneumonia results is not clear. Colonisation of the tracheal mucus may occur (as with toxigenic type D strains in the nose) and some isolates produce fimbriae and may adhere to epithelium. Toxigenic strains of type A and type D cause pneumonia but toxigenic type D strains are cleared faster.

Serum antibodies develop to the somatic antigens on *P.multocida* and can be demonstrated within 12 days of infection. They do not appear to be protective. Antibodies to the toxin can be demonstrated in some cases.

Clinical signs

In acute pasteurellosis affected animals may be lethargic and show dyspnoea, with laboured abdominal type breathing, coughing, slight nasal discharge and fever of 40-41.5°C, 104°-106°F. Mouth breathing and cyanosis of extremities may be seen. Lung sounds are often loud. The clinical signs usually last for 5-10 days and may end in recovery or death but may continue for 3-5 weeks. Recovered animals often remain thin.

Less severe degrees of pneumonia associated with coughing and fever may occur and last for 3-5 weeks. Humane slaughter should be carried out on animals which have collapsed, are lethargic and severely congested with white froth on the lips and low rectal temperatures. Animals which are thin with severe respiratory distress may also be destroyed.

Post-mortem findings

Lesions of enzootic pneumonia are almost always present and lesions of an exudative pneumonia are superimposed on these. Greyish-pink consolidation with reddish atelectic areas is found in the anterior lobes and, in severe cases, in the diaphragmatic lobes as well. Lesions often have a yellowish outline and a fibrinous pleurisy is often present. Congestion of the carcase is frequently seen and froth is commonly present in the trachea. Oedema of the cut lung tissue is evident. In more chronic cases of pasteurella pneumonia, the cut surface has a granular whitish or greyish appearance.

Histological sections show oedema, congestion and haemorrhage with bronchiolar exudate containing bacteria, macrophages and neutrophils which are also present in the alveoli. The bronchi may be blocked by this material and by desquamated epithelial cells.

Aerobic culture of heart blood and lung lesions usually gives a pure culture of *P.multocida*. Anaerobic cultures may yield *Bacteroides* spp in addition. Examination for *Haemophilus* spp may also yield these organisms. Electrophoretic type 01 has been found consistently in lesions of Porcine Immune Complex Glomerulonephritis and Dermatitis and similar organisms (*Apa* I restriction pattern) have been found in the kidneys in the Porcine Dermatitis and Nephropathy Syndrome (PDNS), but their significance is not yet clear.

Epidemiology

Pasteurellosis is transmitted by aerosol by contact and by ingestion and usually occurs in finishing pigs or breeding stock in herds in which enzootic pneumonia is also present and it is commonest under poor husbandry conditions, e.g. overcrowding, dusty ammoniacal atmosphere, etc. Clinical signs may occur after mixing, weighing, transport or some other stress. *P.multocida* is readily killed by heating to 60°C and survives for less than an hour in aerosols at low humidity but survives for longer at high humidity and low temperatures. Organisms survive for up to 14 days in water, 6 days in slurry and for up to 7 weeks in nasal washings at room temperatures. Transmission between farms is by carrier pigs but restriction endonuclease analysis and ribotyping suggest that introduced types may not persist in the face of a prevalent herd type, however, a single ribotype may be present throughout a breeding pyramid. The role of rodent and bird carriage of *P.multocida* has not been extensively evaluated for pneumonia using modern techniques, but RFLP suggests that rodent strains differ from those in pigs in some farms.

Diagnosis

The clinical signs of fever, dyspnoea, and cyanosis without enteric involvement suggest the acute pneumonic or septicaemic condition and this can be confirmed by the post-mortem examination of dead animals when both gross and microscopic lesions provide further evidence. The presence of chronic coughing, reduced daily weight gain and fever may suggest that chronic infection is complicating enzootic pneumonia. The isolation of *P.multocida* in culture confirms its presence. In the absence of other respiratory pathogens such as viruses, *H.parasuis*, *A.pleuropneumoniae*, *B.bronchiseptica* or enzootic pneumonia, a diagnosis of uncomplicated pasteurella pneumonia may be made.

Treatment

Severely affected animals should be treated parenterally with an antimicrobial such as ceftiofur, penicillin, streptomycin, tetracycline, trimethoprim sulphonamide, ampicillin, amoxycillin, marbofloxacin, tulathromycin or spectinomycin for 3-5 days or as appropriate. Parenteral treatment may be supplemented by medication of the drinking water of the affected batch with water soluble derivatives of the above injectable compounds and doxycycline (not UK). Tilmicosin can be used in feed in addition to those antimicrobials listed above. If feed medication is used, severely-affected animals should be treated parenterally. Long-acting oxytetracycline injections may also be used. All pigs in the same air-space should be treated and the space filled on an all in, all out basis. Antibiotic resistance may occur.

Control

Batches of animals may be treated in feed upon entry to an air space. Control is most efficient if all-in, all-out husbandry is practised. Reduction in predisposing diseases such as enzootic pneumonia by medicating with tiamulin at 40 ppm in feed or by vaccination, may reduce the prevalence and severity of disease.

Whole cell killed vaccines (where available) may prevent severe disease from occurring, particularly in older finishing pigs. Vaccination with toxoid vaccines has been shown to reduce the severity of pneumonic pasteurellosis and may be economic.

Husbandry conditions should be improved and dust and ammoniacal levels reduced.

References

Andrews, J.J., Lucas, T.E., Johnson, I. (1988). Prevention and control of experimentally induced *P.multocida* in swine by the use of chlortetracycline in feed. Agri Practice **9**, 33-38.

Bousquet, E., Pommier, P., Wessel-Robert, S., Morvan, H., Benoit-Valjergue, H., Laval, A. (1998). Efficacy of doxycycline in feed for the control of pneumonia caused by *P. multocida* and *M. hyopneumoniae* in fattening pigs. Vet. Rec. **143**, 269-272.

Cameron, R.D.A., O'Boyle, D., Frost, A.J., Gordon, A.N., Fegan, N. (1996). An outbreak of haemorrhagic septicaemia associated with P. multocida subsp. gallicida in a large pig herd. Aust. Vet. J. **73**, 27-29.

Chung, W.B., Backstrom, L.R., Collins, M.T. (1994). Experimental model of swine pneumonic pasteurellosis using crude *A.pleuropneumoniae* cytotoxin and *P.multocida* given endobronchially. Can.J.Vet.Res. **58**, 25-30.

Done, S.H. (1991). Environmental factors affecting the severity of pneumonia in pigs. Vet.Rec. **128**, 582-586.

Isaacson, R.E., Trigo, E. (1995). Pili of *P. multocida* of porcine origin. FEMS Microbiology Letters **132**, 247-251.

Jacques, M., Kobisch, M., Belanger, M., Dugal, F. (1993). Virulence of capsulated and non-capsulated isolates of P. multocida and their adherence to porcine respiratory tract cells and mucus. Inf and Imm. **61**, 4785-4792.

Kobisch, M., Pennings, A. (1989). An evaluation of NobiVac AR and an experimental atrophic rhinitis vaccine containing *P.multocida* DNT toxoid and *B.bronchiseptica*. Vet.Rec. **124**, 57-61.

Mackie, J.T., Barton, M., Kettlewell, J. (1992). *P.multocida* septicaemia in pigs. Aust.Vet.J. **69**, 227-228.

Ose, E.E., Tomkinson, L.V. (1990). Effect of pneumonic pasteurellosis on lung lesions and mortality in *M.hyopneumoniae* infected pigs. Proc. IPVS **11**, 94.

Pijoan, C., Morrison, R.B. and Hilley, H.D. (1983). Serotyping of *P.multocida* isolated from swine lungs collected at slaughter. J.Clin.Microbiol. **17**, 1074-1076.

Thomson, J.R., MacIntyre, N., Henderson, L.E.A., Meikle, C.S. (2001). Detection of Pasteurella multocida in pigs with porcine dermatitis and nephropathy syndrome. Vet.Rec. **149**, 412-417.

Zhao, G., Pijoan, C., Murtaugh, M.P., Molitor, T.W. (1992). Use of restriction endonuclease analysis and ribotyping to study the epidemiology of *P.multocida* in closed herds. Inf. and Immunity **60**, 1401-1405.

Infection with NAD-dependent *P.multocida*

V-dependent *P.multocida* of taxa D, E and F have been isolated from nasal swabs, lungs and joints.

Mannheimia (Pasteurella) haemolytica infections

M.haemolytica has been isolated from septicaemia in piglets, from localised areas of fibrinous pleurisy or pleuropneumonia and from outbreaks of diarrhoea in pigs. Infection in pigs may originate from sheep contact and be *P.trehalosi* (untypable) or of bovine origin and affect bovine leucocytes. Other strains resemble taxon 15 of *A.pleuropneumoniae* closely and should be distinguished from it and from *A.suis*. Infection in piglets may be inapparent.

Local lung lesions, 1 to 2 cm, red with fibrinous pleurisy and petechiation of the affected area are seen in acute cases and these become necrotic, greyish-red, and encapsulated with fibrous adhesions. No clinical signs have been associated with this condition and the local lesions are small and scarce, mostly near the bronchi in any lobe of the lung.

A septicaemic form may occur in piglets particularly when housed in the same airspace as sheep. Fever to 41°C, 106°F and death can occur. Localisation in the joints may result. Carcases of dead piglets resemble those which have died of *Actinobacillus suis* infections but have lung lesions of *P.haemolytica* infection (see above) and may have enteritis. Treatment and control may be necessary and should be as for *A.pleuropneumoniae* or *P.multocida*. Vaccines to many *P.haemolytica* serotypes are available should a problem persist and could be used.

Pleuropneumonia *(Actinobacillus pleuropneumoniae* infection).

Definition

A highly contagious, often fatal, respiratory disease of weaned growing and finishing pigs in which infection of the lungs with *Actinobacillus pleuropneumoniae* causes fibrinous pleurisy, pneumonia with characteristic infarcts and depression of growth rate in chronically affected pigs.

Incidence

A major problem in much of Europe, the USA., Canada and Eastern Asia *Actinobacillus pleuropneumoniae* is present in Britain and the disease was initially described here in 1957 but extensive outbreaks of the type so common elsewhere have only been seen since 1980. Control measures may suppress clinical disease but reports from many countries suggest that 30-50% of all pigs are infected.

Aetiology

The disease is caused by *A.pleuropneumoniae* which forms small translucent mucoid ß-haemolytic colonies around staphylococcal streaks on sheep blood agar. Colonies may be firmly adherent to the agar in freshly-isolated cultures. The organism usually requires NAD (V factor) (Biotype 1).but some strains do not (Biotype 2). It is urease positive, reduces nitrate, ferments D-xylose and ribitol and is indole, citrate, methyl red and VP negative.

The organism produces fine and coarse fimbriae (type 4 fimbriae have been cloned), capsules and secretes toxins. Thirteen major serotypes of Biotype 1 and at least two of Biotype 2 (total 15) have been distinguished based on capsular antigens. Some serotypes occur in both Biotype 1 and Biotype 2.

Four main toxins are produced. Apx 1 has a M.W. of 105-110 kDa, is haemolytic and cytotoxic and is produced by serotypes 1, 5a, 5b, 9, 10 and 11. Apx II has a M.W. of 103-105 kDa, is weakly haemolytic, moderately cytotoxic and occurs in all serotypes except 10. Apx III has a M.W. of 120 kDa, is non-haemolytic, strongly cytotoxic and occurs in serotypes 2,3,4,6, and 8. Apx !V has a MW of 202 kDa and is produced by all serotypes, but only in vivo. A CAMP factor of MW 29 kD which aids haemolysis, is also produced. The genes for all these toxic factors have been cloned, sequenced and recombinant proteins produced. A range of enzymes, adhesive factors and capsular antigens has been identified and cloned and their importance in disease has been studied.

A.pleuropneumoniae is fairly delicate but can survive for 5 days at 18°C particularly in mucopurulent nasal discharge. It is sensitive to drying and may disappear from dry swabs within a few hours. Protection for organisms on swabs requires the use of a transport medium preferably including yeast extract and nicotinamide. The organism survives periods up to 30 days in clean water at 4°C. It is killed by formaldehyde, glutaraldehyde, ethanol, isopropyl alcohol and chlorhexidine.

A.pleuropneumoniae is sensitive *in vitro* to a number of antimicrobials but resistant strains occur. It is sensitive in most cases to penicillin and ampicillin, amoxycillin, tetracycline, tiamulin, ceftiofur, cephalexin, chloramphenicol, florfenicol, enrofloxacin, ciprofloxacin tulathromycin, and trimethoprim sulphonamide.

Pathogenesis

Infection is by aerosol or by contact. The organism enters the upper respiratory tract or oral cavity where it adheres only to the tonsillar epithelium. Tonsillar inflammation may result and infection may be restricted to this site, colonise the middle ear or contribute to lower respiratory tract infection. Experimental studies suggest that the caudal lobes, diaphragmatic and accessory, receive the bulk of aerosolised organisms. Here they attach to the alveolar epithelium possibly by means of fimbriae until the disease process disrupts the lung (1-3 hours). Low numbers of organisms may colonise without effect. The exact cause of the lesions is not yet completely clear, but the production of transposon mutants lacking Apx I and studies with the infusion of toxins suggest that many of the changes described below are initiated by the toxins alone. Cytokines (TNFα, IL-1 and IL-6) are produced by affected phagocytes and effect many of the lesions. The toxins (principally Apx I and Apx III) kill macrophages within 30-60 minutes of exposure and reduce the phagocyte efficacy of neutrophils. The presence of capsules reduces the efficacy of phagocytosis further and protects organisms against the effects of complement. Bacterial numbers increase and they may be found in microcolonies in the lung and in tracheal mucus and mucopus. Toxins are produced during the log phase of bacterial growth and cause the earliest lesions within 3 hours post infection in the peracute form and pronounced lesions by 6 hours post-infection.

Capillary congestion results in marked oedema of both the alveolar wall and the interstitial septum. Lymphatics become dilated with oedema fluid, fibrin and inflammatory cells. Platelet aggregation and neutrophil accumulation exacerbate the alveolar wall damage and this necrosis is followed by pulmonary artery thrombosis. Cytokines such as interleukin 1β and IL8 are produced into alveloar fluids and are accompanied by TNF in the lesions. At any stage from 9 hours onwards *A.pleuropneumoniae* may be found in the blood and can colonise sites such as joints or bone at this stage. Microcolonies of organisms may be seen in affected lung. By 4 days post-infection the lesions, now filled with macrophages and lymphocytes, are clearly demarcated from normal lung. Later, fibrosis occurs and the centre of the lesion becomes greyish and necrotic. Bacteria are common in the lesion at this stage.

A.pleuropneumoniae induces antibodies to its capsule, lipopolysaccharide toxins, outer membrane proteins especially one of 42 kDa and enzymes such as superoxide dismutase and to the iron binding proteins. These antibodies occur in the respiratory secretions as IgA antibodies and in serum as IgG with some IgA. IgM does not appear in high concentration. The antibody neutralises the toxins and allows the successful phagocytosis and killing of organisms. Passive antibody protects against infection and can be demonstrated until at least 4 weeks of age. Active immunity can first be demonstrated 5-10 days after infection and appears to peak 3-4 weeks after infection. Immunity to the homologous serotype appears to be lifelong but disease may occur following challenge with a different serotype. Serotype 2 infections may give rise to protection against other serotypes.

Clinical signs

Acute disease occurs in a non-immune herd or individuals which have not received passive immunity. 15-30% of pigs may suffer depression, anorexia, high fever (41.5°C, 107°F), or laboured respiration, especially after rising to drink or after disturbance. Cyanosis, subnormal rectal temperature and death may follow within 4-6 hours of the onset of clinical signs. Blood stained froth may be seen at the mouth. Some pigs may be found dead and mortality may reach 30-50% of those affected. In the sub-acute form groups of pigs may be affected and are anorexic, fevered, and show respiratory distress, coughing and exercise intolerance. Variable mortality occurs. Recovering animals may cough, and show respiratory distress particularly when disturbed. Exercise intolerance may continue for days and affected animals may have reduced appetites, appear gaunt and hairy, be depressed and show reduced rates of liveweight gain. Non-immune animals of all ages may be affected and abortion may occur in affected gilts or sows. Where infection is enzootic the condition is most common amongst pigs of 6-12 weeks of age. Medication can alter the clinical signs and mortality. *A. pleuropneumoniae* has been involved in cases of otitis media and in arthritis and osteomyelitis.

Humane slaughter should be carried out when blood-stained froth appears at the lips of acutely affected pigs with cyanosis of the extremities and sub-normal rectal temperatures. Chronically-affected animals with very poor bodily condition, continued exercise intolerance and respiratory distress may be killed.

Pathological findings

In most acute cases, the lesions are limited to the thoracic cavity. The nasal cavity and trachea may be filled with blood stained froth and the lungs are congested and oedematous with oedema of the interlobular septae (3-12 hours after onset). Later (12-24 hours) yellowish or blood stained fibrinous exudate appears on the pleural surface over pneumonic areas. Blood tinged fluid may be present in the pleural cavity. Firm, dark red irregular shaped, raised areas may be seen scattered throughout the lung but particularly in the caudal (diaphragmatic) lobes 14-30 hours after onset of clinical signs. These areas may be necrotic in severe cases by 48 hours after onset and occupy about 50% of the lung in fatal cases. In chronic cases, these lesions become encapsulated and greyish in colour. They may be felt as firm nodules at post-mortem or slaughter and allow the presence of the disease to be suspected. The severe fibrinous pleurisy becomes fibrous, and persists until slaughter and may lead to stripping of the pleura. Fibrinous pericarditis and inflammation and haemorrhage of the bronchial lymph nodes occur. Infarcts and alveolar haemorrhages are seen histologically and bronchopneumonia is a feature of affected lung. Infarcts are often surrounded by a prominent ring of dead phagocytes. Micro colonies of the organism are often visible in the alveoli and the organism may be isolated from and demonstrated in the lesions (see Diagnosis).

Epidemiology

The organism spreads from animal to animal by contact, particularly during the oral contact associated with fighting after mixing and by aerosol when 10^4 organisms/ml are needed to cause disease ($!0^2$ for serotype 1). It does not survive long in aerosols unless humidity is high and ambient temperature low, and experiments have only demonstrated transmission for 1 metre. More than one serotype may occur in an animal and up to six serotypes have been identified in a single herd. Disease may be more prolonged and severe where more than one serotype is present and where infection with other agents such as PRRS, PCV2 and PRCV occurs. Low levels of infection may result in active immunity and infection with A. suis in early life may protect animals from disease.

The organism survives for long periods in water (30 days at 4°C), for hours in aerosols, appears to be rapidly killed on drying and to survive for up to four days in lung tissue and discharges at room temperature and for up to one year in frozen lung. It is rapidly killed by disinfectants in the absence of protein. The organism survives in lung lesions in pigs for weeks, and in tonsils for 4-6 months or more. Tonsillar and lung isolates have the same restriction endonuclease analysis pattern.

Spread between farms is mainly by the movement of carrier pigs, followed by transmission on fomites. Aerosol transmission is rare or non-existent. No vectors are known on farm although mice can be infected experimentally.

Different serotypes exist in each country. UK isolates are 27.3% 2, 22.2% 8, 13.1% 3, 14.1% 6, 16.2% 7 with 5, 9, 10 and 12 occurring rarely and 1 and 4 absent. Prevalent serotypes in Great Britain are 3, 6 and 8 while in Ireland 2 is common and 6 absent. Similar pictures exist in the US with 1, 5 and 7 being relatively common, but 2 and 3 are also common in neighbouring Canada. International trade in pigs results in spread of different serotypes.

Diagnosis

The clinical signs of acute and fatal respiratory disease are suggestive. Influenza rarely causes mortality and affects pigs of all ages, while enzootic pneumonia is more chronic. The post-mortem findings of massive pleurisy and pericarditis are suggestive and the firm lung infarcts are characteristic of this disease. Fibrous pleurisy and pericarditis at slaughter with firm nodules representing residual infarcts suggest the past presence of the disease.

Confirmation of the diagnosis is by demonstration of the agent or its products. Samples for examination include nasal swabs, tonsillar swabs or scrapings, bronchoalveolar lavage and tissue from affexcted lung. Culture can be carried out on sheepblood agar with a streak of ß-toxin-producing staphylococcus across the inoculated area. Satellite ß-haemolytic colonies develop. It may be grown on chocolate (altered blood) agar and on selective media containing crystal violet 1 μg, lincomycin 1 μg, spectinomycin 8 μg and bacitracin 128 μg/ml. Isolates may be identified presumptively by possession of urease and CAMP factor and confirmed biochemically. *A. pleuropneumoniae* may occur as biotype 2 (not NAD dependant) and should then be distinguished from *A. suis* , other porcine species of Actinobacillus, and pig isolates of *Mannheimia (Pasteurella) haemolytica*. *Haemophilus parasuis* and NAD dependant actinobacilli such as *A. minor.*, *A. porcinus*, and *A. indolicus* may also be isolated. *A. pleuropneumoniae* may be serotyped by slide agglutination using antibody to capsules, by ELISA, coagglutination, latex particle agglutination, and using labelled DNA probes, ribotyping, PCR and restriction endonuclease analysis.

Antigens may be identified and serotyped in lung tissue by coagglutination tests on extracts, indirect immunofluorescence and immunoperoxidase in tissues and DNA may be identified by single or multiplex PCR using a range of primers. Primers to *apx*IV have been developed to detect all serotypes, and a range of multiplex PCR tests specific to 3 or more serotypes have been described. Antigen ELISAs have also been described, using monoclonals raised to recombinant proteins..

Chronically affected or carrier pigs may be identified by culture of tonsillar swabs or by the presence of antibody in saliva, nasal secretions, colostrum, meat juice or, more usually, serum. Most current antibody tests use ELISAs with capsular antigen, recombinant protein antigens or blocking ELISAs using monoclonal antibodies, but the Complement Fixation Test, radioimmunoassay, latex agglutination tests and 2-mercaptoethanol tube agglutination tests are still used. A wide variety of other tests have been described. Positive titres in agglutination tests may be >1:20, CFT >1:20 and in some ELISAs >1:160. ELISAs using toxins may require confirmation of neutralising ability as antibody to Apx toxins from other species may occur. Most tests are serotype specific.

Treatment

The rapid onset of the lesions and clinical signs mean that treatment of clinically-affected animals may eliminate the organism but may not allow complete resolution of the damage. Both lung damage and fibrinous pleurisy or fibrous pleurisy may persist to affect performance for the remainder of the finishing period and such animals may have persistent exercise intolerance and low average daily gain. Lesions may be colonised by organisms such as *Pasteurella* spp. and *Bacteroides spp* and these may persist after *A.pleuropneumoniae* has been eliminated.

Clinically-affected animals should be treated parenterally with an antimicrobial likely to be effective. Water and food consumption is reduced by infection, making medication of feed and water largely ineffective.

The agents which can be used include penicillin, cephalexin, ampicillin, amoxycillin, oxytetracycline, doxycycline, trimethoprim sulphonamide, tiamulin, florfenicol (and chloramphenicol, not EU). Recently enrofloxacin has been used at 5 mg/kg, danofloxacin at 1.25mg/kg, tulathromycin 2.5 mg/kg, ceftiofur at 3-5 mg/kg and lincospectin. Parenteral treatment may need to be repeated for 3 days. Affected pigs may have to be given water by stomach tube. The remainder of the group can be treated in water or feed with the antimicrobials listed above (where available).

Resistance to antimicrobials varies with their use. In the UK fewer than 10 per cent of isolates were penicillin and tetracycline-resistant in one survey in 1988, but elsewhere resistance has been recorded more frequently. Levels may reach 90% to tetracyclines in countries such as US and Denmark. Japanese studies found resistance to be associated with serotype.

Control

(a)   Treatment

Therapeutic levels of appropriate antimicrobials in feed given at entry to a house may prevent any further disease when used with all-in, all-out stocking of single airspaces or sites. Pulse dosing by treatment for a single day on introduction of new animals to an existing continuous flow system may also reduce or prevent disease. Treatment alone has not been shown to eliminate infection.

(b)   Vaccination

Deaths from pleuropneumonia can be prevented by current vaccines (not UK, 2006) and the extent of lung lesions can be reduced by at least 50% and often more. They may improve days to slaughter by at least 5.5 and daily liveweight gain by up to 100 g. Current vaccines can be made from killed whole cultures harvested young to obtain extracellular products and containing up to 4 serotypes chosen to reflect those present in the herd or country concerned. Where these serotype-specific vaccines are in use, it is particularly important to use diagnostic techniques which determine the serotypes present. Oil adjuvants have been described but modern products contain less irritant adjuvants such as alum suitable for use in young piglets. They are given as two injections two weeks apart to non-pregnant animals no younger than six weeks of age. Vaccine programmes often require the vaccination of the sow to give passive protection and subsequent vaccination of the piglets. Where passive immunity is present (from enzootic infection or vaccinated sows) best results are obtained by vaccinating piglets after the disappearance of maternal immunity. This usually occurs from 4-6 to 12 weeks of age and weaners can be given the first injection at this stage. Unfortunately, this also coincides with a peak in colonisation by *A. pleuropneumoniae* in many herds. The most appropriate time for vaccination in any herd can be identified by serological monitoring to produce a serum profile for the disease. Monitoring for the organism by PCR of nasal or tonsillar swabs can also be used for profiling. Serum profiles can vary from building to building on the same farm. Vaccination prior to entry to a finishing unit can be particularly effective.

Experimental studies have shown that a number of *A.pleuropneumoniae* antigens protect against the disease to some degree and a combination of Apx I, Apx II, Apx III and the 42 kDa outer membrane protein OMP protects against other serotypes. These vaccines are commercially available in many countries of the EU and can be effective aginst a number of serotypes. Gene deleted vaccines have been constructed and tested. Parenteral, aerosol and intraperitoneal routes and a number of adjuvants have been used.

(c)   Isolation: treatment: vaccination combinations

Isolation using all-in, all-out systems within a farm reduces infection but does not prevent it. The use of vaccination or treatment prior to or at the move increases the degree of control. Isowean (PIC) technology using separate site isolation for each stage also minimises disease.

(d)   Eradication

Hysterectomy-derived herds are free of *A.pleuropneumoniae* infection and may be maintained free by isolation. They form a source of disease-free stock for repopulation.

Depopulation of farms, cleaning, disinfection and repopulation with disease-free animals can be carried out. Antimicrobial treatment alone has not been successful in eradication but combinations with vaccination, partial depopulation and removal of serological and tonsillar carriers has been successful. Treatment of the breeding and sucking herds with enrofloxacin was found to eradicate the infection.

References

Belanger, M., Dubreuil, D., Jacques, M. (1994). Proteins found within porcine respiratory tract secretions bind lipopolysaccharides of A. pleuropneumoniae. Inf. and Imm. 62, 868-873.

Bosch, J.F., van den, Jongenelen, I.M.C.A., Pubben, A.N.B., Vugt, F.G.A van, Segers, R.P.A.M. (1992). Protection induced by a trivalent *A.pleuropneumoniae* subunit vaccine. Proc. IPVS 12, 194.

Chiers, K., Haesebrouck, F., Overbeke, I. van, Charlier, G., Ducatelle, R. (1999). Early in vivo interaction of A. pleuropneumoniae with tonsils of pigs. Vet.Micro. 68, 301-306.

Chiers, K., Donne, E., Overbeke, I. van, Ducatelle, R., Haesebrouck, F., (2002). Evaluation of serology, bacteriological isolation and polymerase chain reaction for the detection of pigs carrying A. pleuropneumoniae in the upper respiratory tract after experimental infection. Vet.Micro. 88, 385-392.

Cruijsen, T., Leengoed, L.A.M.G. van, Kamp, E.M., Bartelse, A., Korevaar, A., Verheijden, J.H.M. (1995). Susceptibility to A. pleuropneumoniae infection in pigs from an endemically-infected herd is related to presence of toxin-neutralising antibody. Vet. Micro., 47, 219-228.

Cruijsen, T., Leengoed, L.A.M.G. van, Kamp, E.M., Hunneman, W.A., Riepema, K., Bartelse, A., Verheijden, J.H.M. (1995). Prevalence and development of antibodies neutralising the haemolysin and cytotoxin of A. pleuropneumoniae in 3 infected pig herds. Vet. Quarterly, 17, 96-99.

Duff, J.P., Scott, W.A., Wilks, M.K., Hunt, B. (1996). Otitis in a weaned pig: a new pathological role for A. (H) pleuropneumoniae. Vet. Rec. 139, 561-563.

Frey, J. and 21 others (1993). *A.pleuropneumoniae* RTX toxins: uniform designation of haemolysin, cytolysins pleurotoxins and their genes. J.Gen.Microbiol. 139, 1723-1728.

Gagne, A., Lacouture, S., Broes, A., D'Allaire, S., Gottschalk, M. (1998). Development of an immunomagnetic method for selective isolation of A. pleuropneumoniae serotype 1 from tonsils. J. Clin. Microbiol. 36, 251-254.

Gram, T., Ahrens, P. (1998). Improved diagnostic PCR assay for A. pleuroneumoniae based on nucleotide sequence of an outer membrane lipoprotein. J. Clin. Micro. 36, 443-448.

Guttierez, C.B., Barbosa, J.I.R, Suarez, J., Gonzalez, O.R., Tascon, R.I., Ferri, E.F.R. (1995). Efficacy of a variety of disinfectants against *A.pleuropneumoniae* serotype 1. Am. J. Vet. Res. 56, 1025-1029.

Fussing, V., Barfod, K., Nielsen, R., Moller, K., Nielsen, J.P., Wegener, H.C., Bisgaard, M. (1998). Evaluation and application of ribotyping for epidemiological studies of A. pleuropneumoniae in Denmark. Vet. Micro. 62, 145-162.

Hensel, A., Stockhofe-Zurweiden, N., Ganter, M., Petzoldt, K. (1995). Aerosol exposure of pigs to viable or inactivated A. pleuropneumoniae serotype 9 induces antibodies in bronchoalveolar lining fluids and serum and protects against homologous challenge. Vet. Micro. 47, 27-41.

Jensen, T.K., Boye, M., Hagedorn-Olsen, T., Riising, H.J., Angen, O. (1999). A. pleuropneumoniae osteomyelitis in pigs demonstrated by fluorescent in situ hybridisation. Vet. Path. 36, 258-261.

Larsen, K.V., Dahl, J., Baekbo, P. (1998). Testing of an eradication strategy of a sow herd for A. pleuropneumoniae types 2 and 6 and M. hyopneumoniae involving medication with Baytril IER (enrofloxacin) powder 2.5%. Proc IPVS **15**, II, 249.

Liggett, A.D., Harrison, L.R. and Farell, R.L. (1987). Sequential study of lesions development in experimental *Haemophilus pleuropneumoniae*. Res.Vet.Sci. **42**, 204-212.

Lo, T.M., Ward, C.K., Inzana, T.J. (1998). Detection and identification of A. pleuropneumoniae serotype 5 by multiplex PCR. J.Clin. Micro. **36**, 1704-1710.

Loftager, M.K., Eriksen, L., Aasted, B., Nielsen, R. (1993). Protective immunity following immunisation of pigs with aerosol of *A.pleuropneumoniae* serotype 2. Res.Vet.Sci. **55**, 281-286.

Moller, K., Fussing, V., Grimont, P.A.D., Paster, B.J., Dewhurst, F.E., Killian, M. (1996). *A. minor, sp.nov., A. porcinus, sp. nov.* and *A. indolicus, sp. nov.*, 3 new V factor-dependent species from the respiratory tract of pigs. Int. J. Syst. Bact. **46**, 951-956.

Pijpers, A., Vernooys, J.A.C.M., Leengood, L.A.M.G. van, Verheiden, J.H.M. (1990). Feed and water consumption in pigs following *A.pleuropneumoniae* challenge. Proc. IPVS **11**, 39.

Schaller, A., Djordjevic, S.P, Eames, G.J., Forbes, W.A., Kuhn, R., Kuhnert, P., Gottschalk, M., Nicolet, J., Frey, J. (2001). Identification and detection of A. pleuropneumoniae by PCR based on the gene *apx* IVA. Vet. Micro. **79**, 47-62.

Stevenson, A., MacDonald, J., Roberts, M. (2003). Cloning and characterisation of type 4 fimbrial genes from *A. pleuropneumoniae*. Vet.Micro. **92**, 121-134.

Utrera, V., Pijoan, C. (1991). Fimbriae in *A.pleuropneumoniae* strains isolated from pig respiratory tracts. Vet.Rec. **128**, 357-358.

Glasser's Disease

Definition

An infectious, sometimes fatal, polyarthritis, polyserositis and meningitis of young pigs caused by *Haemophilus parasuis*. Bronchitis and other syndromes may occur in older animals in non-immune herds.

Incidence

Infection occurs in all pig herds worldwide with the exception of a few primary SPF units and in some batches of pigs produced by Segegated Early Weaning (SEW). Isolation studies in several countries suggest 29-30% herds are positve by culture. Clinical disease is sporadic in herds with enzootic infection but has become more important since the appearance of PRRS.

Aetiology

Glasser's Disease is caused by the infection of non-immune pigs with some serovars of *Haemophilus parasuis*. *H.parasui*s is a Gram-negative coccobacillus which requires V factor (NAD) but not X factor. It is not haemolytic. Growth only occurs on blood agar in the presence of a staphylococcal streak. Small translucent l mm colonies develop adjacent to the streak within 48 hours. The organisms produce fimbriae and capsules. The species is currently (2006) divided into 15 serovars 1-15. Serovars 1, 2, 4, 5, 10, 12, 13, 14 are virulent, 15 less so and 3, 6, 7, 8, 9 and 11 appear to be avirulent. Many isolates are not typable. Pathogenic organisms appear to possess a 39 kDa outer membrane protein and a neuraminidase and to be distinct from upper respiratory tract isolates based on Enterobacterial Repetitive Intergenic Consensus-based PCR (ERIC-PCR). A cytotoxin has been described but not defined.

Pathogenesis.

Glasser's Disease can be reproduced by intravenous, intraperitoneal or aerosol infection, but many challenge infections are now carried out by intranasal instillation. As few as 10^2 colony forming units are capable of causing disease with serotype 5 in SPF pigs, but inocula are often larger in experimental infections.

The incubation period may be as little as 12 hours and septicaemia results in fibrinous polyserositis, polyarthritis and purulent meningitis within 36 hours of infection. Aerosol or intratracheal infection can give rise to bronchopneumonia. Organisms appear to colonise the tracheal mucus rather than the cilia and it is rare to see bacteria attached to the cilia. Patchy ciliary loss is seen and a purulent rhinitis develops. *H.parasuis* pneumonias often follow damage such as that caused by swine influenza. Following the acute phase of disease, the serous exudates in the body cavities often organise to leave a fibrous peritonitis, pleurisy or pericarditis which may persist until slaughter and give rise to chronic cardiac failure or strangulation of the bowel.

Immunity to infection develops and is complete to the homologous serovar. A variable degree of protection occurs against other serovars. Passive immunity may protect piglets for up to 4 weeks.

Clinical signs

Outbreaks of the disease occur in young pigs 3-6 weeks of age. A sudden onset with fever (40-41°C, 104-107°F) complete anorexia, shallow, dyspnoeic breathing and extension of the head occurs. There may be a serous nasal discharge and coughing may occur. Lung sounds and pericardial rubbing can be heard by auscultation. Animals become lame and shuffle. All joints are swollen, warm and painful. There may be swelling of the face and one or both ears. Pigs may die within 2-5 days of the onset of the disease and show a red to blue skin discolouration before death. Survivors may develop chronic arthritis, pericarditis and congestive cardiac failure, meningitis or intestinal obstruction after adhesions. Water consumption decreases and there is marked weight loss. Animals of any age may be affected in non-immune herds. Coughing, bronchitis and meningitis may occur in gilts or older fatteners and sudden death has been recorded in this age group.

Clinical signs may be overlooked until signs of chronic disease appear. Animals unable to rise with arthritis, those paralysed following meningitis and animals with chronic cardiac failure or strangulated hernias should be humanely destroyed.

Pathological findings

Suppurative rhinitis is often present. Fibrinous pleurisy, pericarditis and peritonitis are always seen and bronchopneumonia may also occur. Thrombi may be present in these lesions. The spleen and liver may be enlarged and petechial haemorrhages may be seen on the kidneys. There is inflammation of the joints, the joint fluid is turbid and yellowish-green fibrin deposits may be present in the joint cavities. Purulent meningitis is often present. In animals which have died from chronic disease fibrous adhesions are present. Fibrous pericarditis is frequently present and is accompanied by signs of chronic congestive cardiac failure, enlarged heart, pulmonary oedema, enlarged liver and enlarged spleen with excess straw-coloured peritoneal fluid. Pure cultures of *H.parasuis* may be isolated from the nasal cavity, tracheobronchial tree, joint fluids, heart blood or, if meningitis is present, from the cerebrospinal fluid in the acute stages of the disease. Organisms are rarely isolated from the blood and cannot be isolated from the lesions of chronic systemic disease.

Epidemiology

Spread within units is primarily by contact or aerosol. Only a small number of organisms (10^2 - 10^4) is required to initiate infection. Maternal immunity declines after 2-4 weeks and infection commonly occurs at this stage. More than one serovar may occur in a herd and avirulent serovars may be present in the nose and in systemic infections. Spread between units is by the movement of carrier pigs. The organisms are delicate and are easily killed by drying.

Diagnosis

The clinical signs of reluctance to move, lameness and polyarthritis are suggestive of Glasser's Disease but must be distinguished from those of streptococcal joint ill in young pigs and from polyserositis and arthritis caused by *Mycoplasma* spp. in older animals (much milder). The occurrence of fever and the death of the affected animal often suggests Glasser's Disease. When death occurs following meningitis, *Streptococcus suis* Type II should be considered as should Oedema Disease, Talfan and Aujeszky's disease. Post-mortem findings of massive amounts of fibrinous pleurisy pericarditis and, especially peritonitis are particularly suggestive. Confirmation of diagnosis in the acute disease depends upon the isolation of the organism from the lesions. The organism can be recovered most consistently from the nasal passages and less consistently from the trachea. It remains viable in exudates and nasal swabs in Amies transport medium for at least 5 days at 5°C, but recovery is best from freshly killed, untreated animals and fresh specimens. Selective media (chocolate altered blood agar with 10 units bacitracin/ml) or enrichment overnight in broth with added NAD (0.004%) may improve recovery. PCR testing using specific primers is generally more effective than culture, but is not yet widely available. Serotyping by gel diffusion, indirect haemagglutination or RFLP-PCR using the *tbp* gene as one of the virulent serovars is final proof of involvement. This is particularly important in respiratory tract infections. The organism can be demonstrated in fixed tissue using avidin-biotin-linked antibody and by digoxygenin labelled DNA probes. The presence of complement-fixing antibodies to the serovar responsible at titres greater than 1:80 is a useful indicator of herd infection, and antibody can also be detected using ELISA tests.

Treatment and control

Parenteral penicillin, ampicillin, amoxycillin oxytetracycline, ceftiofur, florfenicol, enrofloxacin, danofloxacin, tulathromycin and trimethoprim: sulphonamide may all be used to treat early cases with success. Spread to other animals at risk may be prevented and treatment continued by water medication with one of the above drugs for the appropriate treatment period. Feed medication over the period of risk may prevent disease. Most isolates are fully sensitive to antimicrobials, although trimethoprim sulphonamide resistance has been reported. Killed vaccines containing serotypes 4 and 5 have been produced and may be used to vaccinate sows or piglets. Studies with restriction endonuclease analysis have shown that vaccine failure is associated with infection with serovars not included in the vaccine and successful protection

217

depends upon inclusion of appropriate serovars in the vaccine. Serotypes 4 and 5 are important in most countries surveyed to date and commercial vaccines contain both (Suvaxyn M.hyo-parasuis, Fort Dodge) or 5 (Porcilis Glasser, Intervet) and may protect against 1, 2, 12, 13 and 14 in addition to the homologous strain. Vaccines made from the herd's own organisms are also effective.

Eradication has not been reported, although treatment during segregated early weaning may leave animals uninfected.

References

Bak, H., Riising, H.J. (2002). Protection of vaccinated pigs against experimental infection with homologous and heterologous *H. parasuis*. Vet.Rec. **151**, 502-505.

Kielstein, P., Rapp Gabrielson, V.J. (1992). Designation of 15 serovars of *H.parasuis* on the basis of immunodiffusion using heat stable antigen extracts. J.Clin.Microbiol. **30**, 862-865.

Oliveira, S., Galina, L., Pijoan, C. (2001). Development of a PCR test to diagnose *H. parasuis* infections. J.Vet.Diagn. Invest. **13**, 495-501.

Rapp-Gabrielson, V.J., Kocur, G.J., Clark, J.T., Muir, S.K. (1997). *H. parasuis* immunity in swine after vaccination. J.Vet. Med. **92**, 83-90.

Smart, N.L., Hurnik, D., MacInnes, J.J. (1993). An investigation of enzootic Glasser's disease in a specific pathogen-free grower finisher facility using restriction endonuclease analysis. Can.Vet.J. **34**, 387-490.

Smart, N.L., Miniats, O.P. (1989). Preliminary assessment of a *H.parasuis* bacterin for use in specific pathogen-free swine. Can.J.Vet.Res. **53**, 390-393.

Solano-Aguilar, G.I., Pijoan, C., Rapp-Gabrielson, V., Carvalho, L.F., Winkelman, N. (1999). Protective role of maternal antibodies against H. parasuis infection. Am. J. Vet. Res. **60**, 81-87.

Tadjine, M., Mittal, K.R., Bourdon, S., Gottschalk, M. (2004). Development of a new serological test for serotyping *H.parasuis* isolates and determination of their prevalence in North America. J.Clin. Micro. **42**, 839-840.

Vahle, J.L., Haynes, J.S., Andrews, J.J. (1995). Experimental reproduction of *H. parasuis* infection in swine: clinical, bacteriologic and morphologic findings. J.Vet Diag. Invest. **7**, 476-480.

Vahle, J.L., Haynes, J.S., Andrews, J.J. (1997). Interaction of H. parasuis with nasal and tracheal mucosa following intranasal inoculation of cesarian derived colostrum deprived (CDCD) swine Can. J. Vet. Res. **61**, 200-206.

Tuberculosis

Definition

Tuberculosis rarely causes clinical disease but is a cause for the condemnation of carcases at slaughter when gross lesions are detected and is a potential risk to human health.

Incidence

The incidence has fallen in most developed countries, 0.7% US, 1989 and is now generally so low (0.21% US, 1995) that single infected farms can cause an appreciable rise in cases. Where *M.bovis* and *M.tuberculosis* are controlled in cattle and human populations (UK, US) the incidence of infection with these organisms is very low, but in some parts of Spain, free-living wild boar and the Iberian pig may be infected. Infections with the *M.avium-intracellulare* complex are more common, and reflect environmental exposure.

218

Aetiology

A wide range of mycobacteria has been associated with tuberculosis in pigs. Infections with the *M.tuberculosis:bovis* group and the infections with *M.avium*, its subspecies and *M.intracellulare* are most important for public health. Species can be identified by their DNA sequences and species such as *M. porcinum* and subspecies such as *M.avium* subsp *hominisuis* have now been identified. The organisms are acid alcohol fast, waxy bacteria which can be demonstrated easily in tissue and can be cultured by specialist laboratories.

Pathogenesis

Infection is generally oral and lesions may first be detected histologically in mesenteric and submandibular lymph nodes after 14 days. More often they require 6-10 weeks or even 90-115 days (some *M.avium* strains) Antibodies are produced early in infection but immunity to infection is cell-mediated.

Clinical signs

These are usually only seen in generalised tuberculosis and usually result from infection with mammalian tuberculosis infections such as *M.bovis*. The incubation period is at least 6-12 weeks after which loss of weight, chronic pneumonia or local sinus formation may be seen. Chronic diarrhoea has been recorded in enteric infections. Most infections are only detected at slaughter.

Humane slaughter is indicated when chronic wasting is identified, but infected animals are often destroyed for legislative reasons if detected in life.

Pathology

External changes such as sinuses may be obvious, but the principal findings are whitish or yellowish granulomatous lesions which may be calcified. They may be generalised in submandibular, bronchial and mesenteric lymph nodes, lungs, liver, spleen and kidney and may reach 1-2 cm in diameter, sometimes becoming calcified or necrotic centrally. *M.bovis* and *M.intracellulare* are mainly associated with this type of distribution. Grey, firm, translucent miliary lesions 1-2mm in diameter may be present in the early stages of systemic disease.

Localised tuberculosis usually occurs only in the pharyngeal, cervical and mesenteric lymph nodes. The lesions vary between small yellowish-white caseous lesions and generalised enlargement of the node. Granulomata are often fleshy and are rarely calcified, although calcified lesions are regularly found in Spanish wild boar infected with *M.bovis*. Experimental infections with *M.avium* suggest that infection often occurs at about 8 weeks of age to produce the type of lesions seen at slaughter. 6-10 weeks after infection multinucleate giant cells develop and are the most prominent feature of lesions from twelve weeks onwards. Diffuse infiltrations of epithelioid cells predominate with some caseation and by 18 weeks, encapsulation, necrosis fibrosis and caseation are common. Acid-fast organisms may be seen but may be sparse in some cases.

Epidemiology

Infections with avian bacteria usually originate from infected poultry infections or from contamination of feeders, etc. with bird droppings containing the bacilli. Gross lesions may take at least 85 days to develop. *M.intracellulare, M. avium* and *M. fortuitum* infections appear to have originated in sawdust, peat or kaolin in some outbreaks and are not readily transmitted from pig to pig. In some cases these infections take place in the farrowing house and may also be associated with peat given to piglets. Water may be infected on some farms and *M. xenopi* has been recorded in such incidents. *M. avium* isolates from pigs do not appear to be the same as those found in human infections although the same serotypes are present, restriction endonuclease analysis suggests they are different.

M.bovis infections arise from contact with tuberculous cattle or access to infected milk and may spread from pig to pig. Infection in wild boar has been identified in several parts of Europe and this poses a risk to outdoor pigs as may infection in badgers and the increasing population of wild boar in Britain.

M.avium paratuberculosis infection has been associated with contact with cattle.

All mycobacteria can persist in the environment and flies of a number of species have been found to carry the organisms.

Diagnosis

Tuberculosis is usually detected at slaughter or the post-mortem examination of wasted pigs. Lesions suspected of being tuberculous (granulomas, chronic pneumonia) can be confirmed as such by demonstration of the organism in smears by Ziehl Neelsen staining. Histological examination confirms the granulomatous nature of the lesions and acid-fast (ZN+ve) organisms may be seen. The organism may be demonstrated by culture in specialist laboratories. Mycobacteria are Category 3 pathogens in the EU and may only be grown in registered laboratories and identified to species. These laboratories can now use the polymerase chain reaction (PCR) to identify mycobacterial DNA in tissue or clinical and environmental samples and DNA probes to identify mycobacteria in histological sections. Tuberculosis must be notified to the veterinary authorities in most countries as it is a zoonosis (Bovine Tuberculosis, UK under the Tuberculosis Orders 2006).

ELISA tests have been developed to detect serum antibodies to recombinant mycobacterial proteins but are not yet widely used. Intradermal tuberculin testing may be used on a herd basis with either mammalian or avian tuberculins given intradermally on the ear. Pigs may be negative 6 weeks after infection but positive at 12 weeks. Desensitisation may occur in late cases.

Treatment

Treatment is technically possible for valuable individuals (e.g. rifampicin) but is not practised commercially.

Control

Remove sources of infective material e.g. sawdust or kaolin and prevent access by birds. Pasteurise peat used for piglets. Affected carcases may still be found at slaughter until unexposed stock reach slaughter age. Where *M.bovis* is involved, skin or ELISA testing may reveal infected animals which may be culled. Ensure separation of outdoor pigs from areas contaminated by wild boar or other infected wildlife. Carcases for human consumption may be heat treated.

220

References

Acland, H.M. and Whitlock, R.H. (1986). *M.avium* serotype 4 infection of swine: The attempted transmission by contact and the sequence of morphological changes in inoculated pigs. J.Comparative Pathology **96**, 247-266.
Charette, R., Martineau, G.P., Pigeon, C., Turcotte, C., Higgins, R. (1989). An outbreak of granulomatous lymphadenitis due to *M.avium* in swine. Can.Vet.J. **30**, 675-678.
Klausen, J., Giese, S.B., Fuursted, K., Ahrens, P. (1997). Distribution of serotypes, IS901 and a 40kDa protein in *M. avium* complex strains isolated from man and animals in Denmark. Acta Path. Microbiol. et Immunol. Scand. **105**, 277-282.
Lysons, R.L. (1992). Pigs, peat and avian tuberculosis. Pig Vet.J. **29**, 193-197.
Windsor, R.S., Durrant, D.S. and Burn, K. (1984). Avian tuberculosis in pigs: *M.intracellulare* infection in a breeding herd. Vet.Rec. **114**, 497-500.
Parra, A., Fernandez-Lario, P., Tato, A., Larrasa, J., Garcia, A., Alonso, J.M., Hermoso de Mendoza, M., Hermoso de Mendoza, J. (2003). Epidemiology of *Mycobacterium bovis* infections of pigs and wild boars using a molecular approach. Vet.Micro **97**, 123-133.

Exudative epidermitis (Greasy Pig Disease)

Definition

An acute generalised dermatitis of piglets, characterised by the sudden onset of excess sebaceous secretion and exudation from the skin without pruritis, leading to dehydration, growth depression and death. Infected skin lesions may occur in adults.

Incidence

Sporadic (16.5% herds, UK 1994) but can cause appreciable losses in non-immune herds (35% during the period of the outbreak, 9% over the year in one outbreak). Infection occurs world wide and has been reported from countries in all continents.

Aetiology

Caused by *Staphylococcus hyicus*, which forms non-haemolytic, white, 2 mm colonies on blood agar, pink colonies on MacConkey agar and is coagulase-negative but DNAase positive. It produces capsules, Protein A and pathogenic strains produce an exfoliative toxin of M.W. 29-30 kDa of which at least 4 antigenic types exist (ExhA, ExhB, ExhC, ExhD). At least 6 serotypes and a large number of phage types of the organism exist. The organism is resistant to drying but does not form spores and is readily inactivated by heat. It is sensitive *in vitro* to many antibiotics including penicillins, fluoroquinolones, trimethoprim sulphonamide and cephalosporins. Resistance to these can occur. Toxigenic *S. chromogenes* producing ExhB has also caused the condition.

Pathogenesis

Infection with *S.hyicus* often follows abrasions produced by scratches, bites or rough bedding, e.g. sawdust or rough concrete flooring. Fodder or mange mites may act as irritating agents in the development of the disease. Application of cultures to the skin of gnotobiotic or SPF piglets results in infection and similar lesions can be produced by the subcutaneous injection of culture filtrates containing the exfoliative toxin. Pathogenic strains are encapsulated and resist phagocytosis.

The exfoliative toxins digest desmoglein, which maintains epidermal cell adhesion, and rounding of epidermal epithelial cells occurs within 12 hours of infection and lesions progress with exfoliation (shedding) of epithelial cells, crust formation, exocytosis i.e. neutrophil accumulation in the epidermis, formation of vesicles, formation of pustules and acanthosis. The gross changes of skin reddening are associated with inflammation and excess sebaceous secretion. Microcolonies of *S.hyicus* are present in the skin and a neutrophil response occurs followed by erosion down to the stratum germinativum in some areas. Affected piglets die from dehydration and sometimes from loss of protein. Immunity (either passive or active) protects against the homologous phage type or serotype.

Clinical signs

The disease commonly occurs in piglets of between 7 days and 5 weeks of age. The clinical signs begin with listlessness, a dulling of the skin and the appearance of thin, pale brown flecks or scales on the skin surface. There is often scabbing of the cheeks or knees due to fighting or kneeling on rough floors. Within 3-5 days the scabs become darker in colour and extend over much of the back and discolour the abdomen and axillae. The skin surface becomes covered with exudate which gives it a greasy texture and which matts the hair. There is no pruritis. Bacterial multiplication and dirt caught in the scabs soon give the skin a black colour. Affected animals lose weight rapidly and eventually die, often with a grossly thickened, wrinkled skin. Death normally occurs within 5-10 days. Recovery occurs by healing of the scabs, but takes at least 10 days. Fever is usually absent. Exudative epidermitis usually only affects a few litters on a farm and may not affect all the animals in any one litter. The disease affects younger pigs most severely and up to 90% of those affected may die. When affected piglets are weaned into flat decks with rough surfaces or humid atmospheres, infection may occur and persist in successive batches. Localised lesions may occasionally be seen on older pigs such as gilts or sows as 1-2 cm patches of greasy exudate or areas of ulceration usually on the back or rump, or, possibly in flank lesions. The organism has been incriminated (with trauma and a streptococcus) in ear necrosis and with PCV2, in abortion. It has been identified as a major cause of arthritis in young pigs in Australia.

Humane slaughter is only indicated in young pigs. Piglets with extensive chronic lesions and loss of condition should be destroyed, particularly if they cannot suck.

Pathological findings

At post-mortem examination, pigs are found to be dehydrated and emaciated and the superficial lymph nodes are normally oedematous and swollen. There is usually no food present in the bowel and a white or yellowish-white precipitate may be found in the pelvis of the kidney. Hypertrophy of the sebaceous glands and inflammatory changes are seen in histological sections of the skin. Rete pegs are prominent and microabscesses can be seen in the keratinised layers. Bacteriological examination of the skin usually yields a profuse growth of the staphylococcus and it may also be recovered from the enlarged lymph nodes, and, in some cases from the kidneys or from aborted foetuses. Non-specific organisms may be present in the parenchymatous organs and organisms such as *Pseudomonas aeruginosa* occur in older skin lesions. *Dermatophilus* spp. have been recovered from some lesions.

222

Epidemiology

The disease is introduced to clean herds by infected carriers and first occurs in litters in contact with those of carrier sows. The latter remain unaffected. Infection may persist in improperly cleaned farrowing pens and may even persist in local lesions on older pigs caused by mange or harvest mites. In improperly ventilated flat decks the disease may spread from mildly affected animals and infection may remain on fittings. The progeny of non immune recently purchased gilts are susceptible in a herd where the disease is enzootic. Outbreaks are normally self-limiting lasting 2-3 months but may persist for 12-18 months. *S.hyicus* has been identified on a number of species such as cattle and horses but their role, as sources of disease for pigs, is as yet unknown.

Diagnosis

Diagnosis is normally made on the basis of the clinical signs, and this condition in piglets must be distinguished from parakeratosis (age), swine pox (discrete scabby lesions), dermatosis vegetans (Landrace pigs only) and from mange and other mite infestations (no pruritis). The location of the lesions, their non-circular nature and the age incidence differentiate them from ringworm. Post-mortem and bacteriological findings may provide confirmation. Staphylococci isolated from the lesions may be identified as *S.hyicus* by biochemical tests (such as the API staph system) but virulence, toxin and phage typing is only experimental at present. Multiplex PCR testing can determine the toxin type. In older animals ringworm may resemble the lesions, as may bites, injections, abscesses and abrasions.

Treatment

Early cases may be treated successfully using amoxycillin, ampicillin, fluoroquinolone, ceftiofur and trimethoprim sulphonamide. Lincomycin, tylosin (8mg/kg) and erythromycin were effective at one time but recent sensitivity data suggests that resistance may occur. Affected piglets should be given access to fluid replacers and washed in a solution of cetrimide (Hibitane, Zeneca) or other mild disinfectant. Injections may need to be repeated daily for 2-3 days. Antimicrobial resistance can be present or arise after prolonged treatment.

Control

The disease may be controlled by clipping the teeth of litters at risk, by providing soft bedding, e.g. chaffed straw and removing sharp wood shavings if present. Hygiene, washing of sows into farrowing houses and local treatment of lesions on sows may all reduce infection. Segregation of infected animals before placing in flat decks prevents outbreaks in that type of accommodation and separate airspaces may be helpful as the organism may spread by aerosol. Thorough cleaning and disinfection of accommodation should be carried out between farrowings. Emergency vaccines (autogenous bacterins) have been used to reduce the duration of outbreaks in piglets by sow vaccination and by the vaccination of piglets when infection occurs at weaning. Vaccines made from one strain may cease to work if another virulent strain (exfoliative toxin type, serotype or phage type) is present in the herd or colonises it. Vaccines only protect against the homologous strain.

References

Andresen, L.O. (1998). Differentiation and distribution of three types of exfoliative toxin produced by *S. hyicus* from pigs with exudative epidermitis. FEMS Immunol. Med. Microbiol. **20**, 301-310.

Andresen, L.O., Ahrens, P., (2004). A multiplex PCR for detection of genes encoding exfoliative toxins from *S. hyicus*. J.Appl. Micro. **96**, 1265-1270.

Hill, B.D., Corney, B.G., Wagner, T.M. (1996). Importance of *S. hyicus* subsp *hyicus* as a cause of arthritis in pigs up to 12 weeks of age. Aust. Vet. J. **73**, 179-181.

Sato, H., Tanabe, T., Kuramoto, M., Tanaka, K., Hashimoto, T., Saito, H. (1991). Isolation of exfoliative toxin from *S.hyicus* subsp. *hyicus* and its exfoliative activity in the piglet. Vet.Micro. **27**, 263-275.

Wegener, H.C., Watts, J.L., Salmon, S.A., Yancey, R.J. (1994). Antimicrobial susceptibility of *S. hyicus* isolated from exudative epidermitis in pigs. J Clin. Micro. **32**, 793-795.

Other Staphylococci

S.aureus is the other common pathogenic staphylococcus to be isolated from pigs and can be distinguished from *S.hyicus* biochemically. *S.aureus* can be isolated from swollen ears, umbilical abscesses, vegetative endocarditis, subcutaneous abscesses, foot lesions, arthritis, mastitis, metritis and from enteritis. *S.aureus* strains are known to produce enterotoxin but it has not yet been associated with any specific type of enteritis. Apart from the presence of creamy pus there are few features other than bacterial isolation which lead to suspicion of infection with this organism. *S.aureus* is often sensitive to penicillin, streptomycin, trimethoprim sulphonamide but may be resistant to any of these. A wide variety of other staphylococci have been recorded in pigs but *S.hyicus* is the most important.

Spirochaetal granuloma

Localised areas of ulceration with a blackened weeping crust may occur on the lower margin and tips of the ears and on the neck nearby. Spirochaetes may be seen in smears made from the lesions. Parenteral or local treatment with tetracycline is usually effective.

Swine Erysipelas

Definition

An infectious condition of pigs caused by *Erysipelothrix rhusiopathiae* and characterised clinically by sudden death, fever associated with characteristic diamond skin lesions, arthritis or vegetative endocarditis and by abortion in pregnant sows.

Incidence

Clinical disease is commonly seen in pigs in extensive conditions and strawyards but is less common in housed animals. It is found worldwide. Considered enzootic on 14% farms UK 1994 and re-emerged as a problem in the US MidWest in 2001..

Aetiology

E.rhusiopathiae is a slender, slightly curved aerobic Gram-positive rod forming I mm greyish translucent non haemolytic colonies on blood agar after 24-48 hours incubation. Different colonial types of *E.rhusiopathiae* may be distinguished and at least 28 different antigenic types exist. In general, strains forming smooth colonies and those of antigenic types 1 and 2 are most commonly isolated from the septicaemic form of the disease. "Rough" strains are generally considered to be less virulent. Virulent strains produce a capsule which resists phagocytosis and some produce neuraminidase. Recently the species has been subdivided by DNA relatedness into 2 new species which reflect biochemical and serological characters. *E.rhusiopathiae* comprises serotypes 1, 2, 4, 5, 6, 8, 9, 11, 12, 15, 16, 17, 19, 21 and N and *E.tonsillarum* comprises serotypes 3, 7, 10, 14, 20, 22 and 23 with serotypes 13 and 18 intermediate between them. Some isolates identified as *E. tonsillarum* on serological grounds have proved to be *E. rhusiopathiae* by multilocus enzyme electrophoresis. The organism can live for months or years in animal tissue at +4°C, in frozen materials and is relatively resistant to drying and 0.2% phenol but is sensitive to penicillin, some other antimicrobials and to heat (15 minutes at 60°C).

Pathogenesis

E.rhusiopathiae is present in soil contaminated with faeces and urine from affected or carrier animals and is present on the tonsils of normal animals. Invasion of the susceptible pig by *E.rhusiopathiae* may occur in certain circumstances, especially during hot, muggy weather or in particular fields or buildings. Entry may be through the tonsils, gastrointestinal tract or through minute skin abrasions. In experimental transmission studies, clinical disease has followed the inoculation of scarified skin more repeatably than intravenous or subcutaneous inoculation with pure cultures.

Once invasion has taken place, multiplication proceeds and results in a septicaemia within 1-7 days of infection. Erysipelothrix produces a 64 kDa surface protective antigen (Spa) which appears to protect it against phagocytosis. Septicaemia may be sufficiently severe to cause acute clinical signs or even death, but usually results in fever with subsequent localisation of the organism in the skin, joints or the muscle or valves of the heart to give rise to the chronic form of the disease. The joint lesions begin with an acute synovitis and progress through a fibrinous exudation to a fibrosis. Synovial villous hypertrophy is severe and polypoid, there is diffuse erosion of articular cartilage and the draining lymph node is often enlarged. In the later stages antigen may still be demonstrable but cultivation is difficult. Heart lesions also begin with early inflammatory changes. Abortion appears to be due to fever but the organism has been isolated from foetuses and congenital erysipelas has been recorded. The organism may be found in the anterior vagina in some circumstances. The organism produces a neuraminidase which may be responsible for the changes. Antibody develops to the serotype of organism involved but cannot eliminate the organism from arthritic joint or valvular endocarditis lesions.

Clinical signs

Hyperacute, acute and chronic forms of the disease occur.

Hyperacute form. Sudden death may occur or affected pigs of 55-80 kg. liveweight may be found to be dull, collapsed with a high temperature (41.1-42.8°C, 106-109°F) and often show a scarlet flush on the skin. This form is uncommon in adults.

Acute form. The signs of acute erysipelas vary with the age and the immune status of the animal. In younger pigs such as gilts, fattening pigs and young boars, anorexia, high fever of 41.1-42.2°C, 106-108°F is common and there may be flushing or blotching of the skin and ears. Affected animals may die within 12-48 hours with cyanosis of the ears and body and with dyspnoea. In older pigs, anorexia and thirst are most commonly noted and a high temperature is found. Affected animals may be dull and may be reluctant to move. Piglets may rarely have lesions, but appear relatively normal when infected. Disease in wild boar may be of the acute, cyanotic/congestive type – skin lesions are difficult to detect.

The pathognomonic diamond skin lesions appear within 24-48 hours of the onset of clinical signs. At first they can only be palpated as raised patches along the back or neck but, later, in white pigs, they take on an angry, purplish-red colour. Abortion may occur at this stage in pregnant sows, temporary infertility may develop in boars (possibly a temperature effect) and sows may return to service.

Chronic form. Affected animals may recover completely, but the skin lesions may become necrotic, turn black and slough. The tips of the ears may also be lost. Localisation of the bacteria in the joints may occur and the elbow, hip, back, stifle and knee joints may be affected. Affected joints become hot and painful to the touch but become swollen and firm after 2-3 weeks and may stiffen. Affected pigs become lame and may lose condition.

Valvular lesions may develop in the heart and give rise to a murmur. Sudden death or signs of congestive heart failure, cyanosis, tachycardia, tachypnoea and murmur may occur later, the latter occurring commonly at farrowing in older sows.

Humane destruction is not indicated in acute cases due to the excellent response to treatment but is indicated where chronic arthritis causes severe lameness or ataxia and in chronic congestive heart failure with cyanosis and a subnormal temperature.

Pathological findings

Gross lesions

a.   Hyperacute, Congestion of the carcase and discolouration of the skin may be seen but no specific lesions are present.

b.   Acute. The skin may show purplish discolouration and the ears may be cyanosed. Diamond skin lesions may present. Congestion of the carcase is common and there may be enlargement of the spleen. Lymph nodes may be haemorrhagic and swollen, and ecchymoses may be present under the kidney capsule, pleura, peritoneum and on the heart.

c.   Chronic. Affected pigs may have necrotic skin lesions or enlarged joints. A non-suppurative proliferative arthritis may be found in the limb and intervertebral joints in which thickening of the joint capsule and tags of granulation tissue may be seen. These changes are preceded by inflammatory synovitis and may be followed by erosion of the articular cartilage and ankylosis.

Lesions of an embolic nature may be found in other organs and large granular vegetations may occur on the heart valves.

Histological Lesions

Specific histological features are absent. The vegetations on the heart valves are composed of granulation tissue and connective tissue. The synovial lesions are filled with macrophages and lymphocytes with proliferation of the synovial membrane.

E.rhusiopathiae may be seen as a short, fine Gram-positive bacillus in smears made from heart blood. It can usually be cultured from heart blood, spleen or bone marrow (a long bone is best) in hyperacute and acute cases. Examination of local lesions, e.g. synovial fluid or vegetations may be necessary in chronic cases, but E.rhusiopathiae cannot always be isolated from these. Fluorescent antibody may be used to identify the organism in tissue and may demonstrate E.rhusiopathiae antigen in sites such as joints from which the organism cannot be isolated. Recent methods which release organisms from chondrocytes have improved isolation.

Epidemiology

E.rhusiopathiae is commonly recovered from the tonsils of clinically normal pigs and from other parts of their bodies. It may also be recovered from the ground on farms where clinical disease has occurred. The association with hot weather, viral infection, fatigue, pregnancy and vaccination may be circumstantial. It is now thought that immunity to the local strain of organism is present and that the introduction of susceptible pigs to a contaminated environment, e.g. newly purchased gilts or the introduction of a new strain - with pigs or in fish meal in which E.rhusiopathiae is common may be the cause of outbreaks.

Affected pigs shed the organism in faeces and urine and it can survive on the ground for long periods although there is as yet no evidence for its multiplication in soil. It appears to survive for about 7 days in slurry when distributed on soil. Many birds and mammals may be infected with this organism, and provide a reservoir of infection for the pig population.

Outbreaks of disease are most common amongst pigs kept in poor conditions, in yarded sows, fatteners in irregularly cleaned pens and in batches of recently purchased gilts, especially in hot weather. Recovered animals retain lifelong immunity to the local strain, but remain carriers of E.rhusiopathiae for life. Vaccination may not protect against all 32 serotypes and disease may therefore occasionally occur in vaccinates, although vaccines from types 1 or 2 have recently been shown to protect against serotype 10 (E.tonsillarum).

E.rhusiopathiae commonly (20-50%) contaminates pork and infections in slaughtermen, veterinarians, abattoir workers and butchers are common. The disease in man is known as erysipeloid and is usually localised as inflammation and swelling of a finger.

Diagnosis

Erysipelas should be considered if a high fever of 41.1°C, 106°F or more is found in any fattening or adult pig which has gone off its feed and shows no respiratory signs. The development of the pathognomonic skin lesions in one of an affected group of animals is sufficient to confirm the diagnosis, and erysipelas should be considered in cases where lameness and fever occur together. Sows in difficulties and with fever at farrowing may also be affected.

If post-mortem examination is necessary, a reliable diagnosis can only be made after bacteriological examination in the absence of the pathognomonic skin lesions. Spleen, kidney and a long bone should be submitted for examination and joint fluid, synovial membrane and chondrocytes may also aid diagnosis. Freezing the organ and thawing may improve the isolation rate as may homogenising in serum broth with neomycin, kanamycin and vancomycin. Serological tests for infection in recovered animals are unreliable although a rising titre in an agglutination test using the homologous serotypes and performed with suitable controls is diagnostic. High levels of antibody may be present in joint fluid. The complement fixation test has recently been shown to be reliable. ELISAs have been developed but also requires appropriate antigens such as the Spa antigen or antigen from Serotype 2 which appears capable of detecting antibody to most serotypes. PCRs have been constructed which are both genus-specific and species-specific and these may be used directly on tissue or after enrichment culture to detect the organism.

Treatment

Penicillin is the drug of choice and the response to treatment is normally rapid. It is advisable to give 2 or 3 daily injections to prevent relapse or the persistence of the organism to give chronic infection. Tylosin, amoxicillin, ceftiofur and danofloxacin can all be used. Hyperimmune serum is commercially available for treatment in some countries, but is more expensive than doses of antibiotic. If used, it should be given intraperitoneally or intravenously at the stated dose.

Control

As *E.rhusiopathiae* is widespread in the environment and is carried by clinically normal pigs, its total elimination is not practicable. However, it is advisable to clean out and disinfect the pens of affected animals as high concentrations of virulent bacteria may be present.

Control is normally exercised by prophylaxis and this takes the form of preventing the spread of outbreaks to other susceptible or in contact animals by prophylactic injections of penicillin (short term protection) or hyperimmune serum (medium term protection, about 6 weeks). The latter is of particular value in preventing disease in finishing pigs which will soon be marketed, but the product is no longer available in the UK.

Vaccination is commonly employed to prevent clinical swine erysipelas in breeding stock and in young fattening pigs over 12 weeks of age on farms which have an erysipelas problem. Most commercially available vaccines are formolised whole cultures and include an adjuvant. Vaccination is normally practised in recently weaned pigs (fattener protection) and in gilts or sows before service or, to prevent conception problems soon after farrowing. Immunity lasts for 6 months and regular re-vaccination should be practised. The vaccination of pregnant animals is not recommended with some dead vaccines and all live ones. All boars should be vaccinated at 6 month intervals. Vaccine breakdowns may occur if a serotype with sufficient antigenic divergence from the vaccine is encountered. Some vaccines prepared from serotypes 1 and 2 (those most common in acute disease and belonging to *E.rhusiopathiae*) can protect against serotype 10 (*E.tonsillarum*) but have not been tested against serotype 20.

Vaccines containing serotypes 2 and 10 protect against both *E.rhusiopathiae* and *E.tonsillarum*. Successful vaccination has been carried out using the Surface protective antigen (Spa) produced during log phase, both as native protein and as arecombinant vaccine in a *Lactococcus lactis* vector.

Prevention of human exposure from meat is now required in the EU and carcases with lesions should be destroyed. If detected ante-mortem, it is permissible to keep the animal until safe. As this takes at least 15 days, regulations about holding and moving pigs can be breached.

References

Franz, B., Davis, M.E., Horner, A. (1996). Localisation of viable bacteria and bacterial antigens in arthritic joints of *E.rhusiopathiae*-infected pigs. FEMS Immunol. Med. Microbiol. **12**, 137-142.

Johnston, K.M. Doige, C.E. and Osborne, A.D. (1987). An evaluation of non-suppurative joint disease in slaughter pigs. Can.Vet.J. **28**, 174-180.

Makino, S.I., Okada, Y., Marayama, T., Ishikawa, K., Takahashi, T., Nakamura, M., Ezaki, T., Morita, H. (1994). Direct and rapid detection of *E.rhusiopathiae* DNA in animals by PCR. J. Clin. Microbiol. **32**, 1526-1531.

Molen, G., Soderlind, O., Ursing, J., Norring, V., Ternstrom, A., Lowenhiels, C. (1989). Occurrence of *E.rhusiopathiae* on pork and in pig slurry and the distribution of specific antibodies in abattoir workers. J.Appl.Bact. **67**, 347-352.

Takahashi, T., Fujisawa T., Tamura, Y., Suzuki, S., Muramatsu, M., Sawada, T., Mitsuoka, T. (1992). DNA relatedness among *E.rhusiopathiae* strains representing all 23 serovars and *E.tonsillarum*. Int.J.Syst.Bact. **42**, 469-473.

Timoney, J.F., Groschup, M.M. (1993). Properties of a protective protein of *E.rhusiopathiae*. Vet.Micro. **37**, 381-387.

Yamazaki, Y., Sato, H., Sakakura, H., Shigeto, K., Nakano, K., Saito, H., Maehara, N. (1999). Protective activity of the purified protein antigen of E. rhusiopathiae in pigs. J.Vet. Med. Series B. **46**, 47-55.

Streptococcus suis infections

Infections with *Streptococcus suis* cause septicaemia, arthritis (joint ill) and meningitis in sucking piglets and in recently weaned growing pigs but less commonly in finishing pigs. The organism is found in bronchopneumonia.

Streptococcal infection of young pigs (Joint III)

Definition

A condition of young piglets 7-14 days of age in which septicaemia may cause death or local infections such as meningitis, arthritis or endocarditis.

Incidence

Worldwide.

Aetiology

Most infections are associated with *S.suis* type I but infection with *S.suis* type 2 may also occur in this age group. *S.suis* is described below.

Pathogenesis

Infection is by aerosol, ingestion or contact and invasion may take place through the tonsils (see *S.suis* type 2 below). Bacteraemia may lead to septicaemia or localisation in joints, meninges or heart valves. Animals recover but may remain chronically infected.

Clinical signs

The disease is seen in piglets of 10-14 days of age. Affected animals cease to thrive, become rough-coated and may die. Fever (40.6-41.1°C, 105-106°F) may be present. Later, enlarged, hot, painful joint swellings may be seen or the animals may appear stiff and may be blind or show muscular tremors ending in ataxia or death. Sudden death may occur in endocarditis due to streptococcal infection. Typically, up to 2/3rd of the litter may be affected with one or another form of the disease. Affected pigs rarely recover completely.

Affected piglets respond to treatment, so humane destruction should be carried out on those with paralysis or ataxia after meningitis only when treatment has failed and on chronically stunted or arthritic animals.

Post mortem findings

Few lesions are seen in the septicaemic phase, but a purulent meningitis may be seen where brain involvement occurs and in arthritis the joints are swollen by mucoid synovial fluid and inflamed. In endocarditis, the organisms are a major feature of the histological lesion on the valves. They may be demonstrated by culture and in smears.

Epidemiology

Infection may arise from carrier sows, infected animals within the same airspace (by contact, ingestion or aerosol) and by transfer on needles used for routine injections. Infection may remain in uncleaned accommodation.

Diagnosis

The characteristic spectrum of clinical signs and the age of the affected pigs (10-21 days) is normally sufficient. Bacteriological examination of joint fluid, blood or post-mortem specimens will confirm and distinguish the condition from *H.parasuis* infections.

Treatment and control

Parenteral antibiotic such as penicillin, ampicillin or trimethoprim: sulphonamide for 3-5 days is most satisfactory. Animals with advanced septicaemia, meningitis and arthritis rarely respond and must be nursed by giving milk supplement and water by stomach tube.

Control may be possible in herds with the disease by farrowing sows in isolation and by fumigating the accommodation between animals. Where arthritis is associated with knee damage on floors, additional bedding may prevent the development of the condition. Injection of piglets at birth with long-acting penicillin may prevent disease. Inactivated vaccines have been prepared and used on sows to provide passive immunity to piglets but are often effective only against the homologous strain.

Epidemic streptococcal meningitis

Definition

An epidemic disease of weaned and fattening pigs which occurs after mixing and moving, resulting in sudden death, fever, nervous signs or, in younger pigs, arthritis. Bronchopneumonia is being identified increasingly.

Incidence

Present in all countries of Western Europe, the United States, Canada, Australasia and the Far East. Type 2 is most common worldwide, but changes in distribution may occur and affect the clinical picture in a country as when type 14 became more widespread in the UK.

Aetiology

S. suis is a weakly ß-haemolytic streptococcus which forms clear greyish mucoid colonies 1-2 mm in diameter on blood agar. The cells may appear boat-shaped and produce a polysaccharide capsule and have fimbriae. The capsule has been used to separate isolates into at least 35 serotypes. Virulent strains of *S.suis* type 2 appear to produce two specific proteins, the muramidase related protein MRP of 136 kDa and the extracellular factor (EF) of 110 kDa, and a thiol-activated haemolysin, suilysin. The capsular types appear to be related to DNA structure and 1-8 can be distinguished by restriction endonuclease analysis, although more than one REA type may occur within a serotype. *S. suis* survives in distilled water at 4°C for 1-2 weeks, in nutrient medium at 4°C for 9 months, is relatively resistant to heating, being destroyed only after 2 hours by heating to 50°C and after 10 minutes after heating at 60°C. It is sensitive to a wide range of antimicrobials but least so to aminoglycosides. Resistance has been reported.

Type 1 is consistently associated with piglet infections and type 2 is responsible for about 50% of all invasive infections in older pigs.

Pathogenesis.

S.suis type 2 infects pigs at or shortly after birth from maternal vaginal secretions, skin or tonsils or by aerosol or by contact within 5-25 days of mixing with carrier animals and can infect in the presence of antibody. The organism multiplies in the tonsillar crypts to which it may adhere by means of an adhesin and enters the circulation in some cases to give rise to a bacteraemia. It is taken up by both neutrophils and macrophages. The organism is protected from phagocytosis in macrophages by its polysaccharide capsule and multiplies to give a septicaemia within a few hours. This may kill the animal directly or organisms carried by macrophages may localise in the brain, joints or other areas to produce local lesions. In the brain these take the form of purulent meningitis which is frequently fatal. Otitis interna or media may develop. Immunity develops and includes opsonising antibody to the capsular polysaccharide antigen. Antigens which may be important include the adhesin/haemagglutinin, capsule, 94, 86 and 44 kDa proteins, haemolysin, MRP (136 kDa) and EF (110 kDa) which does not appear to be required for invasion. Deletion mutants suggest that haemolysin, capsule, MRP and EF may not be necessary for disease, although North American studies suggest that virulent strains there have at least some of the suilysin gene..

The organism may survive after clinical recovery in the tonsillar crypts or nose for up to 512 days.

Some serotypes are associated particularly with a particular clinical syndrome (serotype 14 with arthritis) and restriction endonuclease analysis suggests that serotype 2 organisms isolated from meningitis and bronchopneumonia belong to different REA types.

Clinical signs

The incubation period varies from 24 hours to 2 weeks or more. The first signs of an outbreak may be the death of a pig in a good condition. If the pig is seen alive, fever of 40.6-41.7°C, 105-107°F and evidence of septicaemia may be seen. Nervous signs such as incoordination, tremor, paralysis, paddling, opisthotonus and tetanic spasms may be seen in that order before death which may occur within 4 hours of the onset of the clinical signs. Some untreated animals with meningitis may not die. Animals developing the meningitis may be detected early in the condition by the glassy stare, flushed skin and their unsteady gait. Head tilt is sometimes present. Arthritis may occur in younger pigs and occasionally in gilts and sows, and bronchopneumonia may occur. The clinical signs of bronchopneumonia are not distinctive but include fever, raised respiratory rate and bronchial sounds. Disease may occur in animals of any age in susceptible herds but is most common in the 3-12 week age group in herds where the infection is enzootic but is not uncommon in animals up to 6 months of age. Mortality varies from 1-50% in any batch of pigs and in herds with enzootic infection may be 0.5% with 1% morbidity. In Canada, a syndrome has been reported in which neonatal disease is followed by death within 24 hours of birth.

Decisions about humane slaughter are commonly required in this condition. Affected pigs should be treated and their condition assessed after 3 days' treatment and nursing. Those unable to stand or feed themselves as a result of meningitis should be humanely destroyed, as should chronically stunted animals and those with severe chronic polyarthritis. Blind animals and those with head tilt can be left if properly managed.

Pathology

The skin and the carcase may be reddened, lymph nodes are often enlarged and congested and congestion of the parenchymatous organs is common. Fine strands of fibrin may be seen in the peritoneal and pleural cavities. Lung lesions are common in some outbreaks, varying from severe localised pleurisy to pneumonia with congestion and oedema of the interlobular septae. Gross oedema and congestion of the brain may be visible and the cerebrospinal fluid may be cloudy. The cerebellum may herniated through the foramen magnum. Purulent arthritis may be present in young pigs. Histological features of the meningitis include a polymorphonuclear leucocyte infiltration in the meninges and sometimes the ventricles. Cortical necrosis and spongiform changes in cerebellum and brain stem have been recorded. Neuritis of cranial nerves may occur. In treated pigs, the predominant cells in meningitis may be lymphocytes. The organisms may be seen in sections and isolated from the brain and from most organs in untreated animals. Vegetative endocarditis may also be present in chronically-affected animals.

In animals with enzootic pneumonia, *S.suis* type 2 may be isolated from a suppurative bronchopneumonia.

Epidemiology

S.suis infection is spread by contact and to a lesser extent by aerosol and ingestion. Most pigs become infected, but not all develop the disease. Lack of specific immunity is important, but intercurrent disease and environmental factors contribute to the initiation of disease. Once infected, the organism is rarely lost from a herd and more than one type or REA type may be present. Epidemic strains may remain for up to 2 years or change more frequently.

Overcrowding, poor ventilation and mixing of pigs from different litters appear to be predisposing features in a herd. There may be some increase in cases in Autumn and Winter. Although carrier sows may pass on infection to their litters, restriction endonuclease analysis confirms that spread can be both vertical and horizontal within a herd. S.suis persists in the tonsils and may be present in the carcases of slaughter pigs. It can survive in faeces for 104 days at $0^{\circ}C$, 10 days at $9^{\circ}C$ and 8 days at $22\text{-}25^{\circ}C$ and in dust for 54 days at $0^{\circ}C$, 25 days at $9^{\circ}C$ and for less than 24 hours at room temperature. Survival for 6 weeks at $4^{\circ}C$ and 12 days at $22\text{-}25^{\circ}C$ has been recorded in carcases. It is killed in less than a minute by recommended dilutions of most farm disinfectants. It survives on plastic and rubber both directly and in manure and in porcine body fluids. Fomites may contribute to the spread between pens.

Spread between farms is by means of carrier pigs although fomites such as clothing and hypodermic needles may also introduce the disease. S.suis has been isolated from wild boar and from other species but none have been confirmed as vectors nor as reservoir hosts.

Infection occurs in veterinarians, farmers, abattoir workers and butchers and, occasionally in housewives in whom it may cause a fatal meningitis or septicaemia. Antibody and pharyngeal carriage are more common than disease in the exposed human population.

Diagnosis

The clinical signs and post-mortem findings of S.suis infection, particularly the meningitis, are distinctive, but could be confused with those of H.parasuis infection. The organism can be demonstrated in smears of heart blood, C.S.F. or brain tissue, vegetative endocarditis and joint fluid by Gram stain or, more specifically, by immunofluorescence, immunoperoxidase or digoxigenin-tagged DNA probes and can be isolated from these sites in recently dead untreated animals. When sought from the tonsils, a gag should be used and the tonsillar crypts swabbed. The material from tonsillar and nasal swabs should be plated on agar supplemented with 5% horse serum, a selective medium for streptococci (Oxoid SR74, sodium azide, nalidixic acid colestin and crystal violet). and specific hyperimmune serum to the capsular polysaccharide. Halos of precipitate occur around S.suis colonies. Immunomagnetic separation techniques using polyclonal antisera and a species specific PCR have improved the sensitivity of detection.

Isolates may be identified as S.suis biochemically with API strep strips or using starch containing media flooded with iodine to detect amylase Colonies may be identified serologically using coagglutination or by PCR tests specific for types 1, 2 and 9, and then serotyped by capsular typing. Restriction endonuclease analysis patterns may also be used. More than 1 type may be present in a herd.

Serum antibody may be detected using ELISAs with antigens such as capsular polysaccharide but not all pigs are seropositive.

Treatment

Penicillin is the drug of choice in the parenteral treatment of the condition although amoxycillin, ampicillin, cephalosporins, trimethoprim sulphonamide and other antimicrobials may be used except for aminoglycosides such as streptomycin and the tetracyclines. Treatment should be repeated more than once and supportive therapy given. Affected pigs should be removed to a quiet pen and given water and food, by hand if necessary. Paralysed animals rapidly become dehydrated and should be rehydrated using saline given per rectum. Recovery may be faster in a cooler, dryer environment. Other pigs in affected pens may be injected individually or given water or feed medication as described below.

Resistance to penicillin has been described but resistance to ampicillin or amoxycillin is less common.

Control

This may be achieved by:-

1.   Medication

This may be strategic by means of long-acting penicillin given at birth and 10 days post weaning or at entry to the weaner housing or 7 days before the expected peak of the disease. Water medication should be given for 7 days before the expected peak and should be with ampicillin, amoxycillin or trimethoprim sulphonamide.

In-feed medication should be carried out with penicillin. The most effective penicillin and that which survives pelleting heat may be phenoxymethylpenicillin at 75-100 g/tonne although procaine penicillin at 200-300 g/tonne may be as good. Freshly medicated feeds should be used. Tilmicosin has also been used.

2.   Vaccination

Killed and adjuvanted inactivated vaccines are still under investigation and may at times protect completely against the homologous strain when piglets are vaccinated or, passively, after sow vaccination.   Failure of vaccine appears to be due to the use of an incorrect strain or serotype of the organism, and may occur when the dominant restriction endonuclease type is replaced by another after 6-12 months. The MRP and EF proteins, haemolysin, capsule and avirulent strains appear to be capable of producing some degree of protective immunity which is effective against heterologous strains, but no fully protective vaccine has yet been marketed in the UK (2006).

3.   Husbandry measures

Continuous production systems should be avoided, all-in all-out policies followed, batches should be mixed as little as possible and animals should be placed in clean, dry pens with a low slurry level and low humidity.

4.   Eradication

Treatment of herds, removal of carriers and internal isolation are not effective. Medicated early weaning may be effective, but segregated early weaning rarely prevents infection.

5.   Slaughter and restocking

Slaughter and farm disinfection to eliminate residual infection in faeces and dust followed by restocking with meningitis-free pigs is practicable. These can be produced by hysterectomy, by medicated early weaning or by purchase from clean herds.

References

Aarestrup, F.M., Jorsal, S.E., Jensen, N.E. (1998). Serological characterisation and antimicrobial susceptibility of *S. suis* isolates from diagnostic samples in Denmark during 1995 and 1996. Vet Microbiol. **60**, 59-66.

Amass, S.F., Clark, L.K., Wu, C.C. (1995). Source and timing of *S. suis* infection in neonatal pigs: implications for early weaning procedures. Swine Health and Production **3**, 189-193.

Busque, P., Higgins, R., Caya, F., Quessy, S. (1997). Immunisation of pigs against *S. suis* serotype 2 infection using a live avirulent strain. Can J. Vet. Res. **61**, 275-279.

Clifton-Hadley, F.A. and Alexander, T.J.L. (1980). The carrier site and carrier rate of *S.suis* type 2 in pigs. Vet. Rec . **107**, 40-41

Clifton-Hadley, F.A., Alexander, T.J.L., Upton, I. and Duffus, W.P.H. (1984).   Further studies on the subclinical carrier state of *S.suis* type 2 in pigs. Vet.Rec. **114**, 513-518.

Clifton-Hadley, F.A. and Enright, M.R. (1984). Factors affecting the survival of *S.suis* type 2. Vet.Rec. **114**, 584-586.

Gottschalk, M.G., Lacouture, S. (1998). Development of an immunomagnetic method for isolation of *S. suis* serotypes 2 and 1/2 from tonsils. Proc IPVS **15** (3), 158.

Gottschalk, M.G., Lacouture, S., Dubreuil, J.D. (1995). Characterisation of *S. suis* capsular type 2 haemolysin. Microbiol (Reading) **141**, 189-195.

Heath, P.J., Hunt, B.W., Duff, J.P., Wilkinson, J.D. (1996). S. suis serotype 14 as a cause of disease in the UK. Vet. Rec. **139**, 450-451.

Jacobs, A.A.C., Berg, A.J.G. van den, Loeffen, P.L.W. (1996). Protection of experimentally-infected pigs by suilysin, the thiol activated haemolysin of *S. suis*. Vet. Rec. **139**, 225-228.

Johnston, P.L., Henry, N., Boer, R. de., Braidwood, J.C. (1991). Phenoxymethyl penicillin potassium as an in-feed medication for pigs with streptococcal meningitis. Vet.Rec. **130**, 138-139.

McKellar, Q.A., Baxter, P., Taylor, D.J. and Bogan,   J.A.   (1987). Penicillin therapy of spontaneous streptococcal meningitis in pigs. Vet.Rec. **121**. 347-350.

Mogollon, J.D., Pijoan, C., Murtaugh, M., Collins, J.E. (1990). Use of genetic markers in the study of the epidemiology of *S.suis* in a swine herd. Proc. IPVS **11**, 168.

Rasmussen, S.R., Andresen, L.O. (1998). Development of a species-specific PCR assay for detection of *S. suis*. Proc IPVS **15** (2), 92

Sanford, S.E. (1987). Gross and histopathological findings in universal lesions caused by *S.suis* in pigs I and II. Can.J.Vet.Res. **51**, 481-485, 486-489.

Sanford, S.E. and Tilker, A.M.E. (1982). *S.suis* associated diseases in swine. Observations of a 1-year study. J.Am.Vet.Med.Assn. **181**, 673-676.

Thomas, E., Martin, G., voss, B., Boettner, A., Pommier, P., Loehlein, W., Hellmann, K. (2002). A comparative field study of the efficacy of cefquinome and amoxicillin against acute meningitis of weaned piglets. Pig J. **50**, 28-41.

Tikkanen, K., Haataja, S., Finne, J. (1996). The galactosyl (α 1-4) galactoe-binding adhesin of *S. suis* occurrence in strains of different haemagglutinating activity and induction of opsonic antibodies. Inf and Immun. **64**, 3659-3665.

Torremorell, M.P., Pijoan, C. (1998). Prolonged persistence of an epidemic *S. suis* strain in a closed pig population. Vet. Rec. **143**, 394-395.

Walsh, B., Williams, A.E., Satsangi, J. (1992). *S.suis* type 2: pathogenesis and clinical disease. Reviews in Med.Micro. **3**, 65-71.

Williams, D.M., Lawson, G.H.K., Rowland, A.C. (1973). Streptococcal infections in piglets. The palatine tonsil as a portal of entry for *S.suis*. Res.Vet.Sci. **15**, 352-362.
Windsor, R.S. (1977). Meningitis in pigs caused by *Streptococcus suis* Type II. Vet.Rec. **101**, 378-379.
Vecht, U., Wissenlink, H.J., Jellema, M.L., Smith, H.E. (1991). Identification of two proteins associated with virulence of *S.suis* type 2. Inf. & Immun. **59**, 3156-3162.

Streptococcal lymphadenitis, *S.porcinus* infection, Streptococcal abscess

S. porcinus infections cause abscesses particularly in the cervical lymph nodes of pigs in the US and occasionally in Eastern Europe.. The organisms have been identified in other countries but do not seen to cause the same lesions. At least 8 serotypes have been recorded, and infection is transmitted by contact, in drinking water, by scarification or by the ingestion of food contaminated by abscess discharge or infected faeces. Infection appears to cause disease most consistently in pigs aged 28 days or more. The incidence in the US is declining due to medication of feed and the use of inactivated alum adjuvanted vaccines. Most isolates belong to Lancefield's Group E, but P, U and V have also been recorded.

References

Lammler, C., Cirak, N., Smola, J. (1998). Studies on biochemical, serological and further characteristics of S. porcinus. J.Vet. Med. Series B, **45**, 235-243.
Miller, R.B. and Olson, L.D. (1983). Distribution of abscesses and shedder state in swine inoculated with Group E streptococci via routes other than oral. Am.J.Vet.Res. **44**, 937-944.
Miller, R.B. and Olson, L.D. (1983). Frequency of jowl abscesses in feeder and market swine exposed to Group E streptococcus as nursing pigs. Am.J.Vet.Res. **44**, 945-948.
Wood, R.L. and Wessman, G.E. (1984). Immune response of swine vaccinated with a Group E streptococcus whole culture bacterin, Am .J Vet.Res. **45**, 1033-1938.

Lancefield's Group C. and other ß-haemolytic streptococci.

ß-haemolytic streptococci of these groups and especially *S.dysgalactiae* subsp. *equisimilis* (Group C) are commonly isolated from the upper respiratory tract, pharynx, retropharyngeal lymph nodes and genital tract of carrier pigs. They are associated with vaginitis in sows and neonatal septicaemia in newborn piglet, may be isolated from arthritis and vegetative endocarditis in older animals and may be isolated from septicaemia and pneumonic lesions in older, fattening pigs. The bacteria are best isolated in anaerobic conditions and carrier animals may be detected not only by culture but by the demonstration of serum antistreptolysin O antibody.

They may be controlled in the same way as the other streptococci if they appear to give rise to problems on a farm. *S.equi* subsp. *zooepidemicus* has also been recorded.

Enterococcus durans infection

E.durans (Lancefield Gp.D) has been isolated from the intestines and faeces of 3-5 day old piglets with loose watery faeces and has been demonstrated adhering to the villous epithelium. Villous atrophy in the small intestine and epithelial shedding in the large intestine have been described. The condition should be considered when faecal culture or smears demonstrate that the faecal flora is almost entirely streptococcal. Some diarrhoeal isolates have now been grouped as *Enterococcus porcinus* and other adherent strains as *E. villosus*.

References

Cheon, D.S., Chae, C. (1996). Outbreak of diarrhoea associated with *E. durans* in piglets. J. Vet. Diagn. Invest. 8, 123-124.

Drolet, R., Higgins, R., Jacques, M. (1990). Med.Vet.du Quebec 20, 114-115, 118. L'enteropathie associee a *Enterococcus* (Streptococcus) *durans* chez le porcelet.

Anthrax

Caused by *Bacillus anthracis* and rare in pigs. Affected animals may die suddenly, pass bloody faeces or die after swelling of the neck. Recovery may occur. Transmissible to man.

Incidence

Worldwide, rare and sporadic in UK, more common in Southern USA, tropics.

Aetiology

B.anthracis is a large Gram-positive toxin-producing encapsulated rod which grows rapidly to produce large granular medusa-head colonies on a wide variety of media. It forms spores which are resistant to boiling and which persist for long periods (>50 years) in the soil. Sensitive to penicillin and other antimicrobials and to disinfectants such as formaldehyde and glutaraldehyde which kill the spores.

Pathogenesis

Infection is by ingestion and rarely by direct entry through abrasions or by aerosol. Infection in the pig may remain localised near the portals of entry (pharyngeal region and draining lymph nodes and intestine) or become generalised to give bacteraemia and septicaemia. Organisms resist phagocytosis by means of the polyglutamic acid capsule and affect tissue by means of the 3 toxins. Organisms may be shed in urine and faeces and in discharges/blood in dead animals. Recovery and solid immunity may occur but local skin necrosis may remain.

Clinical signs

Septicaemia, pharyngeal and intestinal forms of the disease occur, most commonly as a result of entry of the organism through the tonsils or pharyngeal mucosa.

Pharyngeal form. Oedema and swelling of the neck region associated with dyspnoea and, usually, a fever of up to 42°C, 107°F are the commonest signs noted. Depression, vomiting and inappetence may occur. Death usually follows within a day of the onset of cervical oedema. Blackening and necrosis of the skin over the affected area may occur during recovery.

Septicaemic form. This form is characterised by sudden death and may occur more frequently in young pigs. It is relatively uncommon.

Intestinal form. In some cases, the infection localises in the intestine and digestive disturbance, loss of appetite and the passage of bloody faeces may be seen. Death is uncommon in this form.

A proportion of animals may develop transient fever and then recover.

Severely affected animals should be killed for humane reasons where massive pharyngeal swelling leads to respiratory distress and when collapsed. Chronically affected animals with large areas of necrotic skin should also be destroyed. The disease can be treated but animals are often killed for regulatory reasons.

Post-mortem findings

If anthrax is suspected, the animal should only be opened in order to obtain material for the confirmation of diagnosis and the outbreak should be reported in the usual way. Samples of oedema fluid may be taken with a long needle. However, as the clinical signs of anthrax may be indistinct, and as the disease is an uncommon cause of sudden death in the pig, it may sometimes only be recognised at post-mortem.

Pharyngeal form. Oedema of the cervical region may be obvious when the trachea is exposed at post-mortem. Bloody or clear fluid may be present or the tissues may appear gelatinous. The mandibular and retropharyngeal lymph nodes are usually swollen and reddish in colour. Inflammatory changes of the pharyngeal mucosa may be seen.

Intestinal form. The intestinal mucosa may be covered in diphtheritic membrane and the walls may be thickened with fibrinous adhesions on the serous surface and swelling of the lymph nodes. Copious peritoneal fluid and peritoneal oedema may be present. There may be splenic infarcts.

Septicaemic form. The spleen may be enlarged, but little change may be evident. The carcase is congested and the kidney may be spotted with petechiae and may be pale in colour. The lymph nodes may be engorged.

In animals killed for diagnostic purposes or at slaughter, the changes may be less obvious and petechiation of the kidney, oedematous submandibular lymph nodes or excess blood stained peritoneal fluid may be the only findings.

Epidemiology

Anthrax is relatively rare in pigs, and is normally associated with the ingestion of contaminated feed containing meat or bone meals. Outbreaks may occur where pipeline feeding is practised, as the organism may multiply in the feed. Recovered animals may remain as carriers, and pig to pig transmission may occur. The organism dies out in an unopened carcase within a few days but persists if allowed to sporulate (air, 22°C). Spores persist in slurry, contaminated pens and on clothing and implements and can form a reservoir of infection. Other species may also be affected. Anthrax may affect and kill man.

It primarily affects those cutting carcases and less frequently affects workers in contact or consumers of meat.

Diagnosis

Anthrax may be suspected in life where the pharyngeal form or the haemorrhagic diarrhoea and fever occur. When a case is examined post-mortem, the pathological features described above should suggest anthrax. In known cases the carcase should not be opened and direct smears should be made from blood, but, if negative, any swelling of the neck should be incised and the cut surface of an affected lymph node used to make an impression smear. In the peritoneal cavity, the surface of organs e.g. kidney should be used especially if perirenal oedema or petechiation is present.

Smears should be heat fixed and stained with polychrome methylene blue. The square ended bacilli will be surrounded by a purple-staining capsule. At this stage the State Veterinary Service should be informed and any further samples will be handled by them. The isolation of the 3-5 mm greyish medusa head colonies from swabs or tissue confirms. Handling *B.arthracis* is permitted in the UK only in registered laboratories as it is a Category 3 pathogen.

Treatment

Anthrax responds to penicillin treatment and tetracyclines have been used parenterally and in feed and water.

Control

a)   Technical

The disease may be controlled by vaccination of animals at risk using the Anthrax spore vaccine coupled with medication of affected animals, disinfection with formaldehyde and burning or, formerly, deep burial of the carcases of affected animals. Slurry should also be disinfected and disposed of safely.

b)   Legal obligations

The disease is Notifiable in the UK and in the EU and is controlled by National legislation (Anthrax Orders, 1991, UK). Restrictions of movement and a supervised disposal and disinfection programme will be carried out. This may or may not require the slaughter of the herd.

c)   Commercial requirements

Modern abattoirs are unlikely to accept animals from affected farms and, with no slaughter outlet, the animals may have to be slaughtered after which whole farm disinfection can occur.

References

Edgington, A.B. (1990). An outbreak of anthrax in pigs : a practitioner's account. Vet.Rec. 127, 321-324.

Redmond, C., Hall, G.A., Turnbull, P.C.B., Gillgan, J.S. (1997). Experimentally-assessed public health risks associated with pigs from farms experiencing anthrax. Vet. Rec. 141, 244-247

Cystitis in sows

A group of syndromes associated with a number of different bacteria can be distinguished. One syndrome is, however, particularly striking and will be described separately.

Actinobaculum suis Cystitis and Pyelonephritis

Definition

A syndrome in which a small group of sows or gilts pass bloody purulent urine, often soon after service. They rapidly lose condition and die.

Incidence

Present in all major pig-rearing countries, infection is widespread in Britain (60-90% boars and hog pigs) but outbreaks of the disease are sporadic

Aetiology

Caused by *Actinobaculum suis*, a large Gram-positive rod which occurs in pathological material in characteristic clumps and palisades. Cells bear 2 types of pili. The organism can be cultured anaerobically on blood agar on which it forms dry colonies 2-3 mm in diameter after 3 days' incubation. It can however, be grown aerobically on urea-enriched medium. It is urease positive, liquefies gelatine and ferments maltose, xylose and starch.

Pathogenesis

The organism is widespread in the prepuce of boars and is introduced to the vagina at service but dies out within an hour in most cases. It does not appear capable of colonising the intact urinary bladder of the sow and infection disappears within 3 days of experimental infection in 30% cases. The organism can be isolated from the urine of clinically normal sows in a small number of cases. Colonisation of the bladder is most successful and leads to disease most consistently when pre-existing lesions or infections with organisms such as *E.coli* are present and have damaged the superficial epithelium. *A.suis* adheres to the bladder epithelium by means of pili and splits urea to produce ammonia and raise the pH of the urine to 9.0.

Inflammation of the bladder wall results with loss of epithelium and colonisation by goblet cells. After erosion of the uretero-vesicular valve, infection ascends the ureters and causes a pyelonephritis, tubular damage and uraemia. Inability to retain sodium leads to rises in plasma potassium and sudden death. Circulating antibody can be detected from 3 weeks after infection and lasts 4-9 months.

Clinical signs

In a typical outbreak, a small group of sows or gilts may die suddenly or be found ill, depressed, thirsty with hunched backs and passing blood stained, purulent urine with or without a vulval discharge. Clinical signs may be noted 2-3 weeks after service by a particular boar or may be delayed until farrowing. Affected sows frequently die. Mild cases may occur in which inappetence and vulval discharge is the only obvious sign. Animals with pyelonephritis can be identified by the presence of uraemia.

Humane slaughter should be carried out on chronically-affected animals in poor bodily condition and those which have not responded to treatment.

Pathology

At post-mortem examination one or both kidneys are haemorrhagic with pus, excess mucus and blood in the pelvices. One or both ureters are dilated and filled with pus and the uretero-vesicular valve is often eroded. The bladder wall is grossly thickened, the mucosa is inflamed and covered with excess mucus and any remaining urine is mucopurulent and contains blood. *A.suis* may be demonstrated in Gram-stained smears and on culture of pus from the lesions. Other bacteria may also be present.

Epidemiology

The progeny of an infected sow may be infected from birth, but young boars usuallly become infected from 9-10 weeks of age onwards, frequently from pen floor contamination. Semen is frequently contaminated (50% in some AI studs), but the antimicrobials used in extenders prevent its spread by A.I. Infection frequently follows natural service by a particular boar. Sows in some herds are free from infection, but in others, 10% urine samples may be culture positive. The disease occurs in free-range conditions.

The organism persists on flooring and can be transmitted to clean areas on footwear. It is sensitive to most disinfectants at recommended dilutions. Predisposing factors include multiparity and low water intake.

Diagnosis

This is based on the clinical signs and the history of recent service and is confirmed by the presence of large Gram-positive bacilli in Gram-stained smears of the pus, by immunofluorescence or by the isolation of *A.suis* on urea containing medium or blood agar with 50 µg/ml polymyxin or on nalidixic acid: metronidazole blood agar. Immunofluorescence and culture have similar sensitivity and specificity. Indirect immunofluorescence may be used to detect serum antibody.

Treatment and control

Affected animals may be treated parenterally with penicillin or ampicillin for 7-10 days and this may be effective in the early stages when only the bladder is affected. Recovered sows should be culled. In the later stages, when renal involvement has occurred, treatment is rarely effective. Other sows served by the same boar and the boar itself should be treated parenterally with penicillin and penicillin injections after service should continue for 2-3 weeks after the outbreak has subsided. Enrofloxacin (2.5mg/kg in food for 10 days) or ampicillin 20mg/kg for 20 days have been shown to be effective. It is of advantage to wash out the preputial diverticulum with antimicrobial, but neither this practice nor parenteral or oral medication with tetracyclines or enrofloxacin eliminate the agent completely from sow or boar. Disinfection of contaminated areas and the use of clean boars on gilts may prevent further outbreaks.

241

References

Dagnall, G.J.R. and Jones, J.E.T. (1982). A selective medium for the isolation of *C.suis*. Res.Vet.Sci. **32**, 389-390.

Larsen, J.L., Hogh, P. and Hovind Hougen, K. (1986). Haemagglutinating and hydrophobic properties of *C.(E) suis*. Acta Vet.Scand. **27**, 520-530.

Lawson, P.A., Falsen, E., Akervall, E., Vandamme, P., Collins, M.D. (1997). Characterisation of some *Actinomyces*-like isolates from human clinical specimens: reclassification of *Actinomyces suis* (Soltys and Spratling) as *Actinobaculum/myces? suis* and description of *Actinobaculum schaalii*. Int J. Syst Bact. **47**, 899-903.

Liebhold, M., Wendt, M., Kamp, F.J., Drommer, W. (1995). Clinical and light and electron microscopical findings in sows with cystitis. Vet. Rec. **137**, 141-144.

Ludwig, W., Kirchhof, G., Weizenegger, M., Weiss, N. (1992). Phylogenic evidence for the transfer of *E.suis* to the genus *Actinomyces* as *A.suis* comb nov. Int.J.Syst.Bact. **42**, 161-165.

Wendt, M., Langfeldt, N., Amstberg, G. (1990). Comparison of different methods of detection of *C.suis* infection in sows and boars. Proc. IPVS. **11**, 177.

Wendt, M. (1998). Urinary system disorders in pigs. Proc IPVS **15** (1), 195-201.

Pyelonephritis and cystitis caused by *E.coli* and other bacteria

Definition

Cystitis and pyelonephritis occurs in sows as a result of ascending infection particularly when stalled or tethered and leads to loss of condition, increased frequency of urination and the presence of blood or pus in the urine. It may be fatal.

Incidence

Worldwide and in some situations may be responsible for up to 25% of sow culls.

Aetiology

A wide variety of bacteria have been isolated. 80% are *E.coli* with *Proteus* spp *Pseudomonas aeruginosa*, streptococci and staphylococci in the remaining cases. Uropathogenic E. coli may possess mannose-resistant (P) fimbriae (54.8%), mannose sensitive fimbriae (Type 1) produce aerobactin (45%) and be haemolytic.

Pathogenesis

Infection is ascending with faecal contamination of the vulva often responsible in dry sows and endometritis contributing in recently farrowed sows. Low water intake, reduced frequency of micturition in fat sows or those with leg problems, short sow places with a solid back panel, solid floor or inadequate slats which lead to increased faecal build-up all contribute to the condition where sow stalls are still permitted. In the last third of gestation, mild prolapse of the vagina may occur where the floor slopes too much. Vulval damage in loose housed sows may also contribute to the condition. The organisms multiply in the bladder to give bacteruria which may remain asymptomatic or resolve, but a proportion of cases progress to cystitis with adhesion of the organisms to bladder epithelium, inflammation and eventual erosion of the ureterovesicular valves to give an ascending pyelonephritis, tubular damage and hyperkalaemia leading to sudden death.

Clinical signs

An increased frequency of urination and the presence of blood and or pus in the urine are seen. There may be mucoid discharge of vesicular origin on the vulva and on the tail. The appetite is depressed and the rectal temperature occasionally raised. When pyelonephritis is present temperatures may fall and blood urea rise. Affected animals may die suddenly without clinical signs having been observed, or as a result of chronic disease. Infection may be asymptomatic.

Humane slaughter should be carried out when rectal temperatures fall or at blood urea levels above 15 mmoles/l and when sick animals cannot be nursed.

Pathology

Thickening and inflammation of the bladder mucosa is seen at post-mortem and both the ureters and kidneys may be involved. The bladder contains cloudy purulent urine of which may be of neutral or alkaline pH when opened.

Diagnosis

The clinical signs are sufficiently distinctive to enable a diagnosis of urinary tract infection to be reached. The only confusing condition is the presence of phosphate crystals in the urine, occasionally seen and causing no clinical signs. Crystal deposits as a white crust maybe seen on the vulva. Pus of vaginal origin may cloud the urine in recently farrowed sows.

The organism concerned can often be identified and the presence of *A.suis* should be ruled out. The use of dip slides to enumerate bacteria may be misleading as endometritis may contribute bacteria to the urine and *A.suis* may not be identified.

Treatment

Daily parenteral treatment with tetracyclines, ampicillin, enrofloxacin, other broad-spectrum antimicrobials and with streptomycin may all be of value. Affected sows should be encouraged to drink by placing meal on water in front of them or ion replacers in the water which should be presented in a trough at least 4cm deep.

Prevention

Where stalls are present, they should be cleaned of faeces. Water intake can be encouraged by increasing the salt concentration of the ration to 1% in the presence of water *ad libitum*. The design of sow places should be considered in relation to the size of the animal and sows should be maintained in fair but not fat condition. Sows should be encouraged to rise by feeding them twice daily and ensuring that drinkers are in good working order and delivering water at the correct pressure. AI should be considered, and service and farrowing hygiene improved.

243

References

Brito, B.G.de, Silva Leite, D.da, Linhares, R.E.C., Vidotto, M.C. (1999). Virulence associated factors of uropathogenic E. coli strains isolated from pigs. Vet.Micro 65, 123-132.
Carr, J., Walton, J.R. (1993). Bacterial flora of the urinary tract of pigs. Vet.Rec. **132**, 575-577.
Carr, J., Walton, J.R. (1991). Cystitis and pyelonephritis in pigs. Pig Vet.J. **27**, 122-141.
Madec, F. (1984). Urinary disorders in intensive pig herds. Pig News and Information **5**, 89-93.
Smith, W.J. (1983). Cystitis in sows. Pig News and Information 4, 279-281.
Wendt, M. (1998). Urinary system disorders in pigs. Proc IPVS **15** (1), 195-201.

Miscellaneous bacteria

Aeromonas hydrophila

A.hydrophila has been isolated from cases of enteritis, uterine infections and from lymph nodes. It appears to be associated with an enterotoxin-type watery diarrhoea, especially in young or recently-weaned pigs. Isolates from pig faeces contain virulence factors and A.caviae and A.sobria are also present

Acinetobacter calcoaceticans

Recovered in profuse culture from some cases of rhinitis in piglets and from the trachea in tracheitis. Acinetobacter spp. may cause deterioration in semen during storage or transport.

Arcanobacterium (Actinomyces) pyogenes

A.pyogenes infection produces no specific clinical signs and is found, with other bacteria, such as Bacteroides spp. in abscesses in many parts of the carcase at post mortem examination or slaughter. A. pyogenes is a small Gram-positive coccobacillus which can bind to cells by means of two neuraminidases and a collagen binding protein (CbpA, MW 124.7 kDa) and produces an haemolytic (56 kDa) exotoxin and proteolytic enzymes. It invades damaged tissue, particularly following foot damage and tail biting. It is responsible for most of the abscesses found in the vertebral bodies which collapse and cause the paralysis in spinal abscesses. It complicates chronic pneumonic lesions and is found in enlarged, abscessed head lymph nodes and in the tonsil. It invades and complicates pyelonephritis of any cause. Lesions are frequently identified at post-mortem examination at abattoir.
The organism is present in vaginal discharge, metritis and abortion. A.pyogenes attaches to eggs and may destroy them. Invasion of the foetus does not appear to occur, but it can enter via the umbilicus in neonates to cause umbilical abscesses first seen in 7-10 day old pigs.
A.pyogenes can be demonstrated in Gram-stained smears or isolated as 1mm ß-haemolytic colonies after 48 hours' incubation on horse blood agar. Similar organisms belonging to the genus Actinomyces are currently being identified from the reproductive tract and tonsil but their significance is not yet certain.
Antibody may be detected by indirect ELISA to the 25 kDa protease of A.pyogenes. Penicillin or tetracycline may be used to treat infections. Severe abscessation may not respond readily to treatment.

244

Reference

Hommez, J., Devriese, L.A., Miry, C., Castryck, F. (1991). J.Vet.Med. Series B 38, 575-580. Characterisation of 2 groups of Actinomyces-like bacteria isolated from purulent lesions in pigs.

Bacteroides and diarrhoea

Bacteroides fragilis is a strictly anaerobic Gram-negative rod found in the large intestine. Enterotoxigenic strains have been isolated from diarrhoea in piglets both before and after weaning and have been shown to cause diarrhoea when fed to pigs.

Other species such as *B.vulgatus and Bacteroides, now Prevotella melaninogenicus* have been found in enteritis.

Experimental disease in piglets occurs 2-3 days after inoculation as a watery diarrhoea which lasts 4-6 days and is accompanied by anorexia and dehydration. Natural disease in weaned pigs can only be distinguished bacteriologically but lasts 3-6 days, presenting as soft faeces and diarrhoea accompanied by loss of condition. Pathological findings in piglets include epithelial cell swelling and vacuolation, crypt hyperplasia in the distal small intestine and large intestine and an exfoliative colitis.

B.fragilis and other anaerobic Gram negative rods are also found in abscesses, pleurisy and consolidated pneumonic lesions. Treatment with nitroimidazoles is usually effective as they penetrate the pus. Where they are not available, enrofloxacin or amoxycillin may be of value.

Reference

Duimstra, J.R., Myers, L.L., Collins, W.C. (1991). Vet.Path. 28, 514-518. Enterovirulence of enterotoxigenic B.fragilis in gnotobiotic pigs.

Cilia Associated Bacilli

These organisms have been identified in the tracheas of pigs. They are visible in silver-stained sections as thin bacilli lying parallel with the cilia. They differ from similar organisms found in rats, rabbits, dogs, and cattle, but like them may belong to the Flavobacterium/Flexibacter group which form yellow colonies on isolation. They have been recorded in cases of pneumonia and have been associated with lesions of actve tracheitis..

References

Done, S.H., Higgins, R.J. (1998). Unusual lesions in pigs associated with CAR bacillus-like organisms. Pig J. 41, 127-133.

Hafner, S., Latimer, K. (1998). Cilia associated respiratory bacillus infection and pneumonia in a pig. J. Vet. Diagn. Invest. 10, 373-375.

Nietfeld, J.C., Franklin, C.L., Riley, L.K., Zeman, D.H., Groff, B.T. (1995). Colonisation of the tracheal epithelium of pigs by filamentous bacteria resembling cilia-associated respiratory bacilli. J. Vet Diagn. Invest. 7, 338-342.

Chlamydial infection

Definition

Chlamydia may cause conjunctivitis, pneumonia, pleurisy, pericarditis, polyarthritis, orchitis, infertility and the birth of weak piglets. They can cause enteritis. Many infections are inapparent.

Incidence

Chlamydia are widespread in birds and occur in many mammalian species. Antibody may be widespread (23% slaughter pigs 1966 UK), 46.7% diarrhoeic faeces samples and 72.7% pneumonic lung samples were positive in Germany. Infection is rarely diagnosed in the UK, but has been identified increasingly in the US, especially in enteritis, and infection appears to be widespread.

Aetiology

Chlamydophila spp and *Chlamydia spp* both occur in the pig and are tiny obligate intracellular parasites which occur as an intracellular reproductive form and a resistant extracellular form, the elementary body. The cell wall outer membrane proteins have been used for classification and it is now clear from PCR studies, gene sequences, DNA probes and immunoperoxidase studies that *Chlamydia.suis*, *Chlamydophila pecorum*, *C. psittaci* and *C. abortus* cause chlamydial infections in pigs. *Chlamydophila psittaci* has been confirmed in respiratory and reproductive tract infections using modern methods and *C. suis* and *Chlamydophila pecorum* have been identified in enteric infections. C. abortus is present in some aborted material.

Pathogenesis

Experimental infection of the respiratory tract results in an acute exudative or interstitial pneumonia within 4-8 days of infection. Raised pale red lesions are present in the diaphragmatic lobes and become paler with age. An arthritis may occur at the same time. Venereal infection can lead to persistent infection in sows and orchitis with semen infection in boars. Stillborn piglets and vaginal discharge have also been associated with infection. Infection has been associated with PRRS in the UK. Experimental studies of *C. suis* enteritis show that diarrhoea develops in gnotobiotic pigs within 4-5 days post infection and may last for 8 days. Villous atrophy develops. Antibody develops within 2 weeks of infection.

Clinical signs

A wide range of clinical signs have been recorded, but infection may be asymptomatic. Mucopurulent keratoconjunctivitis in piglets and sows, respiratory distress in weaned pigs, an increase in coughing and arthritis have all been associated with infection or reproduced experimentally. Reproductive disturbances such as infertility, orchitis, an increase in premature farrowings, abortions, stillbirths and a rise in piglet mortality to weaning have all been recorded. Weak piglets may have diarrhoea, and diarrhoea associated with infection may develop in weaned pigs from 4 weeks of age.

Animals with severe respiratory distress or arthritis may require humane destruction.

Pathology

Lesions from which chlamydia may be isolated include pericarditis, pleurisy, enlarged spleens, synovitis, orchitis and dead foetuses and mummified piglets. The most recognisable lesions are probably those in the lung. These occur largely in the posterior lobes as pale red raised areas of consolidation extending deep into the lung. Enzootic pneumonia-like lesions may be produced in the anterior lobes. Oedema, a suppurative necrotising alveolitis and bronchiolitis have been described with penbronchiolar accumulations of plasma cells, lymphocytes and macrophages. In the gut there may be watery colon contents with undigested food, atrophy and multifocal necrosis of the villi of the distal jejunum and ileum and a pseudomembranous colitis in the large intestine. Epithelial cells in infected areas contain the organism which can be demonstrated as clumps of red dots in Kosters-stained preparations, by immunoperoxidase, immunofluorescence or using DNA probes.

Chlamydophila psittaci is a Category 3 pathogen and isolation should only be attempted in a registered laboratory.

Epidemiology

Pigs of all ages may be infected and antibody is widespread in affected herds (49% pigs, 47% herds in Spain, 30% sows in infected herds, Germany). The organisms and antibody to them have been demonstrated in free-living wild boar. Infection can be by aerosol, contact, ingestion or by the venereal route as the agent can be demonstrated in semen (9%). Outside the host the agent is relatively resistant to drying and may survive months in that state. Birds, and to a lesser extent, other mammals, may represent sources of infection.

Chlamydophila psittaci and, possibly, *C. suis*, infect man and pig strains appear to be a cause of chlamydial antibody in pig keepers.

Diagnosis

The clinical signs of reproductive failure, conjunctivitis, raised respiratory rate, arthritis or diarrhoea may suggest the condition. Demonstration of the agent in smears of tissue by Koster' stain only confirms the presence of chlamydia, but immunofluorescence, immunoperoxidase, DNA probes and PCR can identify the organism to species. Isolation from tissue can be carried out on McCoy cells. Serum antibody using complement fixation or ELISAs would confirm infection if rising titres occurred. *Chlamydophila abortus* may be demonstrated in the reproductive tract, *C. pecorum* and *C. suis* in the gut and *C. suis* in conjunctivitis. *C. psittaci* may occur in respiratory disease or more generally.

Treatment

Tetracyclines are the drugs of choice and should be given by the route most appropriate to the age of pig affected. The organism is not eliminated by treatment.

Disinfection and the exclusion of wild birds and rodents may help reduce contamination of the environment.

247

References

Anderson, I.E., Baxter, S.I.F., Dunbar, S., Rae, A.G., Philips, H.L., Clarkson, M.J., Herring, A.J. (1996). Analyses of the genomes of chlamydial isolates from ruminants and pigs support the adoption of the new species Chlamydia pecorum. Int J Syst Bacteriol 46, 245-251.
Camenisch, U., Lu, Z.H., Vaughan, L., Corboz, L., Zimmerman, D.R., Wittenbrink, M.M., Pospischil, A., Sydler, T. (2004). Diagnostic investigation ointo the role of Chlamydiae in cases of increased rates of return to oestrus in pigs. Vet.Rec. 155, 593-596.
Done, S.H., Spencer, Y.I., Bellerby, P. (1998). Pneumonia in the pig: first report of C. psittaci infection in the UK. Pig J. 42, 47-53.
Nietfeld, J.C., Leslie-Steen, P., Zeman, D.H., Nelson, D. (1997). Prevalence of intestinal chlamydial infection in pigs in the midwest as determined by immunoperoxidase staining. Am J Vet Res 58, 260-264
Pospischil, A.; Thoma, R., Schiller, I., Sydler, T., Guscetti, F., (1996). Chlamydia in pigs. Pig J. 37, 9-13.
Popischil, A., Wood, R.L. (1987). Intestinal Chlamydia in pigs. Vet. Pathol. 24, 568-570.
Rogers, D.G., and Anderson, A.A. (1996). Intestinal lesions caused by two swine chlamydia isolates in gnotobiotic pigs. J Vet Diagn Invest 8 , 433-440
Rogers, W.G., Andersen, A.A., Hogg, A., Nielson, D.L., Huebert, M.A. (1993). J.Am.Vet.Med.Ass. 203, 1321-1323. Conjunctivitis and keratoconjunctivitis associated with Chlamydia in swine.
Rogers, D.G., Anderson, A.A., Hunsaker, B.D. (1996). Lung and nasal lesions caused by a swine chlamydial isolate in gnotobiotic pigs. J Vet Diagn Invest 8, 45-55
Szeredi, L.; Schiller, I.; Sydler, T.; Guscetti, F.; Heinen, E.; Corboz, L.; Eggenberger, E.; Jones, G.E.; and Pospischil, A. (1996). Intestinal chlamydia in finishing pigs. Vet Pathol 33. 369-374.
Wilson, M.R. and Plummer, P.A. (1966). J.Comp.Path. 76, 427-433. A survey of pig sera for the presence of antibody to the PLV group of organisms.
Woollen, N., Daniels, E.K., Yeary, T., Leipold, H.W., Phillips, R.M. (1990). Chlamydial infection and perinatal infection in a swine herd. J.Am.Vet.Med.Ass. 197, 600-603.Vasquez-Cisneos, C., Wilsmore, A.J., Bolle, E. (1994). Experimental infections of pregnant sows with ovine chlamydia strains. Vet Microbiol 42, 383-387.

Corynebacterium pseudotuberculosis

Recovered from the vaginas of healthy sows (Japan).

Coxiella burneti

Antibody has been demonstrated in pigs (11.3% Trinidad) but no clinical signs have yet been reported. It is a zoonosis and may be fatal in man (Q fever).

Dermatophilus spp.

Dermatophilus spp. have been demonstrated in tonsillar material and found in lesions of exudative epidermitis. They are filamentous Gram-positive organisms which break up into coccal bodies and may be seen in Gram-stained smears or isolated on blood agar plates containing polymyxin B as haemolytic colonies after 48 hours' incubation. If suspected, penicillin treatment is of value.

Klebsiella

Klebsiella spp. are present in chronic respiratory tract disease, especially rhinitis, in enteritis and cause mastitis (*K.aerogenes*). Treat as *E.coli*. Often present in sawdust (*K.aerogenes*). Distinguished from *E.coli* by biochemical tests.

Legionella

Antibody to *L.pneumophila* has been demonstrated in the sera of pneumonic pigs in the UK and pneumonia and antibody have been recorded in China.

Melioidosis *(Burkholderia pseudomallei)*

B.pseudomallei is a cause of melioidosis in pigs in tropical and subtropical regions. Infection may be asymptomatic or result in fever, unsteady gait, weakness, nasal discharge and subcutaneous swelling of the limbs. Abscesses occur in lungs, bronchial lymph nodes, spleen and elsewhere in the carcase. The organism may be isolated from lesions in acute cases. Antibody may be detected by CFT and IHA tests. Infection may result from contaminated water or from consumption of infected swill. Tetracyclines or ampicillin may be of value in treatment and chlorination of water supplies may prevent. A zoonosis. Category 3 pathogen only to be handled in secure accommodation.

References

Ketterer, P.J. (1986). Melioidosis in intensive piggeries in South Eastern Queensland. Aust.Vet.J. 63, 146-149.
Najdenski, H., Kussovski, V., Vesselinova, A. (2004) Experimental *Burkholderia pseudomallei* infection of pigs. J.Vet. Med. Series B, 51, 225-230.
Webster, W.R., Shield, J., Arthur, R.J., Blackall, P.J, Thomas, A.D., Spinks, G.A., D'Arcy, T.L., Hoffman, D. (1990). Evaluation of a modified complement fixation test and an indirect haemagglutination test for the sero diagnosis of melioidosis in pigs. J.Clin.Micro. 28, 1874-1875.

Rhodococcus equi

Present in granulomatous lesions in submandibular lymph nodes. Experimental infections with the organism result in severe consolidation and pneumonia of the anteroventral lobes of the lung at 7-10 days post infection which gradually resolved. *R. sputi* has been isolated from mesenteric lymph nodes in Japan. The organism may be cultured from granulomatous nodes or identified using PCR tests for the species and its virulence determinants. Lesions must be distinguished from those caused by mycobacteria.

References

Halbert, N.D., Reitzel, R.A., Martens, R.J., Cohen, N.D. (2005) Evaluation of a multiplex PCR assay for simultaneous detection of *Rhodococcus equi* and the vapA gene. Am.J.Vet.Res. 66, 1380-1385.
Zuik, M.C., Yager, J.A. (1987). Experimental infection of piglets by aerosols of *Rhodococcus equi*. Can J. Vet. Res. 51, 290-296.

FUNGAL CONDITIONS

Ringworm

Definition

Ringworm or dermatomycosis is uncommon in the pig and often causes little effect on productivity but is a source of infection for man.

Incidence

Sporadic worldwide but some species e.g. *Microsporum nanum* do not occur in Britain.

Aetiology and pathogenesis.

Most infections in the UK are caused by *Trichophyton mentagrophytes* but *T.verrucosum, T. terrestre, M.gypseum* and *M.canis* may also occur. *Microsporum nanum* is involved in countries such as Australia and the USA, but not in the UK. Exposure to infectious spores of the dermatophyte directly or following abrasions results in colonisation of the skin and development of the skin lesions. Infection may occur in piglets but only become apparent later. Recovered animals develop immunity.

Clinical signs

T.mentagrophytes infections present as circular areas of brown discolouration on the back or behind the ears. The lesions enlarge gradually and may be greasy in texture. There may be little or no alopecia, skin thickening or inflammation but hairs plucked from the lesion may appear reddish brown or orange along most of their length. The lesions are often seen in weaners and older pigs but may be detected in piglets from affected farms by close inspection.

M. canis can occur in pigs of all ages as reddish spots of variable size on the back and flanks accompanied by small areas of alopecia and slight pruritis.

M.nanum infections often occur behind the ear within a week of exposure as 2-3cm rings or circles of dark, crusty skin, expanding as rings or circles of reddish or light brown scabs which may be raised above the surrounding skin on the back, flanks and, eventually, the abdomen. As in *T.mentagrophytes* infections there is little alopecia or irritation.

Humane slaughter is unnecessary.

Epidemiology

Infected weaner producers may spread infection to fattening farms. Infection may be transferred from pig to pig or from pig to man. Morbidity may reach 100% in some groups of animals. Infection in the form of resistant spores may remain for months on wooden or other pen fittings and has been identified in aerosols. Rats and other species may also carry the infection and be a source of it for pigs. Cattle are the commonest source of *T.verrucosum* and cats are a common source of *M. canis*. Wild boar infected with *Trichophyton sp* have been identified in Italy.

Diagnosis

The clinical signs are extremely suggestive. The presence of fungus in hairs plucked from the lesion may be confirmed by microscopic examination and scrapings and hairs may be cultured and the organism responsible identified. Common conditions with which ringworm may be confused include pityriasis rosea in which expanding rings of reddish-brown dermatitis are found usually on the skin of the belly and thighs of young pigs. Swine pox lesions on the skin of the belly may also resemble ringworm lesions in their early stages. Exudative epidermitis lesions in older pigs must also be distinguished from those of ringworm.

Treatment

If found, topical treatment with enilconazole or natamycin may be adequate. Topical treatments may be ineffective unless greasy lesions are cleaned first with a disinfectant such as cetrimide, or better still, hexetidine. Systemic treatment with griseofulvin will certainly be effective at 10 mg/kg griseofulvin daily for 7 days (not food animals, EU). Disinfection of buildings with formaldehyde, hypochlorite or detergents should be carried out. Steam and phenolic disinfectants have also been used. If rats or cats are suspected of introducing infection, they should be controlled or treated as appropriate.

References

Pittman, J.S., Roberts, J.D. (2005). Rinworm in lactating sows. (J.Swine Health and Prod. **13**, 86-90.
Wilkinson, J.D. (1985). Ringworm in pigs. Proc.Pig Vet.Soc. **12**, 103-107.
Gonzalez, J.F.C., Barcena, M.C.A., Gomez, F.R., Amigot, J.A.L. (1995). An outbreak of dermatophytosis in pigs caused by *Microsporum canis*. Mycopathologia **129**, 79-80.

Yeast infections

Infections with *Candida albicans* occur in chronic gastroenteritis in piglets 5-14 days of age and are often secondary. Piglets may be dull, may vomit and have a chronic diarrhoea which has failed to respond to antimicrobial treatment. Some may die. 2-5 mm circular whitish lesions may be seen on the tongue and hard palate. A chronic enteritis may be seen and yeasts may be demonstrated in histological sections and by culture. In cutaneous candidiasis, a moist grey exudate may appear on the surface of the skin of the abdomen and legs with eventual skin thickening and hair loss. Cleaning of skin with detergent or hexetidine-based shampoos may remove the lesions. Nystatin, miconazole and amphotericin B may be used to reduce clinical signs, but not in food animals (EU). Other yeasts may be involved. The lipid dependent skin yeast *Malassezia sympodialis* (58%) and *M. slooffiae* (30%) have been recorded from pig skin and ears

Other systemic mycoses

Mucormycosis may occur in piglets and be a cause of chronic enteritis and gastritis in piglets and Cryptococcus infections may cause pneumonia in areas where the organism is present (Not UK). Zygomycetes infections have been

251

identified in the USA in antibiotic unresponsive diarrhoeas in piglets aged 10-28 days. Catarrhal to fibronecrotic gastroenteritis with histological evidence of the invading fungi was recorded.

Reference

Reed, W.M., Hanika, C., Mehdi, N.A.Q. and Shackelford, C. (1987). Gastrointestinal zygomycosis in sucking pigs. Am.Vet.Med.Assoc. **191**, 549-550.

MYCOTOXICOSES

Mycotoxicosis of pigs occurs as a result of fungal growth on damp feed or the inclusion of affected grain etc. in the ration. A number of moulds have been incriminated but the following toxins produce the most clearly defined syndromes.

Zearalenone Poisoning (Vulvo vaginitis in sows)

Definition

The ingestion by sows in late pregnancy of zearalenone (Fusarium F2 toxin) present in spoiled wheat or barley in feed may result in the birth of small litters, stillborn and weak, splay-legged piglets. Vulval enlargement may occur in the sow and other female stock on the same ration. The subsequent breeding behaviour of such females may be affected.

Aetiology

Barley or other grains harvested or stored under moist conditions or treated with propionic acid may be contaminated with fungi of the genus Fusarium (e.g. *F.culmorum, F.graminearum*). These produce a number of toxins including the oestrogenic toxin zearalenone and deoxynivalenol (vomitoxin).

Pathogenesis

Zearalenone is absorbed from the ration where some may be in the form of zearalenone glycosides and is detectable in the plasma for 5 days after last administration either as zearalenone or as α-zearalenol. It is excreted in the urine for up to 5 days after last administration bound to glucuronic acids and is passed out in faeces where bacteria may break it down. It has an effect on reproductive functions, may reduce the activity of 3 α-hydroxysteroid dehydrogenase and depress plasma LH levels. Experimental studies have shown effects on non-pregnant gilts, on embryonic mortality after service and on sows in the last two weeks of pregnancy. Effects appear to depend upon levels of pure compound. They are summarised below:

Age   Threshold level   Effect

of Zearalenone

Prepubertal gilts gilts >3 weeks old	1-3 ppm 3-5 ppm	Mammary enlargement, vulval swelling, ovarian and uterine swelling and uterine oedema
cycling gilts	3-5 ppm	Enlargement and oedema of uterus, retention of corpora lutea, anoestrus for up to 50 days. Lengthening of cycles. Spontaneous return to oestrus 45 days after removal of zearalenone.
Sows 2-15d. post service	5-30 ppm 60 ppm+	No effect on embryos. Complete embryonic failure
Mid-term	3-5 ppm	Some reduction in weight of uterus and foetuses
14 days prior to farrowing	3-5 ppm	Birth of weak and splay-legged piglets, vulval enlargement in piglets.
Lactating sows	3-5 ppm	Weaning: Service interval extended.
Boars	3-5 ppm	No effect on semen quality or slight rise in abnormal sperm.

Clinical signs

Enlargement of the vulva with eventual prolapse and some development of oedema around the teats may be seen in gilts and sows within 14 days of changing to contaminated feed. In addition to vulval swelling, small litters may be produced and conception rate may be reduced with extension of weaning to service intervals. Sows in the last third of gestation may come into milk early and may give birth to substandard litters composed of fresh, stillborn piglets and a mixture of weak and splay-legged piglets. The weak or splay-legged piglets grow weaker as the toxin is secreted in the milk and they may die of starvation. Any survivors may be normal by 10-14 days of age. In some accounts, rectal swelling and oedema of the prepuce have been described in males. Spermatogenesis has been said to be affected but this effect appears not to be permanent. In females an increase in returns to service and other reproductive changes has been reported. The weaning to service interval is extended, but puberty in the gilt and subsequent fertility does not normally appear to be affected provided that zearalenone is withdrawn 14 days before service. Offspring of affected sows have delayed first oestrus, first conception and lengthening of first weaning to service interval in some cases. There is no effect on growth rate.

Splay legged or weak or wasting piglets may be destroyed humanely as may animals with irreparable vulval damage after prolapse.

Pathology

Affected females may have enlarged vulvas, sometimes with prolapse and there may be mammary enlargement most obvious at slaughter. The uterus is heavy and may be turgid and in served gilts or sows corpora lutea of pregnancy may be present with degenerating blastocysts from 14-35 days post-service.

Epidemiology

Zearalenone levels are highest in grain when rain occurs at the end of the ripening period. Both barley and maize can be affected and zearalenone can also be found in whole maize and corncob silage. Disease can occur outside the affected area following trading of affected grain.

Diagnosis

The presence of vulval enlargement and oedema of mammary tissue and the presence of mouldy grain in the ration indicate that an outbreak of stillbirths and splay leg may be caused by this toxin. The absence of virus antibody and the demonstration of toxin in the feed, milk, plasma or faeces (by feeding trials in 8-10 week gilts, thin layer chromatographic analysis, direct competitive ELISA or by cell culture assay) would confirm. Analysis of bile of slaughtered gilts and sows for zearalenone glucuronide can confirm its role in reproductive disorders.

Treatment

The vulval enlargement and the piglet mortality soon disappear if a normal, clean ration is fed. Zearalenone levels in tissues may be reduced below the level of detection within 14 days and all clinical signs have normally disappeared 3-4 weeks after mouldy feed is discontinued. Recent studies have shown that antibody to zearalenone can be produced and vaccination can increase the rate of zearalenone excretion. None of the feed treatments appear to inactivate the toxin in feed. Safe levels of presence of zearalenone may be as low as 10 ppb but are generally regarded as much higher (see table). Products intended to detoxify grain may result in clinical improvements to reproduction.

References

Diekman, M.A., Long, G.G. (1989). Blastocyst development on days 10 or 14 after consumption of zearalenone on days 7-10 after breeding. Am.J.Vet.Res. 50, 1224-1227.

Edwards, S., Cantley, T.C., Rottinghaus, G.E., Osweiler, G.D., Day, B.N. (1987). The effect of zearalenone on reproduction in Swine I. Theriogenology, 28, 43-49.

Edwards, S., Cantley, T.C., Day, B.N. (1987). The effects of zearalenone on reproduction in swine II. Theriogenology 28, 51-58.

Etienne, M, Jemmali, M. (1982). Effects of zearalenone (F-2) on oestrus activity and reproduction in gilts. J.Anim.Sci. 55, 1-10.

Miller, J.K., Hacking, A., Gross, V.J. (1973). Stillbirths neonatal mortality and small litters in pigs associated with the ingestion of fusarium toxin in pregnant sows. Vet.Rec. 93, 555-559.

Pestka, J.J., Liu, M.T., Knudson, B.K., Hogberg, M.G. (1985). Immunisation of pigs for production of antibody against zearalenone. J.Food Protection 48, 953-957.

Vomitoxin (Deoxynivalenol)

Ingestion of vomitoxin results in vomiting, feed refusal and growth depression. Vomitoxin (deoxynivalenol) may also be present in zearalenone-contaminated feeds and is a 12, 13 epoxytrichothecene. It has been recorded in feeds at concentrations of 0.1-42 ppm but levels rarely exceed 3-10 ppm. Up to 65% of deoxynivalenol present in the pig diet may be absorbed. At 1-2 ppm food refusal can occur initially although animals may become accustomed to it and growth becomes almost normal. At higher levels of 12-20 ppm, vomitng occurs within 5-15 minutes and complete feed refusal follows. Growth depression is the major clinical finding and there are no effects on reproductive behaviour not attributable to reduced feed intake. Vomitoxin is rapidly absorbed, rapidly distributed to all tissues and rapidly excreted unchanged so that plasma is negative within 12-24 hours of withdrawal. Vomiting may be associated with serotonin metabolism and there is an effect on growth other than that caused by depression of feed intake. It is excreted at very low levels in the milk. Residues may occur in kidneys for up to 3 weeks after withdrawal. Inactivation of deoxynivalenol by heating with aqueous sodium metabisulphite has been described. Contaminated feed must be destroyed.

References

Prelusky, D.B., Trenholm, H.L. (1993). The efficacy of various classes of anti-emetics in preventing deoxynivalenol-induced vomiting in swine. Natural Toxins 1, 296-302.
Rotter, B.A., Prelusky, D.B., Pestka, J. (1996). Toxicology of deoxynivalenol (vomitoxin). J. Toxicol. and Env. Health 48, 1-34.
Young, L.G., McGirr, L., Valli, V.E., Lumsden, J.H. and Lun, A.(1983). Vomitoxin in corn fed to young pigs. J.Anim.Sci. 57, 655-664.
Young, J.C. Trenholm, H.L., Friend, D.W., Prelusky, D.B. (1987). Inactivation with sodium metabisulphite. Agricultural & Food Chemistry 35, 259-261
Veno, Y., Ed. Trichothecenes, chemical, biological and toxicological aspects. Elsevier (1983).

Aflatoxicosis

Definition

A syndrome in which reduced growth, weight loss and inappetence, jaundice and death results from liver damage caused by the ingestion of feed contaminated with *Aspergillus flavus* aflatoxin.

Incidence

Rarely diagnosed in the UK where import restrictions are placed on aflatoxin levels in feeds (Aflatoxin Orders) but more common in countries where maize and groundnut meal are common ingredients of the diet.

Aetiology and pathogenesis

Aspergillus flavus or *Aspergillus parasiticus* may contaminate feed components such as maize or groundnut meal and the aflatoxin produced may be present at levels of 360-3422 ppb Aflatoxin B1 which can cause clinical signs. Liver damage includes fatty change, lobular necrosis with an increase in basophilic cells at the periphery of the lobule, bile duct proliferation and, in chronic cases, cirrhosis. The hepatocytes may be variable in size with increased staining of the nuclei. Death may occur in a few days following ingestion of more than 0.2 mg aflatoxin Bl per kg. The L.D.50 is 0.6 mg/kg and levels of 0.4 mg/kg almost always produce clinical signs. 0.1 mg/kg (100 ppb in feed) has been reported to be a 'no effect' level with a safe level of 0.05 mg/kg.

Aflatoxin is excreted in urine as B1, B2, M and G forms. There may be immunosuppression.

Clinical signs

These may appear within 6 weeks of a change to the contaminated ration and consist of depressed growth rate, inappetence, arched back and apathy. Jaundice, ataxia and convulsions may occur before death. Sows may lose their milk or abort. The growth rate of surviving piglets is depressed. Mange and other diseases may become more common.

Humane slaughter is commonly required in field outbreaks and severely jaundiced or stunted animals should be destroyed.

Pathological findings

Jaundice of the carcase is prominent and the liver may be white, tan, or bright orange in colour. There may be oedema of the wall of the gall bladder in acute cases and the whole liver is friable with much blood in the sinusoids. The blood fails to clot and serous or bloody effusions may be present in the thoracic and abdominal cavities. In addition, bleeding into a number of other organs may occur and petechiae and ecchymoses may be present on serous or mucous surfaces. Liver changes including centrilobular necrosis, bile duct proliferation and fatty change may be seen, followed later by regeneration.

Epidemiology

Associated with groundnut meal or maize which has been spoiled in cobs in drought years or stored in moist conditions. In all countries, aflatoxicosis may follow poor storage of complete feed in contaminated feed bins

Diagnosis

A history of introduction to a particular food or batch of feed is of value. It may be possible to confirm that aflatoxin is present in samples of the feed. The clinical signs, post-mortem and histological findings may suggest a diagnosis of aflatoxicosis. Levels of liver enzymes such as alkaline phosphatase serum aspartate transferase and serum glutamyl oxaloacetic transaminase may be raised. Creatine kinase levels are depressed. Aflatoxin levels should be measured in the feed where possible using ELISA, thin layer chromatography HPLC or cell culture toxicity methods. Aflatoxin B1 can be detected in fresh and dried meats at levels of 0.13-0.26 mg/kg.

Similar conditions include warfarin poisoning which is not accompanied by growth depression, phenol-type poisoning, leptospirosis and acute copper toxicity.

Treatment

None. Remove suspect ration. Feed a high protein, aflatoxin-free ration. Most ration components are screened for aflatoxicosis now and the importation of contaminated feed is now prohibited in the UK. A maximum level of 20µg/kg has been imposed by the EU. Hydrated sodium calcium aluminium silicate added to feed can reduce the adverse effects and feed supplementation with Vitamin A, Vitamin E, folic acid or lysine have been reported to reduce its effects. None prevent absorption and growth depression entirely.

256

Reference

Cook, W.O., Alstine, W.G. van., Osweiler, G.D. (1989). Aflatoxicosis in Iowa swine: Eight cases (1983-1985). J.Am.Vet.Med.Ass. **194**, 554-558.
Harvey, R.B., Huff, W.E., Kubena, L.F., Corrier, D.E., Phillips, T.D. (1988). Progression of aflatoxicosis in growing barrows. Am.J.Vet.Res. **49**, 482-487.

Ergot Poisoning

Ergot (*Claviceps purpurea*) on grain or on pasture may be an uncommon cause of agalactia and the birth of small, weak, shortlived or dead piglets. There may be no enlargement of the teats and udder at parturition and repeat oestrus may occur in affected sows and gilts. On rare occasions, the gangrenous form may appear, and extremities such as the ears may become dry or gangrenous. In most cases, little or no abnormality may be seen in growing pigs other than some growth depression. Up to 1g ergot/kg may be fed without effect, but at 2 g FCR may be adversely affected. Above this level, food refusal, restlessness and aggression may be seen.

The agalactia does not respond to oxytocin treatment and the gangrenous lesions must be differentiated from those of swine fever, salmonellosis and erysipelothrix infection. Removal of the source of ergot in the feed leads to the resumption of milk flow within 48 hours in affected sows.

Humane slaughter may be indicated when gangrene has developed or if piglets cannot be nursed successfully.

Reference

Blaney, B.J., McKenzie, R.A., Walters, J.R., Taylor, L.F., Bewg, W.S., Ryley, M.J., Maryam, P. (2000). Sorghum ergot (Claviceps Africana) associated with agalactia and feed refusal in pigs and dairy cattle. Aust. Vet. J. **78**, 102-107.

Mycotoxic nephropathy (Ochratoxicosis)

Definition

A syndrome in which decreased rate of daily liveweight gain, tubular degeneration and interstitial fibrosis of the kidney result from the ingestion of mouldy rations containing Ochratoxin A and other mycotoxins. The lesions are normally only seen at slaughter but an acute syndrome, perirenal oedema, may occur in recently weaned pigs.

Incidence

First seen in Denmark in the kidneys of slaughter pigs, Ochratoxin A and the changes in pig kidney have now been identified in many countries including the U.K., Eire, U.S.A., Australia, Canada, Poland, Germany and Hungary. In 1000 sows surveyed in the U.K. in 1984 20% had demonstrable ochratoxin A but only one had levels above 24 µg/kg.

Aetiology and pathogenesis

Ochratoxin A, citrinin and oxalic acid are produced by *Penicillium viridicatum* in mouldy rye and barley and by fungi such as *Aspergillus ochraceous* in maize. The levels necessary to cause disease differ between pure compound and levels in natural feed . In the latter, levels of 200 ppb appear to cause disease but levels of up to 4000-7000 ppb have been reported. At 200 ppb or more clinical signs may appear within 3 weeks. Decreased glomerular filtration rate and impaired proximal tubular function result from the administration of Ochratoxin A. Urinary glucose and protein levels of the urine rise and the concentrating power of the kidney is lost. Ochratoxin is immunosuppressive and may affect semen quality.

Clinical signs

Few, other than reduction appetite and in the rate of daily liveweight gain, polydypsia and polyuria in fattening and adult pigs. In recently weaned pigs, subcutaneous oedema, ataxia, stiff arched back and distention of the lumbar part of the abdominal wall may be seen followed by death in 1 or 2 days. Mortality may reach 40-90% of affected batches. A possible decline in semen quality has been reported. Ataxic pigs should be slaughtered humanely.

Pathology

In the chronic form, the kidneys are enlarged and pale with an uneven surface. There is degeneration of the proximal tubular epithelium and interstital fibrosis. Glomeruli may be hyalinised. The acute form is less clearly associated with ochratoxin as perirenal oedema and changes such as those described for the chronic form can result from poisoning by weeds in the U.S. Meat from affected pigs contains ochratoxin.

Epidemiology

Has been identified in Eire following feeding with wet-stored barley. In Denmark where the incidence is recorded, the rate per 100,000 seems to vary with the year, and clear associations between wet years, late harvests and organically grown grains and high feed levels have been found. Ochratoxin A is present in a wide range of pig-derived foods such as sausage, black pudding and liver products.

Diagnosis

The clinical signs of increased thirst and polyuria may suggest ochratoxicosis and the finding of enlarged pale kidneys may also suggest the presence of the condition. Reduced levels of renal phosphoenol pyruvate carboxykinase (70-80% reduction) and a similar reduction in gamma glutamyl transpeptidase have been shown to occur and can be used for diagnosis.

Confirmation is by the demonstration of Ochratoxin A in feed, plasma or tissues using ELISA or High Pressure Liquid Chromatography (HPLC) assays. Levels in feed >200 ppb lead to growth depression and mild renal lesions. Those >1,000 ppb may lead to polydipsia and >4,000 ppb to full clinical disease. Levels in tissue vary and even in grossly affected kidneys may not be high. Levels of >2 ng/ml blood indicate potential ochratoxicosis in a herd and levels in excess of 45 ng/ml have been recorded. Levels up to 98 ppb in liver and to 89 ppb in kidney have been recorded.   Safe levels for human consumption are considered to be <25 ppb (Denmark).

Treatment and control

Ochratoxin is cleared from the body within 3-4 weeks if contaminated feed is withdrawn (9 days in one study when 3.0mg/kg had been given). Supportive therapy can be given. Bin hygiene helps prevention but none of the feed treatments save 10% activated charcoal appears to reduce effective feed levels.

References

Biro, K, Barna-Vetro, I., Pecsi, T., Szabo, E., Winkler, G., Fink-Gremmels, J., Solti, L. (2003). Evaluation of spermatological parameters in ochratoxin-challenged boars. Theriogenology, **60**, 199-207.
Frohlich, A.A., Marquardt, R.R., Clarke, J.R. (1997). Enzymatic and immunological approaches for the quantitation and confirmation of ochratoxin A in swine kidneys. J. Food Protection **60**, 172-176.
Holmberg, T., Breitholtz-Emanuelsson, A., Haggblom, P., Schwan, O, Hult, K. (1991). Mycopathologia 116, 169-176. *Penicillum verrucosum* in feed of Ochratoxin A positive swine herds.
Madsen. A. (1980). Pig News and Information 1, 335. Ochratoxin A - a mycotoxin in feeds and pigs.
Madsen, A., Mortensen, H.P., Hald,B. (1982). Acta.Ag.Scand. 32, 225-239. Feeding experiments with Ochratoxin A contaminated barley for bacon pigs. I. Influence on pig performance and residues.
Mallmann, C.A., Santurio, J.M., Baldissera, M.A., Mickwitz, G.von (1994). Determination of ochratoxin A in blood serum of pigs by using thin layer chromatography. Revista de Microbiologia **25**, 107-111.

Fumonisin toxicity (Porcine Pulmonary Oedema Syndrome)

Definition

Fumonisin causes reduction of feed consumption, mild respiratory distress and death from pulmonary oedema at high levels.

Incidence

Fumonisin can be identified in maize grown in most parts of the world, but the clinical syndrome is only identified when high levels are fed. It has been identified in France, Germany, the USA, Hungary, Thailand and South Africa.

Aetiology

Fumonisin is produced by *Fusarium moniliforme* and *F. verticilloides* growing on maize. The principal toxin involved is fumonisin B_1, although similar effects have been shown for B_2.

Pathogenesis

Fumonisin B_1 acts to inhibit sphingosine and sphinganine N-acetyl transferase. At low levels <23 ppm in feed, liver damage develops and at higher levels of >32 and 175 ppm in feed, acute pulmonary oedema develops followed by death. Fumonisin is excreted at 21% (in urine), and 58% (faeces) of feed levels but enterohepatic circulation takes place. Excretion is virtually complete 3 days after withdrawal of contaminated feel.

Clinical signs

Clinical signs begin about 5 days after the first ingestion of contaminated feed with depression and a rapid decrease in feed intake. Watery diarrhoea has been described and there is a progressive increase in respiratory rates (to 60-100 per minute) with cyanosis of the mucous membranes. At low levels of fumonisin intake, the only clinical signs may be those of a progressive hepatic disease, although feed levels of 10 ppm depressed gain by 11% in one study. At higher levels the reduction in feed intake is followed by mild respiratory distress, pulmonary oedema and death. Piglets from sows receiving contaminated feed (300ppm fumonisin B_1) developed pulmonary oedema within 7 days of birth. Piglets of lactating sows are unaffected. Humane slaughter should be carried out when pulmonary oedema is first noted.

Pathology

The major pathological findings are the presence of severe oedema of the lung and pleural effusions (up to 0.5L). The lungs are heavier than normal and there is interlobular and alveolar oedema. Flluid in the interlobular septae is proteinaceous. Hepatic changes are always present. Membranous material is present in the hepatic sinusoids, and there are multilamellar bodies in hepatocytes, Kupffer cells, pancreatic acinar cells and pulmonary macrophages. Oedema and haemorrhages of the heart muscle have been described as have haemorrhages in the adrenal cortex. Brain changes including malacia have been recorded.

Diagnosis

Diagnosis is based on the clinical signs, the rise in liver enzymes and the tissue and serum sphinganine : sphingosine ratio. The gross and microscopic pathological findings support the diagnosis but confirmation depends upon the demonstration of fumonisin by HPLC in feed or in tissue.

Treatment and Control

There is no treatment and control depends upon screening feeds and destroying contaminated batches.

References

Becker, B.A., Pace, L., Rottinghaus, G.E., Shelby, R., Misfeldt, M., Ross, P.F. (1995). Effects of feeding fumonisin B_1 to lactating sows and their suckling pigs. Am.J.Vet. Res.56, 1253-1258.
Done, S.H. (1995). A new and emerging disease, fumonisin toxicity. Pig J. 34, 134-140.
Haschek, W.M., Motein, G., Ness, D.K., Harbin, K.S., Hall, W.F., Vesonder, R.F., Peterson, R.E., Beasley, V.R. (1992). Characterisation of fumonisin toxicity in orally and intravenously dosed swine. Mycopathologia 117, 83-96.
Riley, R.T. and 10 others (1993). Alteration of tissue and serum sphinganine to sphingosine ratio: an early biomarker of exposure to fumonisin-containing feeds in pigs. Toxicological and Applied Pharmacology 118, 105-112.

Mycotoxin control

1. Mycotoxin-free feed should be used wherever possible. Analysis for mycotoxin is necessary to prove absence, but visible mould is a guide to the presence of mycotoxins

2. The EU requires mycotoxin containing feed to be destroyed, but makes an exception for aflatoxin contaminated feed which can be diluted with uncontaminated feed down to the no effect levels by a few specialist, licensed companies.

3. High protein, activated charcoal, and high (2.5 ppm) selenium have been reported to protect.

4. Ammonia, calcium hydroxide, sodium hydroxide and sodium calcium aluminosilicate treatments of feed have been reported to reduce mycotoxin levels, but have little effect in practice.

5. Prevention using mould inhibitors should be considered where mould damage may occur after harvesting. Calcium propionate, sorbic acid and propionic acid may all be used. Rapid drying of grain may also arrest the development of moulds.

6. Routine bin hygiene.

PARASITIC DISEASES

Parasitic disease in the pig is caused by 3 main groups of organism: the helminth parasites (nematode worms and cestodes especially tapeworms or flukes); protozoa, primarily coccidia but also including flagellates and trypanosomes and the arthropod ectoparasites. The parasitic diseases of pigs considered here in detail are those important in large scale pig rearing and particularly those which occur in housed pigs. Porcine parasites may cause syndromes which are recognisable clinically or pathologically, but most require laboratory examinations such as microscopy to confirm the presence and identity of the agent concerned. Isolation and culture of the agent is rare, but specific identification is becoming more feasible by means of serological and DNA techniques. Parasitic infections are generally resistant to antimicrobials and this may be of value when an unknown syndrome develops. Resistance to anthelmintics has been recorded.

1. ENDOPARASITES

Helminthosis in the pig seldom appears as clinical disease in Britain and the EU where the majority of animals are kept on concrete for much of their lives or are subject to parasite control programmes. It is a potential problem in pigs housed outdoors and the current importance of extensive systems in the UK makes it even more important. Its importance is chiefly economic with subclinical infections delaying the achievement of marketing weight and being responsible for poor food conversion rates.

References

Hale, O.M., Stewart, T.B. and Marti, O.G. (1986). Pig News and Information 7, 439-441. Endoparasite effects on performance of pigs.
Nansen, P., Roepstorff, A. (1998) Worm infections in pigs a general review with particular reference to epidemiology and control. Proc. IPVS 15 (1), 159-165.

Hyostrongylosis

Definition

Primarily a disease of sows and hardly ever found in housed growing pigs. It is characterised by anaemia, inappetence, and loss of weight and may contribute to the 'thin sow syndrome'.

Incidence

28% of sows were found to be infected in a recent survey but less than 1% of growing pigs. 1994 figures UK suggest 47% breeding herds infected but only 25% finishing herds. Similar figures have been found for organic farms in Denmark.

Aetiology and life cycle

Hyostrongylus rubidus occurs in the stomach. The adults are less than 1 cm long, slender and reddish, and are found closely applied to the gastric mucosa. The eggs are thin shelled and typical of strongyles. They develop on the ground into infective L3 larvae in about 7 days. The remaining (parasitic) moults occur in the gastric glands following ingestion of the third-stage larva. The prepatent period is about 15 days to first egg production with highest levels reached at 22 days post-infection.

Pathogenesis

The pathogenesis depends upon invasion of the gastric glands with resulting loss of parietal cell function. Macroscopically the mucosa has a cobble-stone or morocco leather appearance and a diptheritic membrane may form in heavy infections, with detachment of the mucosa and ulceration. Protein leakage from the gastric lesions and increases in plasma pepsinogen both occur.

Inhibition of larvae in the mucosa is a common phenomenon in this infection, and development of the inhibited stages with effects on the gastric mucosa occurs after farrowing. This resumption of development appears to have a hormonal basis, and to be related to lactation. It may also occur after therapy with an anthelmintic not effective against inhibited larvae.

Clinical signs

The clinical disease is seen predominantly in the lactating sow where marked weight loss is observed despite adequate feeding: this weight loss continues after the litter is weaned. In typical cases the sow is thin, shows pallor of visible mucous membranes and skin and, although diarrhoea is not present, the faeces may be dark intermittently. In chronic cases affected animals become dull, lethargic and may have a depraved appetite.

Experimental studies with moderate infections suggest that growth in weaners may be depressed by 8% compared with controls and that crude protein is less well utilised, that faecal nitrogen is greater and that a worse nitrogen balance occurs than in uninfected animals. Meat quality may be adversely affected.

Infertility manifested by reduced fecundity and irregular returns to oestrus, especially after farrowing, have been reported in sows with high *Hyostrongylus* egg counts. Birth weights may be reduced by 15% and survival and weaning weights are also reduced.

Epidemiology

Hyostrongylosis often appears when sows and gilts have been turned on to permanent pig paddocks with the boar between litters. Studies with pasture in the South of England suggest that larvae can develop to the infective stage from May to October. These infective larvae survive best on herbage and may survive for 10 months. Eggs do not hatch and produce infective larvae at 4°C but do so between 10°C and 27°C. Drying kills eggs and developing larvae and frequent freezing and thawing also does so. In spite of this, overwintering can occur. Heavy stocking of pasture to give bare earth reduces larval survival. Transmission can occur in housed pigs but infection is confined to outdoor animals in most cases.

Diagnosis

Diagnosis is based on clinical signs of weight loss and a history of poor food conversion rates in sows and gilts which have previously grazed on permanent pasture. The presence of infection may be suspected when the gastric lesions are seen and worms may be identified in digests of gastric mucosa. Faecal egg counts and plasma pepsinogen levels are useful aids to diagnosis.

Treatment and control

See below.

References

Connan, R.M. (1967). Observations on the epidemiology of parasitic gastroenteritis due to *Oesophagostomum spp.* and *H.rubidus* in the pig. Vet.Rec. **80**, 424-429.

Davidson, J., Murray, M. and Sutherland, I.H. (1968). *H.rubidus: A* field study of its pathogenesis diagnosis and treatment. Vet.Rec. **83**, 582-588.

Roepstrff, A., Murrell, K.D. (1997). Transmission dynamics of helminth parasites of pigs on continuous pasture: *Oesophagostomum dentatum* and *H. rubidus*. Int. J.Parasitol. **27**, 553-562.

Rose, J.H. and Small, A.J. (1982). Observations on the development and survival of the free-living stages of *H.rubidus* both in their natural environments out of doors and under controlled conditions in the laboratory. Parasitology **85**, 33-42.

Stewart, T.B., Hale, D.M. and Martin, O.G. (1985). Experimental infections with *H. rubidus* and the effects on the performance of growing pigs. Vet. Parasitol. **17**, 219-227

Oesophagostomosis

Definition

Oesophagostomum infection may cause diarrhoea but is more frequently associated with poor weight gain, and, in sows, with reduced productivity.

Incidence

Oesophagostomum occurs worldwide. It is least common in intensive SPF units in any country and most common in conditions of poor hygiene both indoors and outdoors where effective control is not practised. Surveys in Denmark suggest that infection is present in 8% sows in large indoor intensive herds and 50% in small indoor and all outdoor herds. Infection was enzootic in 42% breeder finishing units, 12.5% weaner producers and 22.4% finishing units. 20% of sows, 14% finishers and 5% weaners on organic herds in Denmark were infected in 1999. Similar figures have been recorded elsewhere in Europe. It is seldom present in sufficient numbers to cause the clinical disease characterised by diarrhoea and weight loss.

Aetiology and pathogenesis

Two species of Oesophagostomum are involved, *O.dentatum* and *O.quadrispinatum*. The adult worms are about 1.5 cm long and occur in the colon and caecum. The life cycle is direct, infection occurring by ingestion of the third stage larvae which enter the mucosa of the caecum and proximal colon where they remain for at least 2 weeks. Here they moult to become fourth stage larvae which complete their development in the lumen, taking a further 3 weeks. The prepatent period for monospecific infections of both species is 17-19 days and 18-24 days (mean 20.2 +/-1.4days) for mixed populations. In very heavy infections , this may be extended to 27-33 days. Populations of *O. dentatum* are most common in the proximal third of the colon and the preferred habitat of *O. quadrispinatum* is slightly more proximal to this. The lesions seen and the diarrhoea appear to result from the tissue damage and the subsequent infection with bacteria such as campylobacters and spirochaetes. Immunity, diet, competition between the two species, sex ratio and numbers of larvae in the infecting dose all influence the location of the worms, their size, fecundity and the infectivity of the subsequent generation larvae.

Clinical signs

In heavy infections, which are comparatively rare in the U.K., the principal clinical sign is soft faeces or diarrhoea. The main effect of the parasite is a subclinical one, usually associated with reduction in weight gain and poor milk yields of sows (in conjunction with *H. rubidus* it can contribute to the 'thin sow syndrome'). Performance of litters from infected dams is impaired as reflected by the litter size, birth weights, growth and food conversion. Growth may be depressed by 13% and feed conversion raised by 15%.

Pathology

All that may be seen at post-mortem examination may be a diffuse enteritis in the colon and caecum but the mucosal surface may bear nodules containing larvae. These should be distinguished from the enlarged lymphoid diverticulae present in normal animals and made prominent from the serosal surface by any inflammation. Adults may be seen on the surface of the mucosa and larvae may be seen in histological sections.

Epidemiology

The infective larvae do not survive on dry concrete or through a Danish winter on pasture and theoretically this disease can be prevented under conditions of good husbandry. However, despite the high proportion of pigs housed in ideal conditions, infections with *Oesophagostomum* remain common. Eggs require moisture (100% humidity is best) and a minimum temperature of greater than 10°C and usually 15-17°C for infective larvae to develop. Outdoor development of infective larvae takes place largely between April and November with 3-10% of all eggs reaching the infective stage within 1-5 weeks. Indoors, where development occurs all the year round, 70-90% of eggs reach the infective stage within 1-2 weeks. All may survive for up to 20 weeks. Third stage larvae may migrate from faeces for 80-150cm under conditions of high humidity and up to 50% migrating larvae will enter parasite free faeces at 14 days of age if available. Eggs are usually killed within 7-14 days in slurry or manures (ensiled).

The 'periparturient rise' in sows is an epidemiological phenomenon based primarily upon Oesophagostomum infection. During the first half of pregnancy, the burdens of adult worms are low, but in the second half, the egg count begins to rise, reaching a maximum during lactation. At weaning there is an abrupt drop to the low level of early pregnancy. The importance of the phenomenon is that piglets are born into a highly infective environment. It has been shown that the rise can be eliminated by the application of a single dose of anthelmintic one week before farrowing (see control section). Wild boar and rats may be infected.

Diagnosis

Currently based on the identification and enumeration of eggs from faeces, and on the recovery of adults from the intestinal contents and mucosa. PCR techniques have recently been described which confirm the presence of *Oesophagostomum sp* and distinguish between the two species regardless of stage of development. ELISAs using L4 antigen or a 30kDa antigen can detect serum antibody specific to *O. dentatum* as soon as 7 days after infection.

Herd monitoring of faecal egg counts every 6 months sampling 10 growers (10-12 weeks) 10 finishers (5-6 months), 10 gilts and dry sows and 10 lactating sows allows the level of herd infection to be monitored.

Treatment and control

See below.

Effective cleaning under most indoor regimes reduces transmission to a minimum.

References

Barutzki, D. (1990). On the development of *O.quadrispinulatum* Proc. IPVS **11**, 310.

Cannon, R.M. (1967). Observations on the epidemiology of parasitic gastroenteritis due to *Oesophagostomum spp.* and *Hyostrongylus rubidus* in the pig. Vet.Rec. **80**, 424-429.

Joachim, A., Daugschies, A., Christensen, C.M., Bjorn, H., Nansen, P. (1997). Use of random amplified polymorphic DNA polymerase chain reaction for the definition of genetic markers for species and strains of porcine Oesophagostomum. Parasitol. Res. **83**, 646-654.

Kendall, S.B., Small, A.J. Phipps, L.P. (1977). *Oesophagostomum sp.* in pigs in England. J.Comp.Path. **87**, 223-229.

Kraglund, H.O., Roepstorff, A., Gronvold, J. (2001). The impact of season and vegetation on the survival and development of O. dentatum larvae in pasture plots. Parasitology **123**, 415-423.

Larsen, R.H., Christensen, C.M., Lind, P. (1997). Serological assays for the identification of O. dentatum infections in pigs. Res Vet. Sci. **63**, 5-10.

Pattison, H., Thomas, R.J., Smith, W.C. (1980). The effect of subclinical nematode parasitism on digestion and performance in pigs. Anim.Prod. **30**, 285-294.

Pattison, H., Thomas, R.J. and Smith, W.C. (1980). A survey of gastrointestinal parasitism in pigs. Vet.Rec. **107**, 415-418.

Roepstorff, A. (1997). Helminth surveillance as a prerequisite for anthelmintic treatment in intensive sow herds. Vet. Parasitol. **73**, 139-151.

Thomas, R.J. and Ferber, M. (1985). The epidemiology of helminthiasis in pigs. Proc.Pig Vet.Soc. **12**, 50-55

Ascariosis

Definition

Infection with *A.suum* is widespread but causes few clinical signs. The main importance of ascariosis is as a cause of condemnation of livers and 'plucks' (heart and lungs) due to the lesions produced by migrating larvae.

Incidence

A. suum occurs relatively commonly in growing pigs and sows in all parts of the world (47% of breeding:finishing herds infected UK 1994, 25% finishing herds). Milk spot livers (the consequence of larval migration) are commonly detected at slaughter at frequencies related to control programmes and management.

Aetiology and pathogenesis

The adults occur in the small intestine and may be up to 40 cm long. The life cycle is direct with infection resulting from the ingestion of eggs containing second stage larvae. The development of the egg to the infective second larval stage depends on temperature (15°C minimum, 30-33°C optimum) and relative humidity (minimum 80%) and takes 2 months outdoors and 2-4 weeks indoors in the U.K. although this may be reduced indoors or in hotter climates. After ingestion, second stage larvae hatch and enter the mucosa of the pig caecum within 3 hours of infection and migrate to the liver within 6 hours of infection where they moult then migrate to the lungs, reaching them 5-8 days post-infection to enter the tracheobronchial tree after a further moult to fourth stage larvae and are coughed up and swallowed to mature in the small intestine. Transient lesions develop in lung and liver but resolve within 40 days. The pre-patent period is 40-53 days. Immunity can develop but may take some time. Both cellular and humoral immunity, including IgE has been demonstrated and is not dependent upon the presence of adult worms. In immune pigs larvae may be prevented from penetrating the gut wall or be stopped in the liver or lung. In some cases liver lesions may occur. Experimental studies suggest that damaged infective eggs, or ultrasonicated extracts of second stage larvae, larval cell walls and intestinal aminopeptidase from larvae may stimulate protection. When large numbers of eggs are ingested, fewer adults are found in the intestine than in infections with small numbers of eggs.

Clinical signs

Clinical signs of intestinal infection are rarely observed even in heavy infections. Growth rate may be reduced by 2-10% and food conversion by 5-13% following experimental infections and reduction in the digestibility of food has been demonstrated. Occasional animals may develop jaundice and some of these may die.

A moist cough, "heaves", may occur during the migration stage, about a week after infection. The role of ascarids in this cough is not clear, but it can be reproduced experimentally. Affected pigs appear hairy, may develop congested extremities and even die.

Humane slaughter is indicated in obstructive jaundice but even severely congested pigs with respiratory distress recover rapidly in the migration stage and should be given symptomatic treatment.

Pathology

Icteric pigs may be found to have bile ducts stuffed with adult ascarids. Normally, lesions are only incidental findings at post-mortem. They consist of the 'milk spot liver' in which whitish fibrous or fleshy lesions up to 1 cm in diameter occur on the liver surface and local petechial haemorrhages occur in the lung. The lung lesions occur during migration and resemble petechiae but consist of worm tracks filled with debris and the occasional larva. Mild hyperaemia of the small intestinal mucosa may be noted where adult worms are located. Occasionally large clusters of worms plug the intestinal lumen.

Epidemiology

In pigs at pasture in the UK infective eggs gradually rise in numbers developing only between June and September to give peak numbers in early autumn. Development occurs indoors from April to October but may extend beyond this in moist warm conditions or in heaps of warm damp material. This is reflected in the 5.4 times greater risk of Ascaris infection in sow herds using straw. Transmission rarely occurs between adults and offspring with short weaning periods because of the time required for the development of the eggs. Their persistence in suitable conditions for up to 7 years means that weaner-weaner transmission can occur in uncleaned pens. Amplified Fragment Length Polymorphism (AFLP) confirms the relationship between worms in an area or herd and suggests that carrier pigs are the main rote of transmission to new herds. Man and sheep may also become infected after eating infective eggs and human infections can occur after eating raw liver. Human infections with adult worms have been shown by mitochondrial DNA analysis to be *A. lumbricoides* where exposure to *A. suum* is also common, although *A. suum* may be responsible for infections in areas where *A. lumbricoides* is absent.

Diagnosis

Clinical signs are variable and difficult to correlate with significant levels of infection. Transient coughing and, later a high egg count in pigs newly moved into contaminated pens, the presence of icteric pigs with no fever and post-mortem or slaughter findings of milk spot liver or ascarids in the intestine are indications for treatment or that treatments given have not been effective. The eggs of *Ascaris suum* are round, rough shelled and 45-85 um in diameter. They may be identified in faeces by flotation methods.

ELISAs for serum antibody have recently been described using L2/L3-ES (excretory fluid from cultured larvae) as antigen and represent an accurate measure of the presence of eggs in faeces for weaners and finishers, but less so for sows, where antibody is more common than the presence of eggs. The ELISA has been found to detect herd infections more easily than faecal egg counts.

Control

Control is difficult because of the adhesive nature of the egg and its longevity on the ground (up to 5 years). In premises where ascariosis is a continuous problem, thorough cleaning of farrowing and fattening quarters with detergent or hot washing soda should be combined with anthelmintic treatment of the sow stock. The use of a horticultural flame gun has given good results in reducing the numbers of ascarid ova on concrete floors and thorough drying may also be of value. Pressure washing without drying may enhance survival. Composting of manure may destroy eggs but requires long periods (30 days at 37°C) or temperatures of 55 °C for 5-75 minutes or of 60°C for 1-8 minutes and they may be killed by some proprietary disinfectants such as oocide (Dupont). Methods of treatment are given below.

Stocking clean farms may be achieved by treatment with an avermectin accompanied by thorough cleaning and disinfection of the pigs prior to movement.

References

Bernado, T.M., Dohoo, J.R., Ogilvie, I. (1990). A critical assessment of abattoir surveillance as a screening test for swine ascariasis. Can.J.Vet.Res. **54**, 274-277.
Dangolla, A., Willeberg, P., Bjorn, H., Roepstorff, A. (1996). Association of *A. suum* and *Oesophagostomum spp* infections of sows with management factors in 83 Danish sow herds. Prev. Vet. Med. **27**, 197-209.
Graasenbeek, C.P.H., Borgsteede, F.H.M. (1998). Studies on the survival of *A. suum* eggs under laboratory and simulated field conditions. Vet. Parasitol. **75**, 227-234.

Lind, P., Eriksen, L., Nansen, P., Nilsson, O., Roepstorff A. (1993). Response to repeated inoculations with *A.suum* eggs in pigs during the fattening period II: specific IgA and IgM determined by ELISA. Parasitol. Res. **79**, 240-244.

Murrell, K.D., Eriksen, L., Nansen, P., Slotved, H.S., Rasmussen, T. (1997*). A. suum*: a revision of its early migration path and implications for human ascariasis. J. parasitol. **83**, 255-260.

Nejsum, P., Frydenberg, J., Roepstorff, A., Parker, E.D.Jr (2005). Population structure in *Ascaris suum* (Nematoda) among domestic swine in Denmark as measured by whole genome DNA fingerprinting. Hereditas (Lund) **142**, 7-14.

Nilsson, O. (1982). Ascariasis in the pig. An epizootiological and clinical study. Acta.Vet.Scand. Supplement **79**, 108 pp.

Roepstorff, A. (1998). Natural *A. suum* infections in swine diagnosed by coprological and serological (ELISA) methods. Parasitol. Res. **84**, 537-543.

Roepstorff, A., Murrell, K.D., Boes, J., Petkevicius, S. (2001). Ecological influences on transmission rates of Ascaris suum on pastures. Vet.Parasitol. **101**, 143-153.

Urban,J.F., Alizadeh,H., Romanowski, R. (1988). *A.suum*, development of intestinal immunity to infective second stage larvae in swine. Exp. Parasitol. **66**, 66-77.

Lungworm (Metastrongylosis)

Definition

Lungworm infection of the bronchioles of the lung may give rise to coughing, depression of growth and emphysematous lesions of the periphery of the diaphragmatic lobe of the lung in pigs housed outdoors.

Incidence

Present in all parts of the world. Rare in the UK. for many years, the recent increase in herds with access to pasture has led to its reappearance and it was enzootic in 20% breeder finisher herds in the UK in 1994..

Aetiology and pathogenesis

Metastrongylus apri (elongatus) and *M.pudendotectus* are white in colour and measure up to 48 mm. The live in the bronchi or bronchioles of the posterior part of the diaphragmatic lobes of the lungs. Eggs measuring 40 x 50 um contain first stage larvae and are thick walled. They are coughed up, passed out in the faeces and ingested by earth worms at temperatures >0°C in which they moult to produce the infective third stage larva (L3) at temperatures above 9°C. Infected earth worms are ingested by pigs and the L3 larvae enter the host caecal and colon wall and move in lymphatics to the mesenteric lymph nodes where they form L4 and then to the lungs to become L5 and mature to produce patent infection after 20-24 days.

Following heavy experimental or field infection, severe cellular reaction to aspirated eggs may occur in the small bronchioles and marked lymphoid and muscular changes have been recorded. Some degree of immunity appears to result from infection.

M.salmi, *M.confusus* and *M. asymmetricus* may occur in wild boar.

Clinical signs

Heavy infections are characterised by coughing and dyspnoea in weaned and growing pigs but adults are largely resistant and heavy infections are rare and cause only an intermittent husky cough.

Post-mortem findings

These are restricted to the lungs and consist of consist of scallop-shaped raised pale areas of emphysema on the edges of the caudal part of the diaphragmatic lobes. When these portions of the lung are cut off and squeezed gently the worms may be seen as white threads, or when full of eggs, coloured brown. There may be hypertrophy of the bronchial muscles, and the bronchi contain neutrophils, eggs and adults when examined histologically. Bronchial lymph nodes may be enlarged and white spots 0.5-1 cm in diameter may be present on the liver.

Epidemiology

The earthworm vector is essential and infection is most common in pigs housed outdoors on pasture where up to 10% earthworms may be infected. Pigs with access to outdoor concrete yards may be infected by eating wandering earthworms. Breeding stock or finishers originally reared outdoors may also be infected. Infection may persist for 2-3 years in individual earthworms in a pasture. Wild boar and feral pigs can carry and spread infection.

Diagnosis

Infection may be suspected in outdoor pigs or wild boar on clinical grounds and confirmed by identifying the embryonated eggs in faeces or the characteristic lung lesions at slaughter.

Control

Heavily contaminated pasture may need to be cropped for 2 or 3 years and pigs may have to be housed or yarded to prevent re-infection after treatment. Treatment is described below.

Trichuris suis infection.

Definition

T. suis infects the porcine large intestine of weaned pigs to cause inflammation and contribute to the colitis syndrome. Mild diarrhoea and reduced weight gain may result.

Incidence

Worldwide, most common in systems where hygiene is poor and where control programmes are not in place. Considered enzootic in 15.8% breeding finishing farms UK 1994, but absent from all finishers. More common in free range pigs (37.5%) than in conventional herds (11.1%) The Netherlands, 2001-2002.

Aetiology

Trichuris suis is 3-4 cm in length (males) and 6-8 cm (females), pearly white in colour and the anterior two thirds of the body is thin and hair-like and the posterior third is much thicker (0.65 cm). The eggs are 60 x 25 μm in size and are shed in the faeces where they become infective after 3-4 weeks and can remain infective for up to 11 years. Worms live for up to 5 months.

Pathogenesis

Infection is oral and the eggs hatch to release the first stage larvae which enter the large intestinal crypts and go through 4 moults in tissue before the posterior portion reaches the surface of the mucosa two weeks later. The prepatent period is 6-8 weeks. The mucosal damage which results is colonised in experimental infections by small spirochaetes and other bacteria (see Spirochaetal Diarrhoea) and severe enteric disease has also been associated with *C.perfringens* type A colonisation. Susceptibility to infection declines with age.

Clinical signs

Affected pigs show few clinical signs. In heavy experimental infections, loss of condition and mild diarrhoea may develop 6 weeks post infection. Occasionally there may be bloody diarrhoea, but this is frequently the result of complicated infections. Treatment is usually effective and only in severe debility with dysentery should euthanasia be considered.

Pathology

Lesions are confined to the caecum and colon. In light to moderate infections in high health pigs, the mucosa is raised and may be mildly hyperaemic. The thickened posterior portion of the adult worms may be seen protruding from the mucosa and remains in place in freshly killed animals in spite of rinsing. Where secondary infection, proliferative enteropathy, spirochaetal diarrhoea, swine dysentery or salmonella infection occur, the mucosa may become necrotic. In histological sections the worms may be seen in section in the mucosa.

Epidemiology

T. suis is present in domestic pigs and wild boar but can infect man. The life cycle can take place both indoors or outdoors, although in temperate conditions eggs may not be infective until the soil warms. The worms are often present in small numbers in adult pigs and lay eggs sporadically, but the ability of the eggs to survive means that high numbers accumulate if pasture is not cleaned or rotated.

Diagnosis

The clinical signs are not distinctive, although the presence of *T. suis* should be considered in any mild diarrhoea or even dysentery of older weaned pigs and adults. The presence of eggs in faeces is not an absolute indicator of infection in an individual, as coprophagy can lead to passive excretion for up to 5 days. The identification of the worms in the large intestine by their characteristic morphology is confirmatory and they may be present in histological sections. Serum antibody can be detected by ELISA using a 20 kDa secretory glycoprotein antigen from culture fluids of adult worms.
Treatment and Control

See below.

References

Beer, R.J.S. (1973). Studies on the biology of the life cycle of *Trichuris suis*. Parasitology **67**, 253-262.

Hill, D.E., Romanowski, R.D., Urban, J.F. Jr. (1997). A *Trichuris* specific diagnostic antigen from culture fluids of adult worms. Vet. Parasitol. **68**, 91-102.

Pedersen, S., Saeed, I. (2002). Host age influence on the intensity of experimental Trichuris suis infection in pigs. Parasite, **9**, 75-79.

Roepstorff, A., Murrell, K.D. (1997). Transmission dynamics of helminth parasites of pigs on continuous pasture: *A. suum* and *T. suis*. Int. J. Parasitol. **27**, 563-572.

Rutter, J.M. and Beer, R.J.S. (1975). Bacteria and worms in colitis. Infection and Immunity **11**, 395.

Other Infections

Strongyloides ransomi infection occurs mainly in very young piglets and weaners. Though recognised as a pathogen in the United States and Europe, it has never been recognised in clinical disease in the UK. *A.ransomi* adult females 3.3-4.5 mm in length are found in the small intestine and pass thin shelled eggs containing larvae into the intestinal contents (45-55 by 26-35 µm) and faeces. Eggs hatch to first stage larvae which may develop into free living males and females or, within a day, into infective larvae. Larvae enter the host through the skin, the oral cavity via the colostrum and transplacentally. All but colostral larvae (which mature directly) enter tissue and migrate to the gut where they produce a patent infection within 4-8 days.

Anorexia, listlessness, anaemia and diarrhoea may be seen. The presence of larvae in the sows' colostrum or milk and of adults in the intestines of piglets 14 days of age can be used to confirm a diagnosis. Free living forms of this parasite exist and it is particularly associated with warm unhygienic conditions.

Reference

Murrell, K.D. and Urban, J.F. (1983). Induction of immunity to transcolostrally-passed *S.ransomi* larvae in neonatal pigs. J.Parasitol. **69**, 74-77.

Kidney worms (Stephanurus dentatus) do not occur in the UK but are important causes of liver and kidney condemnation from the southern USA to southern Brazil and in other subtropical areas. Eggs are passed in the urine, larvae hatch in the soil and may persist there or in earthworms to be ingested. They migrate to the liver and remain there to produce abscesses before migrating to the ureters as adults 2-3 cm in length. Patency takes 9 months to 1 year. Clinical signs are not seen in adult animals and diagnosis depends upon finding eggs in urine or lesions in liver and kidney post-mortem. Infection in growing pigs may result in depression of growth by up to 25% and of feed conversion by 9%. Worms and larvae may be eliminated by single injections of ivermectin.

Trichinosis. An infection of porcine muscle with the larvae of *Trichinella spiralis* (and some other species of Trichinella) which causes no clinical effects on the pig but represents a major zoonotic hazard to those consuming under-cooked pork or imperfectly cured products. Infection occurs in all European countries with wild boar populations and in Asia, North and South America and Africa.

T. spiralis is considered to be absent from Northern Ireland and has rarely been identified in Great Britain in spite of the examination of pig carcases for export. Recent serological surveys (1994) suggest that it is absent. Infection can be detected using trichinoscopy, muscle digestion or stomaching using diaphragm, neck muscle or tongue and, more recently ELISA methods, using excretory antigen and monoclonal antibodies on serum or tissue extracts (meat juice). Antigen is present in the blood for 1-4 weeks and 10-14 weeks after infection. RAPD PCR methods have been used. The most common method of transmission is rat-pig-rat but cannibalism by pigs may maintain disease once introduced. Transmission may also occur where uncooked pigmeat is fed back to pigs and where home killing of pigs or the consumption of undercooked wild boar meat is common. In countries such as The Netherlands which are essentially *T. spiralis*-free, the sampling of foxes which act as reservoirs of *T. britovi* has been suggested as being of greater value than trichinoscopy. Albendazole has been shown to eliminate larvae at 10 mg/kg.

References

Kapel, C.M.O., Webster, P., Pozio, E., Henriksen, S.A., Murrell, K.D., Nansen, P. (1998). *T. spiralis, T. britovi*, and *T. nativa*: infectivity, larval distribution in muscle and antibody response after experimental infection of pigs. Parasitol. Res. **84**, 264-271.

Knapen, F. van (1998). European proposal for alternative Trichinella control in domestic pigs. Fleischwirtschaft **78**, 338-339.

Rodriguez, E., Nieto, J., Rodriguez, M., Garate, T. (1995). Use of random amplified polymorphic DNA for detection of a *T. britovi* outbreak in Spain. Clin. Infect. Dis. **21**, 1521-1522.

Ollulanus worms may be found in gastritis in pigs where the animals have been in contact with cats. It has been recorded in continental Europe.

Fasciola hepatica can occur in grazing pigs and cause severe liver lesions, particularly in young pigs.

Hepatitis cysticercosa is occasionally seen in the U.K. The condition results from the ingestion of onchospheres of *Taenia hydatigena*, where there is mass migration through the liver tissue toward the capsule. It usually occurs as single cases.

Finally, the pig may be infected by ***Cysticercus cellulosae***, which is important in public health. It is not of any clinical importance in the pig itself. The latter has not been recorded in the UK for many years.

Anthelmintic Treatment and the Control of Helminthosis in the Pig

Treatment

A variety of compounds is available for treating helminth parasites in the pig. The spectrum of activity of each compound differs and the species of worm present should be determined before anything more than emergency treatment is attempted. The actual choice of compound used will depend upon:

1.   The species of helminth present (multiple infections are common).

2.   The spectrum of activity of the compound and whether active against both adults and larvae.

3.   The presence or absence of resistance in the helminth population present.

4.   The route of administration required by the farm management system.

5.   The products available to fulfil (4). Different countries have registered or marketed different products.

6.   Any side effects.

7.   Any safety requirements and the capacity of the farm and its staff to meet them.

8.   The withdrawal period.

9.   The cost.

Anthelminthics may be given to pigs as pour-ons or as injections to individual pigs known to be heavily parasitised. In-feed formulations are usually either a powder, liquid, pellets or granules and palatability of the product is important. As with all in-feed drugs, the main problem is to ensure adequate uptake of medicated feed in *ad libitum* feeding systems. Some products have different feed inclusion rates to deliver a fixed dose in mg/Kg to animals of different body weight and feed intake per Kg. Continuous low level medication is sometimes practised to ensure an adequate uptake and compounds administered in this way may prevent economic loss and the establishment of patent infections but protection may cease when they are withdrawn.

At least 4 distinct compounds are registered for use in the U.K. Most are effective against the adult stages of the common helminths but some lack activity against individual species. Activity against larvae is less complete and some products are also ovicidal. The table given below lists the compounds which have been shown to be effective and indicates the form in which they can be administered. Their availability UK is indicated by product names for each class but withdrawal and exact doses recommended for each product are not given and can be found on data sheets and package inserts. The same applies to other countries. The Compendium of Data Sheets for Animal Medicines 2006 was the source for the UK data. Where a product is known to be effective but is not registered for pigs, the cascade system should be employed in the UK. but is limited to products available for food animals and 28 day withdrawals are required.

Compounds available for treatment and suggested treatment schedules:

Compound	Effective against	Route	Dosing Regime	Brands (UK)

		Feed	Continuous	None UK 2006
Thiabendazole	Adult H,O,T,S Larval H,O.T.S Adult and Larval H,O		Single	
Ivermectin	Adult H,O,S,M,A Larval H,O,S,A Some activity T	Injectable Feed	Single	Ivomec injection for pigs Ivomec Premix for pigs (to 100 kg) 100 µg/kg. 7 days and transfer to clear. Panomec injection Merial Alstomec injection (Alstoe Ltd) Animec Injection (Chanelle) Qualmintec (Janssen)
Doramectin	Adult HOTSAM Larval HOTSAM	Injectable	Single	Dectomax injection for pigs (Pfizer), 0.3mg/kg
Cambendazole	Adult A,H,O	Feed	Single	None UK2006
Dichlorvos	Adult H,O,T,A L4 HO,T,A	Feed	Single	None UK2006
Tetramisole	Adult H,O,A,M Larval H,O,A,M	Feed	Single	None UK2006
Levamisole	Adult H,O,A,	Injectable	Single	None UK 2006
Febantel	Adult H,O,A Larval H,O,A,	Feed	5 days	None UK 2006
Thiophanate	Adult H,O,T,A Larval H,O,T,A	Feed	14 days or single	None UK 2006
Flubendazole	Adult HOT(S)AM Larval HOTAM	Feed	Single or 5-10 days	Flubenol Premix (Janssen) (Solubenol water miscible, Janssen, 2006)
Fenbendazole	Adult H,O,T,A,M Larval H,O,T,A,M	Feed	Single course Divided 7d.	Panacur 1.5% pellets (Intervet) Panacur 4% powder (Intervet) Zerofen 4% Powder, Chanelle
Oxibendazole	Adult H,O,A Larval	Feed	10-day course	1.6mg/kg Not UK 2006
Piperazine	Adult A,O	Feed	Single	Not UK 2006
Pyrantel tartrate	Adult H,O,A.	Feed	Single	Not UK 2006

H = Hyostrongylus,   O = Oesophagostomum, T = Trichuris, S = Strongyloides
(S)effective but not claimed UK),   A = Ascaris, M = Metastrongylus

Sample treatment regimes

Sows and Gilts	Treat and wash prior to entering clean farrowing house and again at weaning. Treatment is possible at mid gestation.
Boars	Every 6 months
Growers	Treat on purchase or on entry to clean growing house.
Finishers	On entering clean finishing house and after 8 weeks

Control

These treatments may be used in control programmes which are based upon the ability of the compounds concerned to eliminate most, if not all, of the helminth species present and their larvae. In indoor units with slatted floors, no straw and a regular programme of cleaning and disinfection operating all-in all-out housing policies, helminths may be reduced or even eradicated.

In all programmes, treatment schedules must take account of the possibility that some adults or larvae may survive and that the environment may be contaminated with eggs or larvae. The basic interval between treatments must take into account the prepatent period and be based upon the movement of animals into clean accommodation or uninfected pasture.

If routine therapy is practised, it is usual to carry out a programme which includes regular treatment of the breeding stock as well as the growers and finishers. A popular control programme for outdoor breeding stock is as follows:

Outdoor sows should be treated as above but may require treatment before entering clean paddocks in rotation and monthly between July and October in UK. A sample treatment programme for controlling helminths in pigs at pasture in the UK is to dose in December and repeat the dose 3 weeks later. In June treatment is carried out on 3 occasions and again in October 2 weeks prior to a move to fresh pasture and 1 week after it. This schedule eliminates adult *Hyostrongylus* and *Oesophagostomum* and helps keep larval levels to a minimum.

Specific treatment and control regimes

To prevent milk spot liver in *Ascaris* contaminated accommodation it may be necessary to combine monthly treatment with rigorous hygiene. Eradication may not be achieved for several years. Stocking of clean new premises should only proceed after stock have been treated effectively and then washed clean.

Trichuris may require special treatment e.g., with flubendazole it may be necessary to divide the dose over 7 days.

Metastrongylus may require the use of fenbendazole or ivermectin.

Stephanurus dentatus (adults) are included in the UK claims for doramectin Strongyloides larvae are eliminated from the milk by ivermectin treatment.

References

Barth, D. and Preston, J.M. (1985). Ivermectin against somatic *S.ransomi* larvae. Vet.Rec. 116, 366-367.
Barth, D., Rehbein, S., Reid, J.F.S., Barrick, R.A. (1996). Efficacy of an in feed formulation of ivermectin against adult worms and somatic larvae of S. ransomi. Vet. Parasitol. 65, 89-97.

Rose, J.H. and Small, A.J. (1983). Observations on the effect of anthelmintic treatment on the transmission of *H.rubidus* and *Oesophagostomum spp.* among sows at pasture. J.Helminthology **57**, 1-8.

Taffs, L.F. (1969). Helminths of the pig: pathogenicity diagnosis and control. Br.Vet.J. **125**, 304-310.

Coccidiosis in piglets

Definition

Coccidiosis is most important in the 5-15 day old sucking piglet in which diarrhoea and subsequent growth depression may be accompanied by mortality of up to 20%.

Incidence

Clinical coccidiosis in neonates is present in herds in all parts of the UK. It is massively under reported, but had been identified on 5.3% breeding finishing herds and 6.3% weaner producers in 1994. In The Netherlands 68% farms and 53% litters were infected in 1989 and in Germany, Austria and Switzerland a survey in 2005 found 76% of 324 farms to be infected.. It is present in most pig-rearing countries worldwide and figures from the US and Canada suggest that it may cause disease in 30-60% piglets.

Aetiology

Isospora suis causes coccidiosis in young piglets worldwide. Most species of Eimeria do not occur in, or are of very low pathogenicity for neonates, but some (e.g.*E. polita*) may infect piglets from the sow.

Pathogenesis

Infection with *I.suis* is largely enteric. Infective sporulated *I.suis* oocysts are ingested by piglets from infected faeces and contaminated pen fittings and food. After ingestion the oocysts give rise to sporozoites which infect epithelial cells in the cranial third of the jejunum within 24 hours of infection and produce a first asexual generation of 2-7 merozoites at about 48 hours post-infection. These invade cells to give secondary meronts which give rise to 2-12 large merozoites at 3-4 days p.i and then become 3rd generation meronts which at 4-5 days post-infection give rise to 4-24 small crescent-shaped merozoites. The merozoites invade cells in the distal half of the small intestine to give rise to the sexual stages (micro and macro gamonts) which are mature at 5-6 days post-infection and give rise to multiple microgametes and single macrogametes which, after fusion with a microgamete, give rise to oocysts. Oocysts may be seen in the faeces from 5 days onwards until days 8 or 9 and again from days 11-14 after infection. This second wave of oocysts appears to result from a reappearance of second generation meronts on days 8-9 post-infection and a further crop of sexual stages. In light infections (100 oocysts) up to 3 waves of oocysts have been recorded. Some evidence of extra intestinal infection has been identified, and, in support, most stages of the cycle (from sporozoite to oocyst) have been seen in cultures in swine testicular cells. Oocysts sporulate within 48 hours at 24-27°C (farrowing house temperatures) and may remain infective for more than 10 months. From 1,000-400,000 oocysts per gram of faeces may be passed. Lesions of villous atrophy develop in affected portions of the small intestine by 5 days post-infection to resolve in the absence of other infectious agents by 10-14 days post-infection. Other agents such as rotavirus infection may occur at the same time.

Clinical signs

Faecal changes ranging from transient pasty diarrhoea or whitish faeces to profuse yellowish, watery diarrhoea occur in piglets of 5-15 days of age and are most common at 7-10 days of age. Affected piglets may be thinner than unaffected litter mates and remain gaunt and hairy for some weeks thereafter. Severely affected piglets may die. Mortality rates may reach 20%. The diarrhoea responds poorly to antimicrobial therapy and growth depression occurs in recovered animals. Recently, diarrhoea in the post-weaning period has been associated with *I.suis* infection. Mortality in most indoor units is normally reduced by the provision of electrolytes but may be 20% in outdoor units.

Wasting and moribund piglets should be destroyed, particularly if they cannot be nursed.

Pathology

Carcases of affected piglets may be in poor condition and dehydrated. Gross lesions are restricted to the jejunum and ileum which appear turgid and thickened with a necrotic lining. The intestinal contents may be creamy or watery with flecks of milk and the villi are stunted and local bleeding points and fine fibrino-necrotic flakes may be seen using a dissecting microscope on the mucosa of freshly killed pigs. Histological changes include villous atrophy, increased mitotic activity in the crypt epithelium and the presence of large numbers of coccidial merozoites and male and female gametocytes within vacuoles in the epithelial cells. Oocysts can be demonstrated in colonic contents or faeces.

Epidemiology

Infection has been described both in extensive husbandry systems and indoors. Sows rarely pass *I.suis* oocysts in faeces and the major source of infection for piglets is the faeces of other piglets which contaminates farrowing and rearing accommodation. The high levels of oocysts passed by piglets and their ability to survive for months make environmental contamination important. Carrier sows may, however, be the means of introduction of the disease into clean buildings or farms. Less disease and oocyst shedding has been demonstrated on fully slatted cleaned floors. Eimeria species are carried by sows and may be passed to their offspring. *E.scabra* and *E. polita* infections may occur from 4-8 weeks of age onwards but 96% of piglet infections are due to *I.suis*.

Diagnosis

The clinical signs, especially the age incidence and the failure to respond to antimicrobial therapy may suggest coccidiosis. The presence of coccidial oocysts in the faeces may be suggestive. Faeces from acutely affected pigs may contain few oocysts as the diarrhoea continues between peaks of oocyst shedding, so faeces from less severely affected animals in the litter or 5-10 adjacent litters should also be examined. Samples should be taken in the second and third week of life from 3-5 piglets per litter, grouped on a litter basis and 10 litters sampled. They can be stored at 4°C for several days, but can be submitted without refrigeration and in a sealed container. The sensitivity of detection is improved by flotation and the use of fluorescence microscopy. Other agents such as rotavirus may be present and *Clostridium perfringens* Type A or Type C infections may resemble coccidiosis. The presence of merozoites and sexual stages of coccidia in histological sections, and stained impression smears of jejunal and ileal mucosa, the absence of Clostridia and the failure to respond to antimicrobial treatment confirm the diagnosis. Oocysts may be sporulated in potassium dichromate to confirm the species involved. Cryptosporidia may also be present. PCR has been described and found to be more sensitive than faecal methods.

Treatment and control

Toltrazuril (Baycox Bayer) 20 mg/kg given as an oral suspension by stomach tube on day 3 prevents diarrhoea, prevents oocyst shedding and can maintain piglet growth. Given as a treatment it stops diarrhoea and oocyst shedding, prevents mortality but growth rate in treated animals will depend upon the damage already caused but will be improved. The product is alkaline, and if vomiting occurs, it should be diluted 1:10 with water.

Until this product is registered for pigs (not UK 2006), less effective methods of treatment will have to be used. Trimethoprim sulphonamide may be given by injection or orally to affected piglets and should be supplemented by electrolyte.

The inclusion of an anticoccidial such as monensin at 100g/tonne in sow feed for 7-10 days prior to farrowing and for 2 weeks afterwards will reduce the shedding of oocysts by sows. Similar inclusion rates will reduce shedding by other pigs. Amprolium may also be used to treat affected pigs at 10-20 mg/kg given orally for 4-5 days and reduces oocyst numbers but does not eliminate clinical signs. Treatment should include both clinically-affected pigs and their littermates. None of these products are registered for this use in pigs in the UK. Scrupulous attention should be given to hygiene in control. Sows should be cleaned on entry to farrowing houses which should be disinfected or fumigated with methyl bromide or ammonia (final concentration 2%) to kill oocysts. Steam cleaning at 65°C for 15 minutes and flame guns (safety!) will also destroy oocysts. The disinfectant, oocide (Dupont) can also be used to destroy oocysts.

An experimental vaccine produced from the sporozoite attachment protein has reduced oocyst shedding by 99% when given intramuscularly and orally.

References

Christensen, J.P.B., Henriksen, S. (1994). Shedding of oocysts in piglets experimentally infected with *I. suis*. Acta Vet. Scand. **35**, 165-172.

Driesen, S.J., Fahy, V.A., Carland, P.G. (1995). The use of toltrazuril for the prevention of coccidiosis in piglets before weaning. Aust. Vet. J. **72**, 139-141.

Harleman, J.H. and Meyer, R.C. (1984). Life cycle of *I.suis* in gnotobiotic and conventionalised piglets. Veterinary Parasitology **17**, 27-39

Harleman, J.H. and Meyer, R.C. (1985). Pathogenicity of *I.suis* in gnotobiotic and conventionalised piglets. Vet.Rec. **116**, 561-565.

Joachim, A., Ruttowski, B., Zimmerman, M., Daugschies, A., Mundt, H.C. (2004) Detection of *Isospora suis* (Biester and Murray 1934) in piglet faeces-comparison of microscopy and PCR. J.Vet.Med, Series B **51**, 140-142.

Lindsay, D.S., Current, W.L., Ernst, J.V. and Stuart, B.P. (1983). Diagnosis of neonatal porcine coccidiosis caused by *I. suis*. Vet.Med. S.A.C. **78**, 89-95.

Lindsay, D.S., Ernst, J.V., Current, W.L., Stuart, B.P. and Stewart, T.B. (1984). Prevalence of oocysts of *I.suis* and *Eimeria spp* from sows on farms with and without a history of neonatal coccidiosis. J.Am.Vet.Med.Ass. **185**, 419-421.

Madsen, P., Henriksen, A.A., Larsen, K. (1992). Efficacy of Baycox on *I.suis* coccidiosis in piglets - a pilot study. Proc.IPVS. **12**, 366.

Martineau, G.P., Menard, J., Carabin, H., Villeneuve, A. and Dumas, G. (1994). Strategic control of porcine coccidiosis with toltrazuril. Proc.IPVS. **13**, 243.

Mundt, H.C., Joachim, A., Becka, M., Daugschies, A. (2006). Isospora suis: an experimental model for mammalian intestinal coccidiosis Parasitology Research **98**, 167-175.

Nilsson, O. (1988). *I.suis* in pigs with post-weaning diarrhoea. Vet.Rec. **122**, 310-311.

Nilsson, O., Martinsson, K. and Persson, E. (1984). Epidemiology of porcine neonatal steatorrhoea in Sweden. 1. Prevalence and clinical significance of coccidial and rotavirus infections. Nord.vet.Med. **36**, 103-110.

Stuart, B.P., Lindsay, D.S., Ernst J.V., Gosser, H.S. (1980). *Isospora suis* enteritis in piglets. Vet. Path. I7, 84-93.

Coccidiosis in weaned pigs

Definition

A number of coccidial species may cause enteric infections in weaned pigs kept in unhygienic conditions and cause unthriftiness, diarrhoea and even death.

Incidence

Coccidial infections in older pigs has been recorded from domestic pigs on all continents and in wild boar wherever they occur. 5.3% breeder finisher units and 12.5% weaner producers were considered to be infected in the UK in 1994. A German survey (2004) of 56 farms found 52% infected.

Aetiology

Coccidiosis in older pigs is associated with Eimeria species, *E.debliecki, E.suis, E.perminuta, E.neodebliecki, E.spinosa, E.porci, E.polita, E.scabra* and local species such as *E.szechuanensis*. Most of these species e.g. *E.debliecki* do not occur in, or are of very low pathogenicity for neonates although some, such as *E. polita* may cause disease. Mixed infections are common. In the German survey, positive samples contained *E.polita* (100%) *E. debliecki* (100%) *E. suis* (84%) *E. porci* (52%), *E.perminuta*, (49%), *E. spinosa*, 20%)

Pathogenesis

Eimeria species have an essentially similar life cycle in older pigs to that of I. suis in piglets. *E. neodebliecki* infections develop in the apical cytoplasm of enterocytes in the mid-posterior jejunum. asexual development of two generations of meronts occurs and they may be seen in groups of up to 5 per host cell. The first macrogametes appear at 9 days post infection and infection becomes patent from 6-8 days after infection.

Clinical signs

Wasting and severe, watery yellow diarrhoea have been recorded in gilts, finishing pigs and wild boar infected with *Eimeria* spp. 40% of adult boars in a boar stud developed diarrhoea unresponsive to antimicrobial without loss of condition and associated with *E. spinosa* infection. In experimental *E. neodebliecki* infections, frothy, mucoid diarrhoea occurred 9-12 days post infection. Wasting and moribund weaners or gilts should be destroyed, particularly if treatment is ineffective..

Pathology

Inflammatory lesions covered with foci of pseudomembranous material are present in the mucosa of affected regions of the posterior small intestine. There is moderate villous atrophy and fibrinonecrotic material can be seen at villous tips. The coccidia are frequently visible in the lesions.

Epidemiology

Eimeria species are carried by sows and may be passed to their offspring. *E.scabra* infections may occur from 4-8 weeks of age onwards. Wild boar are frequently infected. Infection and clinical disease usually follows the introduction of naive gilts to contaminated outdoor pens or strawyards. Observation of the reproductive cycle of the sow suggest that infection is most frequent in the service area (82%), is lower in quarantine (50%) and dry sow housing (48%) declines to its lowest point (14%) in the farrowing unit and rises again to its peak 2 weeks after weaning.

Diagnosis

The clinical signs and the failure to respond to antimicrobial therapy may suggest coccidiosis. The presence of coccidial oocysts in the faeces (600,000 opg) may be also be suggestive. Levels in affected intestine may reach 5-6,000,000 opg. The presence of merozoites and sexual stages of coccidia in histological sections, and stained smears of jejunal and ileal mucosa, confirm the diagnosis. Oocysts may be sporulated in potassium dichromate to identify the species involved.

Treatment and control

Trimethoprim sulphonamide may be given by injection or orally to affected pigs.

The inclusion of an anticoccidial such as amprolium at 1 kg premix per tonne or monensin at 100g/tonne in sow feed for 7-10 days prior to farrowing and for 2 weeks afterwards will reduce the shedding of oocysts by sows. Similar inclusion rates will reduce shedding by other pigs. Treatment should include both clinically-affected pigs and the remainder of the group. None of these products are registered for this use in pigs in the UK. Scrupulous attention should be given to hygiene in control. Accommodation should be disinfected or fumigated with methyl bromide or ammonia (final concentration 2%) to kill oocysts. Steam cleaning at 65°C for 15 minutes and flame guns (safety!) will also destroy oocysts. The disinfectant, oocide (Dupont/Antec) can also be used to destroy oocysts.

References

Daugschies, A., Imarom, S., Ganter, M., Bollwahn, W. (2004). Prevalence of Eimeria sp in sows at piglet producing farms in Germany. J.Vet.Med. Series B, 51, 135-139.
Gaudie, C.M., Evans, R.J., Done, S.H. (2005). Coccidiosis in replacement gilts. Vet.Rec. 157, 517-518.
Henry, S.C., Tokach, L.M. (1995). Eimeria-associated pathology in breeding gilts. Swine Health and Production 3, 200-201.
Koudela B., Vitovec, J. (1992). Biology and Pathology of E.spinosa (Henry 1931) for experimentally infected pigs. Int.J.Parasitol. 22, 651-666.
Koudela B., Vitovec, J. (1998). Biology and Pathology of E.neodebliecki (Vetterling 1965) in experimentally infected pigs. Parasitol. Int. 47, 249-256.
Lindsay, D.S., Blagburn, B.L., Boosinger, T.R. (1987). Experimental E.debliecki infection in nursing and weaned pigs. Vet . Parasitology 25, 39-45.
Lindsay, D.S., Ernst, J.V., Current, W.L., Stuart, B.P. and Stewart, T.B. (1984). Prevalence of oocysts of I.suis and Eimeria spp from sows on farms with and without a history of neonatal coccidiosis. J.Am.Vet.Med.Ass. 185, 419-421.
Yaeger, M.J., Holtcamp, A., Jarvinen, J.A. (2003). Clinical coccidiosis in a boar stud J.Vet. Diagn. Invest. 15, 387-389.

Cryptosporidium

Definition

Heavy enteric infections with this sporozoan parasite may cause diarrhoea in young piglets but in older pigs infection may be common, clinically inapparent or associated with diarrhoea.

Incidence

Worldwide with between 5 and 20% of pigs infected. UK figures suggest 6.8% pigs were infected 1991-1997 and infection was highest in growers (20%).

Aetiology and pathogenesis

Cryptosporidia are small coccidian parasites which attach to the brush border of intestinal and respiratory tract epithelial cells and multiply there. New species are currently being identified after sequencing of the genome. Most literature refers to C. parvum, but C. suis has recently been separated (non-transmissible to mice), and C. hominis has been shown to infect pigs experimentally. Oocysts and schizonts of C.parvum are 3-4 µm in length by 0.3 µm. Infection is oral and multiplication on the brush borders of the jejunal and ileal epithelium appears to reach a peak and initiate clinical signs in sucking pigs within 72 hours of infection. The clinical signs appear to be due to the occupation of the absorptive brush borders by large numbers of parasites and the associated inflammation, villous atrophy and crypt hyperplasia. The oocysts are passed out in the faeces from 8-9 days post-infection and remain infective for at least 45 days. Immunity develops and the numbers of organisms rapidly fall after the initial burst of multiplication, persisting on individual cells in the ileum of recovered carrier pigs, particularly on cells of villi adjacent to ileal lymphoid tissue and on the dome cells of the Peyer's patches. In pigs aged 4-8 weeks they may be found throughout the gastrointestinal tract but their role in the associated diarrhoea is not clear.

Clinical signs

282

Most infections are asymptomatic (90% in one study). Clinical signs rarely appear before 3 days of age and are most commonly reported in piglets at 10-21 days of age. Affected piglets are depressed and pass a watery, sometimes brownish diarrhoea which may persist for 3-5 days. The organism can be demonstrated in the faeces of diarrhoeic weaners. Affected weaned pigs are often depressed and anorexic, in poor condition with a rough dirty coat and pasty faeces. Concurrent rotavirus infections can result in more severe clinical signs.

Chronically wasted animals should be killed.

Pathology

Gross changes of inflammation, villous atrophy and fusion and the presence of diphtheresis on the mucosal surface may be seen in both jejunum and ileum. Flattening and alteration of the large intestinal mucosa may also occur. The contents may be watery or blood-stained and contain necrotic material. Cryptosporidia may be seen attached to the brush borders of epithelial cells and lying amongst neutrophils and dead epithelial cells in the exudate in slides made from freshly killed freshly fixed intestinal tissue. In chronically infected, clinically normal pigs they may be seen on eosinophilic cells of the mucosal epithelium particularly in the ileum.

Epidemiology

Cryptosporidial oocysts are resistant to drying and may persist for at least 45 days in pig faeces. They may not die out in slurry for 133-345 days. Epidemiological information may have to be re-interpreted following the new classification. Recent studies using PCR have failed to differentiate adequately between pig cryptosporidia and those present in other species, although there is some suggestion that pig, cattle and human groups of the agent exist. The organism is present in many species including rats and mice and can infect man. In herds in which the infection is enzootic, oocysts may be found in the faeces of pigs of all ages including sows, but infection is most common in weaners and growers (mean age 42.5 days). Infected animals may be parasitised but shed few organisms in the faeces. Antibody can be demonstrated in colostrum.

Diagnosis

The organism can be readily distinguished in formalin vapour-fixed faecal smears stained by a modified Ziehl Neelsen's method using cold carbol fuchsin and 1% acid alcohol. Oocysts appear as 3-4 µm orange-red ovals or circles. In histological sections they are clearly visible on the brush borders of infected epithelial cells. Faecal smears may also be stained by auramine or by fluorescent antibody Antigen ELISAs and DNA probes have been developed by the water industry and techniques of filtration and demonstration in the environment are well developed.

The presence of cryptosporidia in an enteric syndrome does not confirm that it causes the syndrome and other pathogens such as rotavirus, epidemic diarrhoea, *E.coli*, and, especially, *C.perfringens* types A and C should be sought. It may contribute to enteritis when present in large numbers.

Treatment and Control

No treatment has yet been shown to affect the organism in pigs. The oocysts can be destroyed by ammonia and formalin treatment, by hydrogen peroxide and hypochlorite. The propietary disinfectant oocide (Antec International/Dupont) can also be used.

References

Heine, J., Moon, H.W., Woodmansee, D.B. and Pohlenz, J.F.L. (1984). Experimental tracheal and conjunctival infections with *Cryptosporidium sp* in pigs. Vet.Parasitol. **17**, 17-25.

Higgins, R. (1999). Surveillance for cryptosporidiosis. Pig J.**43**, 88-91.

Sanford, S.E. (1987). Enteric cryptosporidial infection in pigs: 184 cases (1981-85) J.A.V.M.A. **190**, 695-698.

Ryan, U.M., Monis, P., Enemark, H.L., Sulaiman, I., Samarasinghe, B., Read, C., Buddle, R., Robertson, I., Zhou, L., Thomson, R.C.A., Xiao, L. (2004). *Cryptosporidium suis, n.sp. (Apicomplexa: Cryptosporidiidae)* in pigs (*Sus scrofa*). J.Parasitol. **90**, 769-773.

Vitovec, J., Koudela, B. (1992). Pathogenesis of intestinal cryptosporidiosis in conventional and gnotobiotic piglets. Vet.Parasitol. **43**, 25-36.

Toxoplasmosis

Infection with *Toxoplasma gondii* is usually inapparent, but may result in abortion, stillbirths and the production of weak piglets. Older pigs may develop clinical signs which include fever, weakness and reduction of weight gain. Toxoplasmosis is a zoonosis.

Incidence

Toxoplasmosis occurs worldwide with prevalences of 2.3% in finishers and 15% in sows and gilts (Illinois, USA), 0.9% and 4.3%(Austria 1992) but higher rates of infection have been recorded in Germany in 2004 where 69% of 94 farms held at least 1 seropositive pig and more than 50% of sows were positive on 23% of farms.

Aetiology and pathogenesis

T.gondii is a coccidian parasite of juvenile cats which produce its oocysts in faeces. Ingestion of oocysts or tissue cysts by pigs results in the release of sporozoites or bradyzoites in the stomach which multiply rapidly in the intestinal epithelium as tachyzoites and can be found in the blood between 108-120 hours, spreading to all parts of the body including the foetus. They may be found in the milk. They encyst to produce tissue cysts. Antibody is produced.

Clinical signs

Infection may be inapparent but abortion may occur in sows infected between days 42 and 50 of gestation and mummified, stillborn and weak piglets may be born following later infections (70-90 days). Congenitally-infected piglets are weak, may develop diarrhoea and ataxia or incoordination. Clinical signs in older animals include anorexia, apathy, fever, cyanosis and hindlimb weakness. Severely affected comatose animals or those with serious incoordination or ataxia should be killed humanely.

Pathology

Affected piglets may have splenic enlargement, lymphadenopathy and there may be grey, white or reddish circumscribed lesions in lungs, liver and kidney. The carcase may be congested or multiple haemorrhages may be present. There is excess pleural and peritoneal fluid. Encephalitis, a catarrhal pneumonia and necrotic lesions in lymph nodes may be present and tissue cysts may be seen in histological sections.

Epidemiology

The prime source of oocysts is juvenile cat faeces but the ingestion of tissue cysts may result from the ingestion of raw meat, other animals such as mice and rats and cannibalism including tail biting (tissue cysts have been found in the tail). Transplacental transmission occurs. Tissue cysts are mature within 103 days of infection with oocysts and are still viable 875 days p.i. Tachyzoites in muscle are not infective for older animals as they cannot pass the stomach acid. Studies of risk factors have confirmed the role of cats (2.5x more likely to be infected where cats present and juvenile cats are worst) and infection studies have shown that feed and soil may contain oocysts and be infective. One oocyst represents an infective dose.

Diagnosis

Toxoplasmosis can be suspected as a cause of abortion in sows and of nervous signs in weak piglets, particularly where cats and their faeces are prominent. The presence of cyanosis may also lead to suspicion. The pathology is suggestive and the identification of tissue cysts confirms the involvement of *T.gondii*. Cysts may be confirmed as those of *T.gondii* by immunoperoxidase, immunofluorescence, ELISA and animal transmission where the cat is twice as sensitive as the mouse. Antibody may be detected by the Sabin Feldman test, indirect haemagglutination, latex agglutination tests and principally by ELISA in serum. Antibody can be detected in serum by blocking ELISA using P_{30} within 2 weeks of infection and lasts for at least 4 months. It can be detected in meat juice prepared from the heart and from tongue or even from pork mince. Antibody is present in transudates from foetuses and confirms transplacental infection. PCR has been used to detect cysts in tissues.

Treatment

Treatment is technically possible but not practised in pigs. Control relies upon the separation of cats from pigs, their pens and their feed, the prevention of cannibalism and control of rodents. Live attenuated, irradiated, rhoptry or ISCOMS vaccines have been tested but are not available UK. The sheep vaccine is not licensed for pigs. Vaccination of cats has reduced infection in pigs.

Tissue cysts in meat remain viable at 5°C but are killed by freezing to -12°C, heating at 70°C or irradiation at 700 Greys.

References

Damriyasa, I.M., Bauer, C., Edelhofer, R., Failing, K., Lind, P., Petersen, E., Schares, G., Tenter, A.M., Volmer, R., Zahner, H. (2004). Cross sectional survey in pig breeding farms in Hesse, Germany: seroprevalence and risk factors of infections with *Toxoplasma gondii, Sarcocystis sp* and *Neospora caninum* in sows. Vet. Parasitol. **126**, 271-286.

Dubey, J.P. (1988). Long-term persistence of *T.gondii* in tissues of pigs inoculated with *T.gondii* oocysts and effects of freezing on viability of tissue cysts. Am.J.Vet.Res. **49**, 910-913.

285

Dubey, J.P., Lunney, J.K., Shen, S.K., Kwok, O.H.C., Ashford, D.A., Thulliez, P. (1996). Infectivity of low numbers of *T. gondii* oocysts to pigs. J. Parasitol. **82**, 438-443.
Dubey, J.P. and Urban, J.F. (1990). Diagnosis of transplacentally-induced toxoplasmosis in pigs. Am.J.Vet.Res. **51**, 1295-1299.
Jones, M.A., Hunter, D.H. (1979). Toxoplasma infection in a newborn piglet. Vet. Rec. **104**, 529,
Lind, P., Haugegaard, J., Wingstrand, A., Henriksen, S.A. (1997). The time course of the specific antibody response by various ELISAs in pigs experimentally infected with *T. gondii*. Vet. Parasitol. **71**, 1-15.
Wingstrand, A., Lind, P., Haugegaard, J., Henriksen, S.A., Bille Hansen, V., Sorensen, V. (1997). Clinical observations, pathology, bioassay in mice and serological response at slaughter in pigs experimentally infected with *T. gondii*. Vet. Parasitol. **72**, 129-140.

Pneumocystis carinii infection

Causes retarded growth and dyspnoea at 4-5 weeks of age lasting for 4-10 weeks with deaths amongst dyspnoeic pigs There is no response to antimicrobial. The lungs are enlarged and do not collapse easily and there are focal brownish areas of consolidation in the cranial lobes. There may be interstitial oedema. Lobular or diffuse interstitial pneumonia with foamy, acidophilic (honeycomb) material and macrophages filling the alveoli. The alveolar septae are thickened by lymphocytes, plasma cells and lymphocytes. Grocott's methenamine silver nitrate staining, Toluidine blue O staining or immunoperoxidase reagents identify *P.carinii* as round or crescent-shaped cysts in the alveoli.
Wasted pigs with severe respiratory distress should be killed humanely.
Infection has been identified in UK, Japan and Denmark but occurs in man and other animal species in the UK. It appears to be secondary to other conditions, especially PCV2 at present.. Human strains appear to differ antigenically (32 and 78 kDa antigens distinct) and genetically (large subunit RNA gene) from those found in pigs

Reference

Bille Hansen, V., Jorsal, S.E., Henriksen, S.A., Settnes O.P. (1990). *Pneumocystis carinii* pneumonia in Danish piglets. Vet.Rec. **127**, 407-408.
Christensen, C.B.Y., Settnes O.P. Bille Hansen, V., Jorsal, S.E., Henriksen, S.A., Lundgren, B (1996). Pnemocystis carinii from pigs and humans are antigenically distinct. J. Medical and Vet Mycology **34**, 431-433

Trypanosomiasis (NOT UK)

A wide variety of Trypanosoma species have been reported to infect the pig. Some infections are inapparent such as *T.cruzi* and *T.rangeli* infections in Venezuela, *T. cruzi* in Brazil, Argentina and Mexico.. *T.evansi* is normally considered non-pathogenic in pigs in India but can cause death after fever, laboured breathing and necrosis of the extremities. An ELISA has been described for antibody detection.
The African trypanosomes have been recorded as causing inapparent infections (*T.brucei, T.b.rhodesiense* in Uganda, *T.b.gambiense* and *T.congolense* in Congo and *T.b.brucei* infection in Liberia where both direct and delayed infection by *Glossinia palpalis gambiense* were demonstrated. Single and mixed infections with *T. brucei* and *T. congolense* have been recorded in Nigeria.

Infection with *T.b.brucei*, *T.congolense* and *T.simiae* can cause disease. *T.b.brucei* causes pyrexia, weight loss, and anaemia with nervous signs in some animals, particularly after relapse. The prepatent phase lasts 4-7 days and acute disease may occur 9-15 days after infection. Chronic infection follows with a fluctuating pyrexia 37.6-41.6°C. Petecchial haemorrhages and plaque-like lesions may develop. Infertility has been recorded in boars.

T.simiae infection is more severe and may cause dyspnoea, inappetence, pyrexia, dullness and abortion in pregnant sows. Death occurs 12-96 hours after the onset of clinical signs. The infections are spread by Glossina sp. principally *G.palpalis palpalis*, *G.pellicera pellicera*, *G.nigrofuscans nigrofuscans* and *G.brevipalpis* from wildlife reservoirs which include the warthog in which infection is largely subclinical. Diagnosis is based on the clinical signs and post-mortem findings of haemorrhages, the demonstration of trypanosomes in the blood and in the cerebral capillaries and C.S.F. Blood smears can be supplemented by the Testryp CATT card test, antigen detection ELISAs and the KIVI system of isolation. Multilocus enzyme electrophoresis may be used to identify species.

Treatment with isometidium chloride 1 mg/kg clears experimental *T.brucei* infections within 72 hours and maintains freedom for 8 weeks and 20 mg/kg diminazeneaceturate (Berenil) has been shown to treat *T.simiae* and to provide at least 17 days' relapse from parasitaemia. T. evansi can also be treated with diminazene acetate, but infection eventually reappears. Affected pigs may not grow at the same rate as formerly. Prophylaxis with Berenil and Antrycide at 3-6 monthly intervals can prevent diease but pigs should be housed in insect-screened buildings.

References

Gill, B.S., Singh, J., Gill, J.S., Kwatra, M.S. (1987). *Trypanosoma evansi* infection in pigs in India.
Onah, D.N., Uzoukwa, M. (1991). Porcine cerebral *T.brucei brucei* trypanosomiasis. Tropical Animal Health and Production 23, 39-44.
Truc, P. and 6 others (1992). Direct isolation *in vitro* of *T.brucei* from man and other animals and its potential value for the diagnosis of Gambian trypanosomiasis. Trans.Royal Society of Tropical Medicine and Hygiene 86, 627-629.

Other protozoa

Balantidium coli occurs in gut lesions but is probably a secondary invader. It multiplies on and may penetrate inflamed mucosa. It occurs most commonly in the caecum and cysts can be found from the middle third of the colon onward. Nitroimidazole drugs eliminate it but cannot be used in food animals (EU).

Blastocystis suis is present on pig farms in Spain where it is most common between 1 and 2 months of age. In Spain and in experimental infection in gnotobiotic pigs it has not been associated with disease, but there are accounts of its presence in catarrhal inflammation of the caecum. The genotypes found in pigs resemble those found in humans.

Giardia lamblia has been identified in the duodenum, jejunum and ileum of recently-weaned pigs without causing clinical signs. The cysts are more common in pens with solid floors and piglets and weaners appear to be infected by the sow.

Sarcocystis infect pigs, cause little if any disease in natural cases but *S.suihominis*. *S.suicanis* and *S.miescheriana* may be noted at meat inspection. Infection is widespread in wild boar in Eastern Europe (primarily with S.

miescheriana). Antibody was found in 72% farms surveyed in Hesse, Germany. Experimental infections suggest that the ingestion of high numbers of cysts can lead to abortion in sows, fever (to 41.5°C) staggering and death in weaned pigs. Meat quality can be affected, with cysts in oesophagus and heart muscle from 60 days post infection. Cysts of *S.miescheriana* took 63 days to become infective for dogs.

References

Dey, S., Khatkar, S.K., Ghosh, J.D., Akbar, M.A. (1995). Clinicohaematologic and serum biochemical changes in piglets experimentally infected with S. miescheriana. Indian Vet. J. **72**, 126-130.

Avapal, R.S., Sharma, J.K., Juyal, P.D. (2004). Pathological changes in *Sarcocystis* infection in domestic pigs (*Sus scrofa*). Vet. J. **168**, 358-361.

Tritrichomonas suis and *T. foetus* have been described separately but are the same organism. They are most common in the large intestinal crypts and may be seen within the crypt lumen as hollow structures. They adhere to mucus and may also be found in nasal washings.

2. ECTOPARASITES

The most important ectoparasites of pigs in the UK are the sucking louse, *Haematopinus suis* and the mange mite *Sarcoptes scabei var suis*. Demodectic mange may also occur in debilitated pigs and biting by the stable fly, *Stomoxys calcitrans* may cause distress to young piglets, especially in hot weather. Ticks may affect pigs kept outdoors.

Lice

Haematopinus suis is the only louse commonly found on pigs in the UK and is most common on the folds of skin of the neck or jowl around the base of the ears, inside the ears, on the insides of the legs and on the flanks. It is a large, yellowish-brown louse (5 mm) which moves about amongst hairs on the pig's skin and may be seen most readily on white pigs.

Life cycle

Eggs are laid on the bristles and appear as a yellow crust which is prominent in black pigs. The eggs hatch into nymphs in 12-20 days. Following two further nymphal stages, the life cycle is completed in 29-33 days. The lice can only live away from the host for 2-3 days. The pig is the only host.

Pathogenesis and clinical signs

In severe infestations, the constant irritation and itching results in scratching and rubbing against gates, rails, etc. and this may lead to damage to the skin. Localised ulceration is found inside the pinna of the ears where lice congregate to feed. Large numbers of lice may cause restlessness and a reduced growth rate. The pig louse may act as a vector for the swine pox virus , *Mycoplasma haemosuis* and has been found to be infected by *Borrelia burgdorferi*.

Epidemiology

Spread of infection is via pig to pig contact. Wild birds may eat lice on pigs outdoors.

Diagnosis

Scratching and the presence of broken hairs and scratches on the skin of the neck and the flank in affected animals may draw attention to the presence of lice. The insects may be seen moving on the skin, especially on white pigs or inside the ears. The presence of nits on hairs also confirms their presence.

Treatment and control

Treatment has been carried out using a wide variety of insecticides, but those most commonly used at present are ivermectin, amitraz and phosmet.

Ivermectin (Ivomec, Panomec, Merial) at 330 µg/kg s/c or orally as the 2% premix for 7 days, doramectin (Dectomax, Pfizer), amitraz (Taktic, not EU) spray and phosmet (Not EU) pour on can be used to eliminate lice from affected animals.

Control can be carried out by the routine treatment of all sows entering farrowing accommodation, boars every 4 weeks and weaners and growers at weaning and during the finishing period together with a mange programme.

Eradication is relatively straightforward and is the preferred option. A whole herd treatment by injection or in feed (ivermectin) should be followed by a second course 18-21 days later. Breeding stock from infected herds should be treated on entry to isolation, treated 18-21 days later, then brought into the herd 7 days after the second treatment. Similar programmes can be carried out using the other agents.

Reference

Davis, D.P. and Williams, R.E. (1986). Influence of hog lice *H.suis* on blood components, behaviour, weight gain and feed efficiency of pigs. Vet.Parasitol. **22**, 307-314.

Mange

Definition

The most common form of mange in pigs is that caused by *Sarcoptes scabiei* var *suis* which burrows in the skin and causes intense pruritis resulting in loss of condition and trauma to the skin, particularly in the region of the ears.

Incidence

The most recent figures (2005) for Great Britain suggest that 23% herds are infected in Scotland and 24% in England. Similar figures from Canada (69% farms), Spain 86.6% herds, 37% pigs, France (56% pigs), Netherlands (5% pigs), Switzerland (10.4% pigs) and US 43% pigs suggest that the disease is common worldwide. Figures from Denmark differentiated between conventional herds (42.5% positive with 30% pigs positive) and SPF farms.

Aetiology

Mange is caused by *S.scabiei*, a small burrowing mite 0.5 mm in length which lives in galleries in the horny skin and feeds on epidermal cells. They are circular and may be identified by the pattern of sucker-and-bristle-bearing legs. In the male this is sucker-sucker-bristle-sucker, and in the female, sucker-sucker-bristle-bristle.

Up to 50 eggs are laid in the burrows before the female dies and they develop through larval and 2 nymphal stages to become ovigerous females, sometimes within as short a period as 10 days, although the normal life cycle usually takes 14-15 days. Multiplication can only occur on the host, although the mites may survive for up to 2-3 weeks in moist places in piggeries etc.

Pathogenesis

Lesions appear at least 3-4 weeks after initial infestation during which period the mites multiply and the host becomes sensitised. The burrowing and feeding activities of the mites cause intense pruritis which causes scratching which in turn results in the liberation of fluid from small vesicles near the burrows of the mites. The serum coagulates and dries on the skin to cause crusts which block the mite burrows 6-7 weeks after infection. Hyperkeratinisation of the skin occurs and connective tissue proliferation follows; lesions tend to be more heavily keratinised in older pigs. This lesion is thought to have an immunological basis and occurs after a period of sensitisation. Bacterial infection may also occur.

Clinical signs

Affected pigs scratch frequently, especially when hot. The first lesions appear as small red papules or wheals and general erythema about the eyes, around the snout, on the inner surface of the pinna of the ears, in the axillae and on the front of the hock and tarsus where the skin is thin. Scratching results in the excoriation of these affected areas and the formation of brownish scabs on the damaged skin. Subsequently, the skin becomes wrinkled, covered with crusty lesions and thickened. The flanks become bare of hair and in badly-affected animals aural haematomas may form as a result of excessive head shaking. Reductions in productivity occur in infected herds. Litter weights may be depressed 10% at weaning, sow feed use per piglet and per kg piglet are both increased by 5-10% and growth rates in finishing pigs are reduced by 5% or more.

Humane slaughter is not indicated as treatment is now completely effective.

Pathology

The hyperkeratotic lesions of mange have been described above. Lesions may be obvious in the ears at post-mortem when the waxy crusts and inflamed internal surface of the pinna can be clearly seen. Localised lesions occur elsewhere on the carcase as small (1-2 mm) round, slightly thickened lesions on rump, flank and abdomen. These can be seen most easily in animals which have been scalded after slaughter, although the scalding and scraping process removes all superficial parts of the lesion and many of the mites. Histological lesions are superficial and processing means that mites are rarely seen, but an eosinophilic vasculitis is present in the dermis.

Epidemiology

Spread of infection is via pig to pig contact; infection of piglets usually occurs from the dam. Infection spreads only slowly from one pig to another and colonisation of a whole group may take weeks. Pigs may contract infection from infected pens after only 24 hours' contact. Mites may survive off the host for up to 3 weeks in the laboratory, but in piggeries, survival has only been demonstrated for 12 days at 7-18°C and 65-75% relative humidity. In warmer conditions, survival is shorter. Infections of man have been reported but disappear once contact with infected pigs stops.

Diagnosis

Scratching and rubbing, broken hairs on the flanks, crusts in the ears, crumpled ears and hyperkeratotic skin all suggest mange. Red, pinpoint lesions on the skin after scalding are 92% specific for mange and are used to score the severity of infection in a herd from 1 (mild lesions on the belly, head and buttocks, 82.5% specific) through 2 (lesions over flanks and back in low to moderate numbers, 98.6% specific) to 3 (severe generalised lesions, specificity 99.5%).

Deep skin scrapings from the anterior portion of the inside of the ears and the face (80% of cases) and the skin of the tarsus (50% of cases) should be examined for the presence of mites, the finding of which is pathognomonic. Mites may be found here and in the axillae in carriers or in affected skin from clinical cases. Prior to scraping, the site should be smeared with 70% glycerine to bind the scraped material. Mites emerge from crusts of skin or ear wax when small portions are subjected to a combination of vibration and heat. Recovery of mites is relatively easy in weaners, but chronically affected sows often have few mites, the lesions being due to an immunological reaction. Where mites do not leave the crusts they may be demonstrated by clearing scabs in 40% potassium hydroxide for 10 minutes. Eggs and mites may be demonstrated by dissolving ear wax in eosin stained ethanol and filtering. Live mites and eggs are white. Sucrose flotation may improve recovery of mites and eggs.

ELISAs using whole mite antigens (from fox mange) can be used to detect antibody. Antibody can be transmitted from sow to piglet, and piglets less than 10 weeks of age may test false positive for infection although maternal antibody has usually disappeared by 5 weeks of age. Specificity of the ELISA is 98% in all age groups, but sensitivity is 80% in weaners, 78% in finishers and only 50% in sows. ELISAs can be used to confirm eradication, but sows may take up to a year to lose antibody after successful eradication.

Other similar conditions include swine pox which causes non-irritant lesions in the young pig, parakeratosis in which loose, dry, crumbly crusts occur with no irritation, exudative epidermitis mostly in young piglets with no irritation, and pityriasis rosea in which expanding ring lesions occur on the belly. Ringworm is rare, see fungi. Mites from old straw, mosquitoes and the Scottish midge may all produce popular lesions which may be confused with those of mange in SPF pigs.

Treatment

Mange may be treated with ivermectin or doramectin. Ivermectin (e.g. Ivomec injection pigs or Panomec, Merial) can be given by subcutaneous injection at 300 µg/kg and kills mites in ears and on skin within 7-14 days. Animals with severe crusty lesions in the ears should be treated again within 14 days as mites persist in the ear wax and such animals may represent a focus of infection. Doramectin has a similar treatment schedule. Ivermectin is also available as a premix for feed inclusion. Amitraz and phosmet were formerly used, but are no longer available

(2006, UK). A single application of phosmet poured on the back with part of the dose placed in the ears where obvious crusts are present, treated the disease. Amitraz solution was sprayed gently with a knapsack or pressure washer. The whole pig was thoroughly treated. Treatment might have to be repeated within 7-10 days in order to kill eggs and larvae. It was particularly important to ensure treatment of ears.

Control

A typical control programme is shown below:

Boars	2-3 monthly intervals
Sows and gilts	at entry to farrowing house
Pigs	after weaning before moving/at moving
Purchased stock	isolate, treat.

With ivermectin, sows and boars may be treated by subcutaneous injection (Ivomec injection for pigs) and weaned pigs using the 2% premix for 7 days. Doramectin may also be used.

In all cases the efficacy of treatment is increased if animals are treated on entry into clean accommodation (rested 3 weeks or cleaned, disinfected and fumigated).

Treated and untreated pigs should not be mixed if best results are to be achieved. Regular treatments will reduce chronic infection and improve productivity. In studies in which ivermectin, doramectin (or phosmet) have been used, an 8-10% improvement in daily liveweight gain and feed conversion efficiency has been gained under many different systems of husbandry. Withdrawal times should be observed.

Eradication

Ivermectin, doramectin (and phosmet) can be used to eradicate mange from a farm, but only by treating all animals at appropriate intervals and by ensuring that treated animals enter cleaned accommodation. Although in theory a single treatment should be adequate, at least two treatments should be given, 14 days apart. Accommodation could previously be sprayed with amitraz (1 g/20 m^2). CNS signs such as head shaking could follow overdosing neonates with organophosphates. When mange has been eradicated, purchased stock should be treated and isolated for 21 days in clean accommodation before being introduced or should be purchased from a mange-free herd. Freedom from antibody and regular clinical and abattoir monitoring may be required to certify freedom from mange. Under the conditions of the Dutch eradication scheme, a certificate of freedom allows trade in pigs from herds inspected every 4 months and using no acaricide.

References

Arends, J.J., Stanislaw, C.M., Gerdon, D. (1990). Effects of mange on lactating swine and growing pigs. J.Anim.Sci. **68**, 1495-1499.

Cargill, C., Davies, P., Carmichael, I., Hooke, F., Moore, M. (1996). Treatment of sarcoptic mite infestation and mite hypersensitivity in pigs with injectable doramectin. Vet. Rec. **138**, 468-471.

Davis, D.P., Moon, D. (1990). Density, location and sampling of S.scabiei (Ascaris, Sarcoptidae) on experimentally infected pigs. J.Med.Entomology. **27**, 391-398.

Firkins, L.D., Jones, C.J., Keen, D.P., Arends, J.J., Thompson, L., King, V.L., Skogerboe, T.L. (2001). Preventing transmission of *Sarcoptes scabiei var suis* from infested sows to nursing piglets by a prefarrowing treatment with doramectin injectable solution. Vet. Parasitol.**99**, 323-330.

Heijden, H.M.J.F.van der, Rambags, P.G.M., Elbers, A.R.W., Maanen, C. van, Hunneman, W.A. (2000). Validation of ELISAs for the detection of antibodies to *Sarcoptes scabiei* in pigs. Vet. Parasitol. **89**, 95-107.

Lee, R.P., Dooge, D.J.D. and Preston, J.M. (1980). Efficacy of Ivermectin against *S.scabiei* in pigs. Vet.Rec., **107**, 503.

Morsy, G.H., Turck, J.J., Gaafar, S.M. (1989). Scanning electron microscopy of sarcoptic mange lesions in swine. Vet.Parasitol. **31**, 281-288.

Sheahan, B.J. (1974). Experimental *S.scabiei* infections in pigs: Clinical signs and significance of infection. Vet.Rec. **94**, 202-209.

Smith, H.J. (1986). Transmission of *S.scabiei* in swine by fomites. Can.vet.J. **27**, 252-254.

Wallgren, P., Bornstein, S. (1997). The spread of porcine sarcoptic mange during the fattening period revealed by development of antibodies to *S. scabiei*. Vet. Parasitol. **73**, 315-324.

Demodectic Mange

Caused by *Demodex phylloides,* a long thin mite (0.25 mm in length). It is present in 10.3% cull sows (GB 1990) and is associated with small reddened or pustular lesions 2-8 mm in diameter on the face and underside of the body which contain from 10,000-500,00 mites. Skins may be damaged by severe infections. There is no treatment and severely affected animals should be killed.

Flies

A number of flies may be found in piggeries. The most important of these is probably *Stomoxys calcitrans* which sucks blood. This species and the non-parasitic *Musca domestica* may disturb piglets and sows and may lead to loss of condition. They breed in slurry and under uncleaned pen furniture and can spread disease within pens. Infected flies have been found considerable distances from piggeries. Flies such as bluebottles (Lucilia sp. and Calliphora sp.) may spread disease from house to house or from farm to farm. They are normally controlled by baiting or sprays.

Ticks

These may occur on pigs from time to time. *Ornithodorus erraticus* occurs in Spain and was a reservoir of African swine fever. *Ixodes ricinus* occurs on pigs in UK and louping ill carried by it has been identified in pigs. This species and *I. hexagonus* have been shown to carry *Borrelia burgdorferi* .

NUTRITIONAL CONDITIONS

Introduction

Nutritional deficiencies and excesses may both give rise to clinical disease in pigs and to reduction in productivity in both growing pigs and in breeding animals. Overt clinical disease frequently results from:

1.   Use of ingredients which have not been analysed so that accurate supplementation can take place. Examples include grains grown on selenium deficient soils and by-products such as bakery waste.

2.   Spoilage of ingredients. This occurs when mould infections attack stored grains and when finished feeds and vitamin:mineral mixes are processed incorrectly or stored beyond their expiry dates.

3.   The inclusion of high levels of normal nutrients as a result of errors in formulation or mixing. These occur most frequently following the addition of incorrect quantities of premix when mixing or the incorrect formulation of the premixes themselves. Occasionally the food itself may contain toxic levels of a nutrient such as salt or selenium.

Overt clinical disease resulting from nutritional deficiency or toxicity is rare as the majority of pigs are fed on standard mixtures supplemented by carefully formulated premixes. Manufactured feeds are carefully supervised by qualified nutritionists and errors in formulation are rare. Most nutritional deficiencies or excesses require time to become apparent and fresh deliveries of feed (which may be normal) reduce the likelihood that nutritional disorders will develop. The following points should be borne in mind when considering a potential nutritional problem:

i)   Nutritional disease giving rise to clinical or pathological signs can be recognised from the descriptions of the appropriate syndromes which follow.

ii)   Nutritional disease should be distinguished from infectious disease and poisonings. Feed refusal or depressed feed intake or growth rate may result from pneumonia or other infectious causes as may reduction in sow productivity.

iii) Nutritional disease frequently occurs in groups of animals fed on the same ration (manufactured feed or premix or raw ingredients) fed on other farms.

iv)   Examination of the feed being given to the animals may reveal physical abnormalities. Samples may be taken for analysis.

v)   There may be a history of prolonged storage of ingredients, of mechanical failure or incorrect incorporation of a particular nutrient or portion of the ration.

The examination of nutritional conditions is based upon the normal nutrient requirements of the pig. These are constantly changing as genetic advances and changes in husbandry develop. One recent change is the manipulation of diets to reduce effluent in terms of volume or nitrogen and phosphorus content and another is the reduction in copper in the EU. The guides to normal nutrient requirements given below are based upon historic requirements supplemented by recent publications and are a guide only

Normal Nutrient Requirements

The figures given here form a basis for assessing the adequacy of a diet in terms of nutrients. For detailed consideration of pig feeding, books such as Practical Pig Nutrition and The Science and Practice of Pig Production (2006) should be consulted. The details of nutrient requirements have been reviewed in the A.R.C. technical review "The Nutrient Requirements of Pigs" 1981 and by the NRC (1998) in the US. Rapidly-growing pigs and those which are ill may have special requirements. Fat levels for lactating sows may be increased in lactation diets.

(a) Major Nutrients

Nutrient	Starter creep (4-28 days)		Standard creep (4 wks - 40 kg)		Grower (40-70 kg)		Finisher (70 kg -)		Gestating sow		Lactating sow	
	Min.	Max.	Min.	Max.	Min.	Max.	Min.	Max.	Min.	Max.	Min.	Max.
DE (MJ/kg)	14.0	15.5	14.0	15.0	13.0	14.0	13.0	14.0	12.0	12.5	13.0	13.5
CP (%)	22.0	25.0	19.0	22.5	17.0	20.0	14.5	17.0	12.0	15.0	15.5	16.5
DCP (%)	18.5	20.0	15.0	16.0	13.5	14.0	11.0	12.0	9.0	9.5	12.5	13.5
Lysine (%)	1.2	1.5	1.0	1.3	0.8	1.5	0.8	0.85	0.60	0.70	0.7	0.8
Meth + cyst (%)	0.88	1.0	0.76	0.9	0.68	0.8	0.58	0.68	0.48	0.60	0.62	0.66
Calcium (%)	0.95	1.1	0.9	1.0	0.8	1.0	0.8	1.2	1.0	1.2	1.0	1.2
Phosphorus (%)	0.85	0.9	.78	0.82	0.6	0.8	0.6	0.8	0.6	0.8	0.8	0.8
Crude fibre (%)	1.0	3.0	2.0	4.0	2.0	5.0	2.0	6.0	2.0	7.0	2.0	6.0
Ether extract (%)	1.0	5.0	1.0	5.0	1.0	6.0	1.0	6.0	1.0	5.0	1.0	5.0

(b) <u>Minerals</u> : inclusion rates per tonne of air-dried mixed diet.

	Suggested in final mixed diet	Indicated as being provided in proprietary trace element
Calcium (kg)	8-12	
Phosphorus (kg)	7-11	4 - 9.2
Potassium (kg)		about 2.5
Salt (Sodium Chloride)(kg)	1.0-2.5	2 - 3.5
Magnesium (g)	400 - 800	10 - 75
Iron (g)	about 80	50 - 400
Zinc (g)	100-150	50-150
Manganese (g)	5 - 40	20 - 60
Copper (g)	3 - 10	5 – 25 (> 12 weeks)
Iodine (g)	0.16 - 0.5	1 - 4
Cobalt (g)	only in Vitamin B12	0.5 - 2
Selenium (g)	0.8 - 1.6	1.2

(c) <u>Water requirements</u>

 Good quality water should be freely available by means of appropriate drinkers to all pigs even when it is provided in the diet. Water points or provision for watering should be available even to pigs normally given wet feed in case of alteration in the dietary constituents or disease resulting in inappetence. Sucking piglets should also have access to water.

Sucking piglets		0.30 - 0.5 kg (51-62ml/kg)
Growing- Finishing pigs:	15.0 kg body weight	1.5-2.0 kg
	90.0 kg body weight	6.0-12.0 kg
Sows: Non-pregnant		6-12.0 kg
Pregnant		10-20 kg
Lactating		25-40 kg

Expressed as minimum requirements in terms of volume and flow rate:

Newly weaned piglets	1.0-1.5 L	0.3L/minute
Up to 20 kg	1.5-2.0 L	0.5-1.0L/minute
20-40kg	2.0-5.0 L	1.0-1.5 L/minute
40-100kg	5.0-6.0 L	1.0-1.5 L/minute
100-180 kg	5.0-8.0 L	2.0 L/minute
Gilts, non-pregnant sows	5.0-8.0L	2.0 L/minute
Lactating	15-30L	2.0 L/minute
Boars	5.0-8.0L	2.0 L/minute

 These requirements may be increased by a number of factors including the salt concentration of the diet, the ambient temperature and the use of leaky drinkers.
The water requirements in the diet expressed as water : dry matter are usually:

Growing pigs	2.5 : 1	(restricted access)
	3.7 : 1	*(ad lib)*
Sows, non-pregnant	2.0 : 1	
pregnant	2.5 : 1	
lactating	3.0 : 1	

(d) Vitamins

	Liveweight and type of pig	Requirement per tonne of mixed dry diet	Normally provided as a supplement
Vitamin A	up to 20 kg	1.98 million i.u. (600 mg or 7.2g beta carotene)	yes
	20-50 kg	1.98 million i.u. (600 mg or 7.2g beta carotene)	yes
	50-90 kg	9.9 million i.u. (400 mg or 4.8g beta carotene)	yes
	sows	6.0 million i.u. (min.700 mg)	
Vitamin D3	up to 20 kg	3.5 mg	
	all other stock	0.2 million i.u. (3.0 mg)	yes
Vitamin E	all stock	10-20,000 i.u. (3.0-6.0 mg)	yes
Vitamin K	baby pigs	300 mg	yes
Thiamine	up to 90 kg	1.5 g	yes
Riboflavine	up to 90 kg	2.5 g	yes
	sows	3.0 g	yes
Nicotinic acid	up to 20 kg	20 g	yes
	20 - 70 kg	14 g	
Pantothenic acid	up to 100 kg	10 g	yes
	sows	10 g	yes
Pyridoxine	up to 90 kg	2.5 g	yes
	sows	1.8 g	yes
Vitamin B12	up to 20 kg	18 mg	yes
	20 - 90 kg	10 mg	yes
	sows	15 mg	yes
Choline	up to 20 kg	800 g	yes
	20-90 kg	850 g	
	sows	1000 - 1900 g	
Biotin	15-90 kg	1 g	
	sows	25 g	yes
Folic acid	growing pigs	1 g	
	sows	5 g	yes
Inositol	Dietary estimates not established		no
Vitamin C			
Essential fatty acids as linolenic acid	up to 30 kg	15 kg	not specifically
	30 - 90 kg	7 kg	not specifically
as arachidonic acid	up to 30 kg	10 kg	not specifically
	30-90 kg	5 kg	not specifically

The figures given above are based on the ARC recommendations (1981) and the NRC recommendations (1998), but there is currently a lively debate about the correct levels of incorporation for many of these nutrients. Industry incorporates many of the minerals and vitamins at levels higher than those recommended (with the exception of phosphorus), and has had to adjust to the reduction in copper levels from growth promoting to nutritional levels. The reviews listed below should be consulted for an expert view of the correct levels for each class of livestock and, particularly, the balance between mineral inclusion and organic or available minerals for any trace element.

References

Nutrient Requirement Standards for Pigs, **BSAS Publications**, ISBN 6906562 42 2

Taylor-Pickard, J.A. (2005). Feeding the modern genotype – trace elements. Pig J. **56**, 179-191.

Whittemore, C.T., Close, W.H., Hazzledine, M.J. (2002). The need for nutrient requirement standards for pigs. Pig News and Information **23**, 67N-74N

Whittemore, C.T.,Green, D.M., Knap, P.W. (2001a). Technical review of the energy and protein requirements of growing pigs: Food intake. Animal Science **73**, 3-17.

Whittemore, C.T.,Green, D.M., Knap, P.W. (2001b). Technical review of the energy and protein requirements of growing pigs: Energy. Animal Science **73**, 119-215.

Whittemore, C.T.,Green, D.M., Knap, P.W. (2001c). Technical review of the energy and protein requirements of growing pigs: Protein. Animal Science **73**, 363-373.

Taylor-Pickard, J.A. (2005). Feeding the modern genotype – trace elements. Pig J. **56**, 179-191.

Nutritional Deficiencies and Excesses

1.   Water

Water Deprivation and Salt Poisoning

Definition

a)   Effects on production

Limited water may cause depression of growth and production. Decreased water intake may result from inadequate supply, (water pressure, number of pigs per drinker, limited access, type of drinker or poorly maintained drinkers), the solids content of the water/sulphates) or disease. Water limitation is particularly important in the farrowing and lactating sow where it has been associated with lethargy and reluctance to rise and leads to increases in piglet mortality and depression of growth in the litter. Ambient temperature is important, as needs increase with rising temperature. Intake varies with the time of day independently of the temperature, peaking in daylight.

In other age groups water limitation may reduce feed consumption and thus growth rate and in adult sows may lead to crystalluria and predispose to cystitis. In post pubertal gilts it may occur in 20-30% of a group and can be detected in individuals by the passage of small quantities of high specific gravity urine (SG >1012)

b)   Clinical disease (Salt poisoning, sodium ion poisoning)

Definition

Excess dietary salt or sudden water deprivation may lead to convulsions and abnormalities of gait and death or recovery within two days of exposure.

Incidence

Occurs sporadically, but may affect large numbers of pigs when water supply to a house is interrupted through cold weather, drought or burst pipes, when a high salt diet is fed or when an outbreak of diarrhoea such as T.G.E. increases water loss. It may also occur in individual pigs which are paralysed or otherwise unable to drink.

Aetiology and pathogenesis

The condition is most commonly associated with water deprivation on normal salt diets but high salt diets such as salted fish, buttermilk or pickling brines also predispose to the condition. The syndrome may follow the ingestion of large amounts of salt on limited water supplies or occur after sudden unrestricted access to water. It is thought that dehydration of tissues and an increase in the sodium content of the brain occur. High sodium levels in the brain inhibit anaerobic glycolysis and acetyl choline esterase levels and appear to be responsible. Sudden rehydration may exacerbate the condition.

Clinical signs

Peracute salt poisoning occurs after the ingestion of massive amounts of salt and results in prostration, running movements, coma and death. Acute salt poisoning following restricted water intake is most common. Pruritis, thirst and constipation are followed 1-5 days later by blindness, lack of interest in food or drink and failure to respond to external stimuli. Affected pigs may bump into obstacles and may circle, pivoting on one foot. Head pressing may occur. Convulsions occur regularly (every 7 minutes). Twitching of the snout is followed by contractions of the neck muscles, holding the head upright and by characteristic backing movements. Seizures last only a short time, but may end in rigidity and coma. Mortality may be high, but is usually 5% or less. Clinical signs may also develop after water is given following withdrawal. Recovered animals may retain abnormalities of gait or remain blind.

Humane slaughter of affected paralysed pigs should not be carried out until after 24-36 hours as many recover.

Pathology

Gross changes are few. There may be congestion of the meninges and plasma sodium levels may be high. The microscopic changes are pathognomonic, and consist of meningoencephalitis with oedema and eosinophil accumulations around the vessels of the cerebral cortex and in the meninges. In later lesions, malacia occurs and cystic spaces are left.

Diagnosis

The history of water deprivation or salty diet usually provides sufficient grounds for diagnosis, and the absence of fever distinguishes salt poisoning from infective causes of meningitis such as streptococcal meningitis but oedema disease (absence of high pitched squeal) or organic arsenical poisoning may resemble it. The histological findings are confirmatory and the presence of high plasma levels of creatinine phosphokinase and sodium (more than 160 m. eq/l.) may confirm. The absence of this level of sodium may only indicate that rehydration has occurred. Brain levels of sodium and chloride are not diagnostic. High salt levels in the stomach contents may also be suggestive. The condition may occur in any pig with chronic disease and inability to reach water.

Treatment

Spontaneous recovery may occur. The feed should be replaced and water intake controlled by giving small amounts at first to unaffected pigs and increasing gradually. Convulsing animals should be allowed to recover naturally, as dosing can lead to inhalation pneumonia. Water should be offered and animals may be sprayed with water. Betamethasone (2 mg/kg) may assist recovery and animals should remain in the dark and undisturbed for at least 24 hours.

Control

Ensure that pigs being placed in new pens can find the drinking water and check supplies, particularly in hot and cold weather. When salty rations such as whey and buttermilk are fed, water must be provided *ad lib*.

References

Almond, G.W., Stevens, J.B., Routh, P.A., Feng, S.M., Hevener, W., Deen, J., Davies, P.R. (1998) Water deprivation in post pubertal gilts: Changes in urine and serum constituents. Proc IPVS **14**, 734.
Marks, S.L., Carr, J. (1989). Water deprivation in weaned pigs Vet.Rec. **125**, 460.

2. Energy
Neonatal Hypoglycaemia

Definition

This condition arises from restriction of food intake in the neonatal pig and may result in death in convulsions. It may be exacerbated by factors such as low environmental temperature and infection.

Incidence

Common in poorly-heated farrowing houses and may be a predisposing factor in many infectious neonatal conditions. Responsible for 40% of all neonatal piglet mortality in the UK.

Aetiology

The prime cause of this condition is an inadequate intake of milk. This may be due to failure of the sow to provide sufficient milk for a number of reasons, including lack of sufficient functioning mammary glands, failure of secretion in case of agalactia, mastitis or systemic illness or for behavioural reasons. Death of the sow may also precipitate the syndrome in neonatal piglets. Failure of the piglet to suck may occur for a number of reasons, including congenital defects such as cleft palate or nervous signs such as splay leg and congenital tremor, infectious conditions such as colisepticaemia or arthritis and mechanical conditions such as foot damage. The presentation of the sow's udder may also be important as may be competition between piglets. Low environmental temperatures may exacerbate the condition and are very important contributory factors both in the UK and elsewhere, particularly at night.

Pathogenesis

The newborn piglet normally possesses carbohydrate reserves in the form of hepatic glycogen stores (10-14 mg/100 g) and blood glucose levels of 80-100 mg/100ml (24 hours after birth). Fructose, the foetal blood sugar, is also present (50-60 mg/100ml) but levels normally decline rapidly. Gluconeogenesis is not efficient until 7 days of age and glycogen reserves become depleted if the milk supply is inadequate. Blood sugar levels then depend upon dietary intake and are unstable. Feeding normally occurs every hour and provides adequate carbohydrate, but, if this pattern is interrupted, blood glucose levels may fall progressively until clinical signs of deficiency appear at a blood-glucose concentration of 50 mg/100 ml.

The original hepatic and muscular glycogen stores may be depleted by delay in parturition. Lower birth weight may cause increased heat loss and difficulty in competing with larger littermates for teats. There is no brown fat so the piglet cannot use fat to generate heat. Low environmental temperature (below 34°C for the single neonate or 25-30°C for the piglet able to huddle) lead to increased utilisation of glycogen reserves in liver and skeletal muscles and to the more rapid development of clinical signs. T.G.E. has also been shown to reduce effective glucose intake and precipitate clinical hypoglycaemia.

Clinical signs

Piglets aged less than 7 days are affected and, at blood glucose levels of 50 mg/100 ml, may show uncertain gait, and later support themselves by placing their noses on the ground and straddling their hind limbs. More severely affected pigs rest on their abdomens but eventually fall on their sides and develop convulsions. These consist of "galloping" of the forelegs, champing and frothing of the jaws in "air hunger" and are accompanied by bradycardia (to 80 beats/min), a decline in rectal temperature, shivering, dullness and, in the earlier stages, a weak squeal. Death normally occurs 24-36 hours after the commencement of the signs.

Animals which have entered a coma from which they cannot be revived by treatment should be killed humanely.

Pathology

Affected pigs have stomachs which are empty or contain a little curd. Blood glucose levels of affected pigs are usually less than 50 mg/100 ml and may be as low as 7 mg/100 ml. Hepatic glycogen is often absent in hypoglycaemic pigs.

Diagnosis

The clinical signs, including the finding of agalactia in the sow should lead to consideration of hypoglycaemia. The involvement of chilling can be confirmed by environmental temperature measurements and observation of the animals. Shivering stops at a body temperature of 34°C.

Other diseases affecting baby pigs should be eliminated, e.g. neonatal septicaemia, neonatal diarrhoea, T.G.E., Aujeszky's disease and bacterial meningitis. Confirmation can be obtained from the response to treatment and from blood glucose and liver glycogen determinations.

Treatment and prevention

Affected animals should be given intraperitoneal injections of 15 ml of 5% glucose solution every 4-6 hours or oral glucose by stomach tube and kept at a minimum of 30-35°C (85-95°F). If the sow is unable to feed them, an artificial sow milk replacer should be given by stomach tube initially or they should be fostered onto another sow. Reduction in draughts and the provision of dry bedding and additional heating for piglets may also improve survival.

References

English, P.R. and Morrison, V. (1984). Causes and prevention of piglet mortality. Pig News and Information 5, 369-376.
English, P.R. and Smith, W.J. (1975). Some causes of death in neonatal piglets. Vet.Annual 15, 95-104.
Losec, G., Herpin, P., Dividich, J. Le(1998). Thermoregulatory responses to the newborn pig during experimentally-induced hypothermia and rewarming. Exp. Physiol. 83, 667-678.

Wasting in recently weaned piglets

Wasting in recently weaned piglets has achieved prominence as a result of the definition of the Post weaning Multisystemic Wasting Syndrome (PMWS) currently (1999) associated with circovirus type II infection. The identification of this syndrome depends upon the presence of the clinical, pathological and virological findings of the syndrome, and is made against a background of loss of condition in recently-weaned piglets due to other diseases, environmental and nutritional factors. Where disease and environmental factors have been ruled out, the composition and freshness of the weaning ration and its presentation should be evaluated, particularly on organic farms and where home mixing occurs. Husbandry factors such as environmental temperature, freedom from draughts, access to water supplies and training to use them should all be considered. Finally, individual low weight or wasted pigs can be nursed in purpose-built incubators with milk diets and adequate temperatures and may then achieve growth rates similar to the remainder of the herd.

The Thin Sow Syndrome

Definition

A syndrome in which heavy weight loss occurs in sows in lactation and early pregnancy followed by failure to regain weight before farrowing again. This may become progressive and result in poor fertility and eventually emaciation and death.

Incidence

Not uncommon, particularly in loose housed sows (including outdoor animals) where individual feeding is not practised. Formerly common in the UK and still common elsewhere in stalled sows of lean breeds

Aetiology

The condition results classically from a combination of parasitism (helminths or mange), low environmental temperatures and inadequate feed intake, particularly during lactation. Weight loss at this time may never be regained. Parasitism is less important in current UK systems where therapy is routinely carried out and feed supply to the group or to individuals is now most important. Bullying may account for individual affected pigs but in the UK with its increasing outdoor pig population, low environmental temperatures are important Outdoor sows require at least 200 kg more feed per sow per year than indoor animals. Indoors the best environmental temperature is 22°C for thin sows in sow stalls and 21°C for sows in moderate condition. Any fall in temperature below this will require extra feed to maintain weight gain in gestation. Sow body condition should be condition score 3/4 or 6/10 (fat depth at P2 16-20 mm) at farrowing and may fall to condition score 2-2-5/4 or 4/10 (fat depth P2 12 mm) at the end of lactation. Unless these criteria are met, total weaning weight of the litter will be reduced, return to oestrus will be delayed and egg numbers will be reduced to give small subsequent litters.

Clinical signs

Emaciation in 30-90% of sows and boars in a herd, associated with hypothermia 36.5-38°C (97-100°F), depraved appetites, restlessness, apathy and later, difficulty in rising. The skin may be dirty and greasy and there may be surface abrasions. As the condition progresses, failure to return to oestrus and permanent infertility may occur.

Humane slaughter is only required in extreme cases of emaciation.

Treatment

Ensure that adequate quantities of food are given to all affected animals and that individual feeding is possible. In loose housing systems, crate feeding or electronic sow feeding may be required. Environmental temperatures should be restored to normal and anthelminthic treatment should be considered. Adequate feed intake during lactation and early pregnancy should be designed to maintain weight of the sow and to increase it by 10-15 kg between litters. This may be done by increasing the energy content of lactating rations with fat or feeding three times daily during lactation. It may be necessary to weigh sows after weaning in order to ensure that adequate weight gain has occurred between lactations, to assign them to groups for feeding at an appropriate level throughout pregnancy or to feed individually to condition. Management systems which feed low protein rations to lean gilts can increase relative fat levels and ensure adequate production during the second parity.

References

Kirkwood, R.N., Nutaru, B.N., Gooneratne, A.D., Blair, R., Thacker, P.A. (1988). The influence of dietary energy intake during successive lactations on sow prolificacy. Canadian J. Animal Science **68**, 283-290.

Johnston, L.J., Pettigrew, J.E., Shurson, G.C. (1997). Sow nutrition and reproduction. Pig News and Information **18**, 61n-64n.

Fat sows.

Sows or gilts may become fat when overfed, when socially dominant in the absence of individual feeding, or when nulliparous. In all cases, the underlying reasons for the fatness should be corrected as herd reproductive performance will suffer.

3. Protein and Amino Acids

The young weaned and actively-growing pig requires 26% crude protein, at 10 kg which should supply the following levels of essential amino acids: Lysine 1.45%, methionine + cystine 0.5-0.6%, L-isoleucine 0.6%, tryptophan 0.18-0.20%, threonine 0.65-0.7%. These figures do not apply to high performance or transgenic pigs or to those receiving porcine somatotrophin in which protein levels of up to 30% may be required. Deficiency of protein or one of the amino acids listed above is first noted as a sub-optimal growth rate in growing pigs. Feed conversion is also less efficient, haemoglobin levels, haematocrit, albumin and serum transferrin levels are all depressed. In sows litter size may be reduced. Analysis of the diet or inclusion of the pure amino acid or a rich source may provide evidence for the causal role of the amino acid. Cystine and methionine deficiency may be a contributory factor in hepatosis dietetica. Diets have been formulated recently to reduce slurry output or nitrogen loss, or contain no fish meal, meat meal or other animal protein or are formulated using vegetable protein only for price reasons or because of organic policies. These diets must be carefully formulated by professionals for recently weaned pigs and may be inadequate in terms of protein and amino acids if formulated by home mixers without expert nutritional help.

4. Minerals

(a) Calcium and Phosphorus

Pig rations should contain at least 0.9% of calcium and 0.7% phosphorus (up to 1% in weaners). High levels of inclusion may be necessary if these minerals are not readily available in the diet. The maximum level of calcium should be 1.0% except for sows where it may reach 1.2%. Absolute or conditioned deficiency of calcium may occur and high phosphorus and low Vitamin D levels may contribute to the latter. The introduction of phytase in diets and dietary policies for the reduction of phosphorus in effluent require expert nutritional input to maintain optimal available calcium and phosphorus for growth and bone strength. Bone strength may be affected before effects on performance are seen, but urinary calcium and phosphorus values alter up to 2 weeks before blood parameters can be detected. Two syndromes are primarily associated with calcium deficiency, rickets in young pigs and osteomalacia in sows.

References

Dritz, S.S., Tokach, M.D., Sargeant, J.M., Goodband, R.D., Nelssen, J.L. (2000). Lowering dietary phosphorus results in a loss of carcase value but not decreased growth performance. Swine Health and Production 8, 121-124.
Hagemoser, W.A., Goff, J.P., Sanderson, T.P., Haynes, J.S. (2000). Osteopenic disease in growing pigs: diagnostic methods using serum and urine calcium and phosphorus values, parathormone assay and bone analysis. (2000) J.Vet. Diabn. Invest. 12, 525-534.

Rickets in Young Pigs

Definition

A syndrome in which rapidly growing pigs cease to grow, may be anorexic, develop lameness and skeletal changes which result in inability to stand and finally, in death.

Incidence

Rare, only likely to occur when home-mixed rations are grossly inadequate. An inherited form has been described.

Clinical signs

Affected pigs are usually 2-6 months of age, may become stunted, anorexic and lame over a period of weeks. In advanced rickets, animals may have obvious signs of skeletal abnormality, such as swollen joints, especially carpal and tarsal, elbow and stifle joints and bowing of the forelegs. Kyphosis may be obvious and affected pigs may be weak, unable to rise without knuckling and may scream weakly if forced to do so. Champing, frothing at the jaws and signs of depraved appetite may also be noted. Temperatures of 39.2-40°C (102.5-104°F)) are not uncommon. Many affected animals adopt a dog-sitting position.

Severely affected animals unable to walk should be destroyed humanely.

Pathology

The carcases of grossly affected animals are emaciated with changes in the skeletal system. Enlarged epiphyses are common in long bones and distortion or collapse of the soft cancellous bone may occur, particularly at the bearing surface of the joints. Pathological fractures of bones of the limbs or ribs may be present and a 'rachitic rosary' is usually present at the costochondral junctions. Histological lesions include enlargement of the epiphyseal plates and widespread deposition of osteoid and failure of even mineralisation. In less severe cases, microscopic lesions may be the only sign that disturbances in ossification are occurring.

Diagnosis

The clinical signs of rickets are distinctive and X-ray examination of bones or post-mortem examination will confirm poor mineralisation. History and the composition of the diet are of value. Plasma calcium levels may vary from 1.58 m mol/1-2.5 m mol/l (normal). Low calcium levels in feed and plasma may suggest primary calcium deficiency but Vitamin D levels in plasma are difficult to obtain in the UK. and a diagnosis of rickets due to Vitamin D deficiency may only be obtained by consideration of the amount entering the diet (minimum requirement 6-11 i.u./kg liveweight/day). Plasma phosphorus levels are low (less than 2.24 m mol/l) in Vitamin D and phosphorus deficiency. The condition must be differentiated from septic arthritis, by the absence of heat and pain in joints, from *M.hyosynoviae* infection (age affected and bony lesions) and osteochondrosis (reduced growth rate).

Treatment

Ensure that the calcium, phosphorus and Vitamin D levels of the finished ration are adequate. Injection of Vitamin D should not be considered until the composition of the ration has been restored to normal for some days. Animals with lesions which include pathological fractures are unlikely to recover or be economic to fatten and should be destroyed.

References

Pepper, T.A., Bennett, D., Taylor, D.J. (1978). Rickets in growing pigs and response to treatment. Vet.Rec. 103, 4-8.
Thompson, K.G., Robinson B.M. (1989). An osteodystrophy apparently caused by vitamin D deficiency in growing pigs. New Zealand Vet.J. 37, 155-157.

Growth depression

Growing pigs fed diets containing Ca:P ratios greater than 2.5:1.0 have reduced daily gain.

Hypocalcaemia and Osteomalacia in Sows

Definition

Hypocalcaemia may result in sudden death at farrowing, protracted farrowings, uterine prolapse and muscular weakness resulting in the adoption of the 'dog sitting' position. It may be accompanied by fever and respiratory distress at this time.

Incidence

May be common but rarely recognised because of lack of sampling of blood calcium levels in farrowing sows.

Aetiology and pathogenesis

Hypocalcaemia results primarily from low levels of calcium in the ration or its poor availability because of high phosphorus levels or for some other reason. Commercial sow diets may contain low levels of calcium and some inclusion rates may be too low. Minimum figures of 0.6% have been considered adequate, but on low cost diets based on vegetable protein, this may be inadequate and a level of at least 0.9% and as much as 1.2% may be required. Low levels of dietary calcium lead to inadequate skeletal mineralisation and inadequate mobilisable calcium reserves at times of peak demand such as farrowing or late lactation. Lowered plasma calcium (normal is 2.5-2.7 m.mol/l in a normal modern hybrid sow) may lead to muscular weakness and problems with cardiac and myometrial function. In heavily lactating young sows or gilts with poor skeletal calcium reserves, this poor calcium status may be sufficient to allow pathological fractures of pelvic bones, femur or, more commonly, the vertebrae of the lumbosacral region. Osteodystrophia fibrosa may also occur and lead to changes in the alignment of the facial bones. Bone mineralisation may decline following restricted exercise.

Clinical signs

Sudden deaths in farrowing sows and the occurrence of a high incidence of prolapsed uteri or weakness and respiratory distress and fever may occur. Affected sows or gilts are usually unable to move their hind limbs and remain sitting or show degrees of posterior paralysis or lameness. Where broken bones are present, crepitus may be felt but the animals frequently guards the break with muscular rigidity or spasm and detection is difficult.

In some cases a large litter will be sucking and the condition may occur where weaning ages are extended in organic programmes without consideration of the calcium intake of the sow/gilt. Occasionally newly-purchased gilts or boars mixed in yards or even finishing pigs will also be affected. Low blood calcium levels (2.0 m.mol/l) are present. Alkaline phosphatase levels are often raised.

Where broken bones are identified, or where animals are unable to rise within 1 hour of treatment, pigs should be humanely destroyed without moving them from the site.

Pathology

Few changes may be seen in animals which die suddenly but in those which have had osteomalacia, brittle bones, with thin cortices and pathological fractures especially of vertebral bodies may be seen. Bone ash levels in rib bones confirm hypocalcaemia.

Diagnosis

The clinical signs of spontaneous fractures, farrowing difficulties or of sows in a dog-sitting position with weakness of the hindlimbs are suggestive. Hypocalcaemia should also be considered in sudden death at this stage. Low plasma calcium levels, low calcium levels in bone ash from tibial bone biopsies or from the third metatarsal of the right front foot, and a low calcium level in the feed will confirm. High osteocalcin levels may indicate osteomalacia in young pigs. Post-mortem examination will allow differentiation of animals with pathological fractures from spinal abscess etc. In sudden death, bone ash will confirm a low calcium status and lesions of gastric torsion, *C.novyi* infection, endocarditis etc. should be obvious. Pigs may develop the dog-sitting position and pathological fractures following electrocution.

Treatment

Intravenous calcium borogluconate will restore affected sows to clinical normality and may need to be supplemented by subcutaneous injections. These should be given to all sows farrowing before the calcium level of the rations can be restored to 1-1.2%. Cull sows unable to rise as soon as practicable.

References

Ayliffe, T.R. and Noakes, D.E. (1985). The effect of oxytocin on the myometrium of the sow during experimentally induced hypocalcaemia. J.Vet.Pharm. and Therapeutics **8**, 212-214.
Combs, N.R., Kornegay, E.T., Lindemann, D.R., Welker, F.H. (1991). Evaluation of a bone biopsy technique for determining the calcium and phosphorus ratio of swine from weaning to market weight. J.Anim.Sci. **69**, 664-672.
Jennings, D.S. (1985). Hypocalcaemia in sows. Proc.Pig Vet.Soc. **14**, 38-40.
Maxson, P.F., Mahan, D.C. (1986). Dietary calcium and phosphorus for lactating swine at high and average production levels. J.Animal Science **63**, 1163-1172.

b) Iron
Piglet Anaemia

Definition

A hypochromic microcytic anaemia of rapidly-growing piglets housed on concrete which results in poor performance and in the deaths of severely-affected animals. It is caused by a primary deficiency of iron in the diet.

Incidence

Rare under modern husbandry conditions but may occur in individual litters or where oral iron dosing is accompanied by diarrhoea. Subclinical disease may occur in outdoor pigs.

Aetiology and pathogenesis

The piglet is born with limited reserves of iron and copper and has a blood haemoglobin level of 120g/L at birth. Within the first 10 days of life, a physiological decline in blood haemoglobin levels to 80 g/L occurs and the correct level is subsequently regained in normal healthy piglets with adequate available dietary iron.

During the first 4 weeks of life, the body weight of piglets may increase five-fold and active haemopoiesis is essential if the normal blood haemoglobin levels of 120-140 g/L are to be regained after the physiological fall. The dietary requirement for iron during this period of life is 15 mg/day, but only 1 mg/day can be supplied by the sow's milk in spite of supplementation of her diet with iron. The remaining requirement is supplied by iron present in the soil ingested by all piglets kept in extensive husbandry systems.

Where animals are farrowed and reared on concrete or outside on iron-free soil or confined in soil-free creep areas, the requirement for iron outstrips the supply and a hypochromic microcytic anaemia develops as the blood haemoglobin levels continue to fall below the physiological low of 80 g/L. They may fall as low as 35 g/L by the age of 3-4 weeks. After this, the intake of creep feed becomes sufficient to supply the dietary requirement for iron and the blood haemoglobin levels normally begin to rise again in deficient pigs. Iron deficiency may reduce gastric and intestinal enzyme secretion and reduce neutrophil levels.

Clinical signs

The clinical signs appear most commonly in piglets of 3 weeks of age, by which time a severe anaemia may have developed, particularly in pigs in good condition. Anaemia may also occur in newborn animals as a result of navel bleeding or intrauterine anaemia.

Affected pigs may be plump, although their growth rate is up to 10% less than that of normal pigs. They appear pale, the ears, belly and the mucosae may be yellowish in colour. There may be oedema of the head and forequarters. Thin, pale, hairy pigs are more commonly seen. Diarrhoea is common, but the faeces are normal in colour. Affected pigs are lethargic and when disturbed, show dyspnoea and a prominent apex beat. Severely affected piglets may die suddenly. Not all pigs in an iron-deficient litter may show clinical signs of the disease.

Humane slaughter is only indicated when animals are emaciated.

Post mortem findings

The carcases of affected pigs are pale, with thin watery blood and oedema of the muscles. Fluid exudates in the body cavities are common. The liver is enlarged in all cases and is a mottled greyish-yellow colour, due to fatty change. The heart is flabby and enlarged and there may be signs of enteritis.

Diagnosis

Diagnosis in piglets is based on the clinical signs outlined above and upon the history of no access to iron. Thrombocytopaenic purpura may also produce pallor and anaemia as may eprythrozoonosis, but these often produce jaundice. Navel bleeding and haemorrhage from castration, tail docking or internal injury may also occur. These are often individual rather than herd problems. Infections such as *C.perfringens* Type C and coccidiosis can cause anaemia as a result of blood loss. In older pigs pallor and anaemia can result from a number of conditions including bleeding from wounds, as a result of warfarin poisoning, gastric ulceration, proliferative intestinal adenopathy and a number of other conditions.

The diagnosis may be confirmed in piglets by the finding of low blood haemoglobin levels (below 70 g/L) in the third week of age and, in clinically affected animals, 40 g/L or less. A better indication is the red cell count which is less than 5 million per µl, and may be as low as 3 million per µl. The red cells are hypochromic and reduced in size. A rapid method of assay is to bleed from an ear vein into haematocrit tubes. Anaemic pigs may have a haematocrit of 10% or less compared with the normal 28-30%.

Treatment and control

Supplementation of the sow's diet cannot raise piglets' liver iron levels at birth or increase the amount of iron in the milk so piglets must be provided with 15 mg of iron per day to prevent the occurrence of anaemia. This may be provided in the following ways:

(i) Intramuscular injection with iron dextran complex, or gleptoferron or other chelates

This is the most satisfactory method of prevention and treatment. For prevention, piglets should be injected in the neck rather than the hind limb at 1-3 days of age with at least 200 mg of elemental iron. As the available preparations differ in their iron content, always follow the manufacturer's recommendations; 2 ml is the most common dose. Recently 200 mg in 1 ml have been given into the neck muscles where 3 week weaning is practised and there is evidence that, where creep feed is available, only 100mg is required.

None of the preparations at present on the UK market appear to cause adverse reactions, but animals which have died may show yellowish staining of the hind limb muscles and brownish inguinal lymph nodes for some time after the injection in the hindlimb. This is normal. Fatal reaction to iron injections may indicate a low selenium or Vitamin E status in the piglets. Some preparations also contain cyanocobalamin (Vitamin B12) as an additional aid to haemopoiesis. Injection should be delayed during clinical infection with PRRS.

(ii) Oral iron supplements

Iron preparations are available in several forms, some of which are pastes containing various forms of reduced iron, usually as the citrate or fumarate given by individual oral dosing to piglets at birth and 14 days of age.

Granules containing iron dextran may also be given under lamps in the creep feed and pastes containing iron dextrans are also available for oral therapy. Recently soluble products for water medication have been used in piglet drinkers. In a few cases, farmers may wish to provide iron by including soil, peat or coal in the pen. The oral preparations suffer from the disadvantages that they may be missed out, that they are labour intensive, that, if given when diarrhoea is occurring, the iron may not be absorbed and that, if given in excess, they may cause diarrhoea. This is especially so with crude ferrous sulphate which may still be in use on some farms. Recent studies have suggested that supplementation of the sows' feed with iron allows the piglets to ingest sufficient iron from her faeces of which they eat approximately 10 g per day. This practice has recently been shown to produce uneven uptake and to be inferior to parenteral administration.

(iii) Complex iron: copper deficiency

If iron therapy alone does not appear to cure the condition, copper supplementation may be necessary in addition. This is an unusual occurrence and is rarely necessary.

References

309

Caperna, T.J., Failla, M.L., Steele, N.C., Richards, M.P. (1987). Accumulation and metabolism of iron dextran by hepatocytes, Kupffer cells and endothelial cells in the neonatal pig liver. J. Nutrition 117, 312-320.
Daykin, M.M., Griffiths, A.J., Towlerton, R.G. (1982). Evaluation of the parenteral iron requirement of early weaned pigs. Vet. Rec. 110. 535-537.
Gleed, P.T., Sansom, B.F. (1982). Effects of feeding lactating sows on iron rich diet on piglet haematology and growth rates. Vet.Rec. 111, 136-139.
Larkin, H.A. and Hannan, J. (1983). Gastric structure and function in iron deficient piglets. Res. in Vet.Sci. 34, 11-15.
Larkin, H.A. and Hannan, J. (1984) Intestinal absorption and structure in iron deficient piglets. Res. in Vet.Sci. 36, 199-204.

Excess iron

High levels of iron in the diet may reduce phosphorus absorption and result in rickets in growing piglets, so iron levels should not exceed 4 g/Kg.

c) Copper

Deficiency. Few clinical signs other than anaemia, an increase in stillbirths, leg weakness, paresis/paralysis and ataxia have been directly related to copper deficiency, but experimental studies demonstrate cardiac enlargement, associated with failure to cross-link new collagen, increases in mitochondrial numbers and accumulations of glycogen. These are reflected in disturbances of conduction. The trend towards reduction of metals in effluent is beginning to affect formulation in some countries and low levels may become more common, increasing the frequency of deficiency.

Supplementation. Copper has been commonly included (usually as copper sulphate) in growing pig rations at levels of 50-175 ppm, but are now limited to 25 ppm in feeds for pigs over 12 weeks of age (EU). Copper, iron and zinc metabolism are linked and high levels of zinc (as in post-weaning scour medication) may reduce liver copper as may iron. The use of organic copper complexes can supply adequate copper for growth even at levels within the new restrictions.

Toxicity. Copper toxicity may occur at 500 ppm or more and clinical signs include inappetence, depression of condition and weight gain, blackened faeces and diarrhoea, jaundice and the accumulation of copper in the hepatocytes of the liver which is yellow brown and fragile. Clinical signs disappear within 2 weeks of feed withdrawal.

References

Pletcher, J.M. and Banting, L.F. (1983). Ataxia and posterior paresis in copper deficient weaners. J.South African Vet.Assn. 54, 43-46.
Pritchard, G.C., Lewis, G., Wells, G.A.H. and Stopforth, A. (1985). Zinc toxicity, copper deficiency and anaemia in swill fed pigs. Vet.Rec. 117, 545-548.
Wildman, R.E.C., Medeiros, D., Hamlin, R.L., Stills, H., Jones, D.A., Bonagura, J.D. (1996). Aspects of cardiomyopathy in copper-deficient pigs. Electrocardiography, echocardiography and ultrastructural findings. Biol Trace Element Res. 55, 55-70.

(d) Zinc

Parakeratosis of Swine

An absolute or conditioned deficiency of dietary zinc may result in depression of growth and the development of non-inflammatory proliferative lesions of the epidermis resulting in hyperkeratisation.

Incidence

May occur in subclinical forms in rapidly-growing pigs. The overt clinical form is rare.

Aetiology

Zinc may be deficient in the diet but in most cases absorption is inadequate due to interference from high levels of dietary phytic acid from soya, from wheat bran or from calcium. Rapid growth, low dietary concentrations of unsaturated fatty acids, dry feeding *ad libitum* and infections resulting in diarrhoea and malabsorption may all precipitate the condition.

Supplementation of the diet with linolenic acid appears to prevent the condition; zinc deficiency may produce its effect by reducing the biosynthesis of essential fatty acids and appears to produce its skin effects by damage to desmosomes linking cells and reducing keratohyalin synthesis.

Clinical signs

The condition occurs in pigs 2-4 months of age, appearing within 15-21 days of the introduction of a deficient diet and associated with depression of the rate of growth. Small erythematous areas develop on the ventral surface of the abdomen and inside the thigh. They become papules and then become elevated and scaly. The pastern, fetlock, knee and hock develop these crusty lesions which may spread to the shoulders and other areas of the body. Lesions are symmetrically distributed and are usually dry and crumbly. Cracking may occur, resulting in exudation of serum and secondary infection. Irritation is not a feature of this condition. Growth may be depressed and feed conversion efficiency reduced. Plasma levels down to 7.5 µg/ml may be found. Long-term feeding studies suggest that the effect of deficiency on reproduction is to increase problems at farrowing, increase stillbirths and lower litter weights to 2 weeks of age.

Pathology

Changes are restricted to the skin. There is a subacute to chronic non-inflammatory change in all layers of the skin except for the stratum lucidum. Keratinisation is incomplete and the stratum corneum is irregularly thickened and the cells within it retain their nuclei. The rete pegs penetrate more deeply into the dermis, there is an increase in the number of basal cells and dilation of the sweat glands and hypertrophy of sebaceous glands occurs. Parakeratosis of the oesophagus has been described in experimental situations and may occasionally be seen in natural cases.

Diagnosis

The age of the pigs affected and the distribution, texture and appearance of the lesions is suggestive of zinc deficiency. A skin biopsy may be of value in confirming diagnosis, serum zinc and alkaline phosphatase levels may be low. The lack of irritation and the absence of mites from skin scrapings differentiate the condition from sarcoptic mange. Exudative epidermitis usually occurs in younger pigs and is often associated with mortality.

Treatment

A dietary level of zinc of 100 ppm will restore health within 10-40 days. Supplementation of the rations with zinc carbonate, or sulphate should not exceed 200 ppm final zinc concentration. Toxicity due to excess zinc in the ration is difficult to produce as the diet is refused at high zinc levels but may be associated with copper deficiency. The therapeutic use of zinc oxide to 5,000 ppm does not appear to cause toxicity, but may cause accumulation of zinc in tissues.

References

Hill, G.M., Miller, E.R. and Stowe, H.D. (1983). Effects of dietary zinc levels on sows' health and productivity of gilts and through two parities. J.Anim.Sci. 57, 114-122.
Hain, J.D., Baker, D.H. (1993). Growth and plasma zinc responses of young pigs fed pharmacologic levels of zinc. J.Anim.Sci. 71, 3020-3024.
Kalinowski, J. and Chavez, E.R. (1986). Low dietary zinc intake during pregnancy and lactation in gilts. Canadian J.Animal Sci., 66, 201-216.

(e) Selenium

(i) Deficiency

Cereals grown in selenium-deficient soils and some cereal varieties may contain less than the optimum level of selenium for animal growth. The addition of selenium to such diets to give a final concentration of 0.8-1.1 ppm increases growth rates in weaned pigs and reduces the Incidence of hepatosis dietetica, diarrhoea, gastric ulceration and iron toxicity following iron injections. Selenium uptake is most efficient in the organic form (as methionine Se, cysteine Se) but inorganic selenium can also be absorbed.

Selenium levels in plasma are related to plasma glutathione peroxidase (GSH Px) activity and low levels of this enzyme indicate selenium deficiency. Serum levels of less than 0.025 ug/ml and liver levels of less than 0.10 mg/kg indicate selenium deficiency.

Studies of glutathione peroxidase levels suggest that selenium uptake may be inhibited by wheat bran and selenium excretion may be reduced by riboflavin in the ration. A genetic predisposition to low blood selenium has been detected and normal blood selenium levels fall at about 3 weeks of age in the absence of supplementation. Lesions of selenium deficiency are similar to those of Vitamin E deficiency and the complex is considered below under Vitamin E deficiency.

(ii) Selenium toxicity

High levels of selenium may be present in the diet through the consumption of poisonous plants such as *Astragalus sp* and, more commonly, through the erroneous inclusion of high levels of selenium in mineral and vitamin premixes for pigs. Levels greater than 5-6 mg/kg (5 g/tonne) may induce toxicity and levels of 6.2, 8.1 and 17.2 mg/kg respectively were toxic when given to growing pigs. Earliest signs can occur within 5-7 days of exposure and include reduction in feed intake followed by forelimb weakness, tremor, hyperaesthesis, recumbency, paresis and death. Hair loss, blanching of the coronary band and cracking and shedding of the hooves may be seen in chronic cases which may present as lameness. Vesicular diseases should be considered during the diagnosis of this condition, as the lesions resemble those on the coronary band and the sloughing of the hooves which occur in Swine Vesicular Disease or Foot and Mouth Disease. Sows fed 2 mg/kg for the last part of gestation produce litters with high levels of stillbirths, and pre-weaning losses and piglets have haemorrhagic lesions of the anterior wall or sole of the feet. Animals which are recumbent should be destroyed humanely.

Affected animals have a symmetrical focal polio encephalo-malacia and lesions affect the ventral grey matter particularly at the lumbar and sacral enlargement. High levels of tissue selenium can be demonstrated (normal liver 0.7-1.8 mg/kg dry matter, kidney 5.0-11.5 mg/kg).

Withdrawal of toxic feed is the only appropriate treatment and a 60 day period on normal feed should be observed before slaughter. Recovery from nervous signs in mobile pigs may take 2 months.

Reference

Chavez, E.R. (1989). Selenium nutrition of pigs; a review. Pig News and Information 10, 167-171.

Mensink, C.G., Koeman, J.P., Veling, J., Gruys, E. (1990). Haemorrhagic claw lesions in newborn piglets due to selenium toxicosis during pregnancy. Vet.Rec. 126, 620-622.

Oldfield, J.E. (1985). Some implications of selenium in pig nutrition. Pig News and Information 6, 419-424.

Panter, K.E., Hartley, W.J., James, L.F., Mayland, H.F., Stegelmeier, B.L., Kechele, P.O. (1996). Comparative toxicity of selenium from seleno DL methionine, sodium selenite and Astragalus bisulcatus in pigs. Fundamental Appl. Toxicol. 32, 217-223.

Penrith, M.L., Robinson, J.T.R. (1996). Selenium toxicosis with focal symmetrical poliomalacia in postweaning pigs in South Africa. Ond. J.Vet. Res. 63, 171-179.

Stave, H.D., Eavey, A.J. Granger, L., Halstead, S., Yamini, B. (1992). Selenium toxicosis in feeder pigs. J.Am.Vet.Med.Assoc. 201, 292-295.

5. Fats

A deficiency of essential fatty acids may result in the development of a scaly skin, particularly in adults. A weekly dose of cod-liver oil (10 ml per animal) is usually sufficient to correct this. The minimum levels of linolenic and arachidonic acids are given in Table C. These acids may also be essential for adequate prostaglandin formation.

Indigestible fats in poor quality waste fat may result in diarrhoea when they are incorporated in feeds at high levels.

Oxidised fats and those containing high levels of polyunsaturated fatty acids (PUFA) may reduce the plasma levels of vitamin E

6. Vitamins

Vitamin A (Retinol) Deficiency

Definition

The absence of Vitamin A from the diet, its presence at low levels or poor absorption of the vitamin causes infertility and the birth of weak or non-viable piglets with congenital defects to sows with poor body reserves of the vitamin. Nervous signs, skin changes and reduction in the rate of bone growth may all occur in growing pigs.

Incidence

Rare now, but may occur in herds where home-mixed rations are given. Subclinical disease may be more common.

Aetiology and pathogenesis

Vitamin A is normally included in pig rations at levels of 3-9 million i.u. per tonne and can be produced in the liver from dietary carotene obtained from grass meal or fresh yellow maize. The presence of unsaturated fatty acids in the ration and the pelleting of feed may cause the destruction of Vitamin A incorporated in the ration and lead to the presence of low dietary levels of the vitamin. Vitamin A is necessary for the formation of visual purple, for normal bone growth, especially the remodelling of bones, for the normal development and function of secretory and epithelial cells and for normal embryological development. Uncontrolled bone growth in the spinal cord and cranium produces nervous signs associated with a rise in C.S.F. pressure. Clinical signs appear after 4-5 months on a deficient ration.

Clinical signs

Nervous signs such as incoordination, tilting of the head and eventual paralysis of the hind limbs with dog-sitting occur in growing pigs in which skin changes, especially splitting of the tips of the bristles, may occur. Sows, and, in particular, gilts, may produce stillborn or moribund piglets at full term in the most severe form of the disease. Stillborn piglets may have ascites and moribund animals are listless, weak and lie on their sides around the sow, making weak, paddling movements and squawking plaintively. Stronger animals may burrow in the bedding. Eye changes may be seen ranging from microphthalmia in all moribund piglets to minor iris or sclera defects in mildly affected animals.

Animals unable to walk should be destroyed humanely.

Pathology

In young growing pigs with posterior paralysis, demyelination of the spinal cord may be found. Signs that increased intracranial pressure may have occurred may also be present. In congenitally-affected piglets, oedema of the subcutaneous tissues is prominent and the body cavities are filled with sero-fibrinous fluid. Kidney abnormalities are common and the livers are yellowish grey (stillborn) or congested (moribund). There may be epithelial hyperplasia of the acini of the salivary glands, alveoli, bronchioles and renal tubules. Cerebellar hypoplasia and cardiac defects have been recorded. Plasma Vitamin A levels should exceed 7-8 ug (15-20 i.u.) per 100 ml. Normal sera contain about 23 ug (50-60 i.u.) per 100 ml. Liver should contain 60 ug (120-130 i.u.) per g, but clinical signs may not develop until levels of 2-5 ug (4-10 i.u.) per g are reached. C.S.F. pressures, normally 80-125 mm water rise to 200 mm or above.

Diagnosis

Based on history of home-mixed rations with no added Vitamin A, clinical and post-mortem findings and confirmed by analysis of liver biopsies or samples for Vitamin A.

Treatment and control

Commercial rations normally contain adequate Vitamin A, but home-mixed feed should be examined for Vitamin A content. If the condition is diagnosed, affected animals or those at risk can be treated parenterally with fat-soluble vitamins. Parenteral multivitamin and oral supplements also exist. Dose according to data sheet.

References

Brief, S., Chew, B.P. (1985). Effects of Vitamin A and B carotene reproductive performance in gilts. J.Anim.Sci. **60**, 998-1004.
Goodwin, R.F.W. and Jennings, A.R. (1958). Mortality of newborn pigs associated with a maternal deficiency of Vitamin A. J.Comp.Path. **68**, 82-95.

Vitamin A toxicity

If Vitamin A levels in the ration are high for long periods of time, lameness, decreased bone weight and depression of performance may occur. Diarrhoea has been described. Short limbs, reduced long bone length flattening and caudal rotation of the humeral head and distal femoral condyles with narrow metaphyseal growth plates in the vertebrae may all be present. Liver Vitamin A levels are high.

References

Coates, J.W., Holbek, N.E., Beames, R.M., Puls, R., O'Brien, W.P. (1998). gastric ulceration and suspected vitamin A toxicosis in grower pigs fed fish silage. Can. Vet. J. **39**, 167-170.
Doige, C.E., Schoonderwoerd, M. (1988). Dwarfism in a swine herd : suspected Vitamin A toxicosis. J.Am.Vet.Med.Ass. **193**, 691-693.

Vitamin D

Rickets

Rickets has been discussed under hypocalcaemia, but, if dietary calcium and phosphorus levels are adequate, treatment with parenteral ADE preparations such as those listed above, may be used as an aid to recovery. A hereditary form of rickets has been described (see Congenital and Hereditary Conditions).

References

Pepper, T.A., Bennett, D., Taylor, D.J. (1989). Rickets in growing pigs and response to treatment. Vet.Rec. **103**, 4-8.
Thompson, K.G., Robinson, B.M. (1988). An osteodystrophy apparently caused by Vitamin D deficiency in growing pigs. New Zealand Vet.J. **37**, 155-157.

Vitamin D poisoning

Vitamin D poisoning has been identified in both commercial and companion pigs when excessive amounts of the vitamin are included in rations.. A reduction in food intake occurs, anorexia, weight loss/reduction in growth rate develop and pigs become lethargic, polyuric and polydypsic. Vomiting, tremor and tenesmus have been recorded and it may be lethal. Metastatic calcification may occur in kidneys, lung and heart. Diagnosis is based on the presence of hypercalcaemia

315

and raised plasma vitamin D levels. Treatment is symptomatic with corticosteroid or non-steroidal anti inflammatories for companion animals and a normal diet for all. Recovery normally occurs within 3 weeks.

Reference.

Wimsatt, J.D., Marks, S.L., Campbell, T.W., Johnson, J.D., Nachreiner, R.F. (1998). Dietary vitamin D toxicity in a household of pot-bellied pigs (Sus scrofa). J.Vet. Intern. Med. **12**, 41-44.

Vitamin E

Vitamin E Deficiency

Definition

Low dietary levels of Vitamin E (α tocopherol) are associated with a number of syndromes including hepatosis dietetica, nutritional muscular dystrophy (white muscle disease), mulberry heart disease, hertztod, yellow fat disease and infertility.

Aetiology

Caused by a deficiency of Vitamin E in the ration and exacerbated by low selenium, methionine and cystine levels and high fat levels in the diet. Oxidised fat, copper and the wet storage of cereals may all reduce the Vitamin E levels of diets. Only α tocopherol can be used by the pig and the descriptions which follow relate to this form of Vitamin E.

Pathogenesis

Alpha tocopherol acts both as an antioxidant and as a stabiliser of membrane lipids. It becomes bound to the membranes of mitochondria and microsomes. A specific loss of membrane bound arachidonic and linolenic acids occurs in Vitamin E deficiency and this is associated with low dietary levels of these acids. Selenium is related to this process in that it forms part of glutathione peroxidase, an enzyme which acts on oxidised polyunsaturated fatty acid radicals. Selenium therefore has a sparing effect on Vitamin E, the action of which in turn is related to methionine and cystine levels. Vitamin A is also spared by Vitamin E and is more rapidly destroyed in its absence. The major clinical signs of this complex deficiency appear to result from the effects on energy metabolism. The cells most severely affected in the pig are hepatocytes and muscle cells in the heart and skeletal muscles.

Vitamin E is normally present in cereal grains but can be destroyed if polyunsaturated fats, e.g. from fish oils, linseed oil or, mouldy or spoiled grain are included in the ration. Propionic acid treatment of barley may be important in the aetiology of the condition in the UK. The presence of low levels of selenium in grain grown on selenium deficient soils may exacerbate the condition and the now common practice of adding high levels of fat to rations may also be important.

Clinical signs

Sudden death is most commonly seen. Piglets affected by muscular dystrophy may be dyspnoeic with normal body temperature and no signs of enteritis. Clinical signs may appear in a few piglets in a litter at about 2 weeks of age. In older pigs, sudden deaths may occur after handling and affected animals within a group may show some signs of circulatory embarrassment such as lethargy, cyanosis and dejection. Muscle tremor may occur, especially at the shoulders. There may be stiffness, a limp or recumbency. In conditions such as dietosis hepatica and herztod, there may be evidence of poor growth rate. Anaemia may develop. Low levels of dietary Vitamin E may also depress fertility, increasing weaning to service intervals and reducing the percentage of returns to oestrus.

Affected pigs are rarely observed in life so humane slaughter is not usually required.

Pathology

Affected piglets with muscular dystrophy are in good condition and there may be some oedema of the subcutaneous tissues and pericardial fluid is commonly found. There is pulmonary oedema and the heart is enlarged. Pale, yellowish streaks are usually present on the ventricular walls. Fresh haemorrhagic streaks may be seen beneath the endocardium. The liver may be pale and there may be excess peritoneal fluid.

In older pigs, post-mortem features include heart lesions resembling those in piglets, necrosis of the liver which is pale and mottled or haemorrhagic. In long-standing cases where methionine and cystine deficiency may also occur, regeneration of liver lobules may be seen on the surface as reddish spots or tags in a yellowish liver. Rupture of the liver may occur, there may be an obvious fissure with an attached blood clot and the abdomen may be filled with blood. Gastric ulceration may be prominent. Oedema of the mesentery of the colon may be present. Muscles, especially the adductor muscle group in the hind limb, may be white or pale in colour. Lesions are often symmetrical. Adipose tissue may be yellow (steatitis or yellow fat disease). The liver changes are often described as "hepatosis dietetica".

Histological findings include hyaline degeneration of individual muscle fibres both in the myocardium and in the longissimus dorsi, leg muscles, diaphragm and intercostal muscles. Where lesions precede degeneration of the arterioles and the presence of microthrombi may be seen, particularly in the cardiac muscle and in the liver.

Diagnosis

The clinical signs and post-mortem findings may suggest a diagnosis of one of the entities associated with Vitamin E deficiency (see hepatosis dietetica and mulberry heart). Confirmation depends on the demonstration of low dietary levels of alpha tocopherol. A level of 10 i.u. (60 mg)/kg dry matter [10,000 i.u. (60 g) per tonne] is considered adequate in sow feed and a minimum of 15 i.u. (5 mg)/kg dry matter (1,500 i.u. (5g) per tonne) in rations for pigs up to 90 kg. Histories of storage of grain in propionic acid, etc. are suggestive.

Levels of serum enzymes such as S.G.O.T., creatinine phosphokinase, ornithine carbamyl transferase and lactic dehydrogenase may all be raised in affected animals and levels of plasma α tocopherol are less than 1 mg/L (normally in excess of 1.8mg/L). Response to α tocopherol treatment is confirmatory although selenium may also have some effect.

Treatment

Parenteral treatment with α tocopherol or α tocopherol-selenium preparations is of value in affected groups of animals. Vitamin E is also available as a component of the fat soluble vitamin mixtures. Pregnant sows may be injected in order to reduce mortality in their litters, but for a period of 3-4 weeks, newborn piglets should be treated at birth until increased feed levels of the vitamin have raised maternal and foetal α tocopherol levels.

Control depends upon ensuring that adequate levels of dietary Vitamin E are present in the final ration. Vitamin E should be included at five times the fat percentage of the ration measured in mg/kg feed is usually adequate, but, where actively oxidising fats are present, up to 20 times the fat percentage may be needed.

Vitamin E/Selenium Deficiency Related Syndromes

1. **Steatitis (Yellow Fat Disease)**

Yellow-brown discolouration of the fat may be seen in pigs at post-mortem examination or slaughter. This is due to the inclusion of high levels of unsaturated fatty acids in the feed (often from byproducts) with a low level of Vitamin E. Vitamin E supplementation prevents the problem.

2. **Hepatosis dietetica**

This may occur in young growing pigs usually 3-4 months of age. Affected pigs may be depressed, vomit or stagger but are usually found dead. At post-mortem examination the livers are enlarged, mottled and may have bled into the peritoneal cavity. The lesions appear to be lobular in section with pale, haemorrhagic and apparently normal lobules. Microangiopathy underlies the changes and there may be evidence of muscular dystrophy.

The condition is associated with selenium deficiency more closely than with Vitamin E but both substances may be deficient and rations should be examined for both. A vegetable protein source such as soya and the use of high percentages of wheat offals with associated selenium-retaining bran and high fat may all predispose. Treat by injection and then correct the ration formulation.

3. **Mulberry Heart Disease**

Definition

A syndrome in which acute heart failure and sudden death occur sporadically, usually in large fattening pigs with no history of stress. It can, however, occur in pigs from birth to adulthood.

Incidence

Common in Britain at present, occurs in some herds as sporadic deaths, particularly when least cost rations are used.

Aetiology and pathogenesis

Feeding propionic-acid-treated barley appears to predispose to the condition and Vitamin E deficiency appears to be involved. Toxic products of bacteria may contribute to the syndrome. Heredity may play a part as Landrace pigs have been said to be susceptible. In most cases selenium levels appear to be normal but tissue Vitamin E levels are low even when dietary levels are apparently adequate. The syndrome develops as a result of congestive heart failure, coupled with hydropericardium.

Clinical signs

Pigs of any age may be affected, but the condition occurs commonly in 20-50 kg animals. Affected pigs are anorexic and depressed with muscle weakness and lowered body temperature. They may become cyanotic before death which occurs within 24 hours of the onset of the clinical signs. Recovery has been recorded, but mortality is usually 100%. Humane slaughter is rarely possible.

Pathology

The carcase is usually in good condition with fluid and shreds of fibrin in all body cavities. The liver is enlarged and mottled. The pericardial cavity is full of gelatinous fluid and fibrin and the surface of the heart is streaked with haemorrhages running from base to apex. Similar haemorrhages occur in the endocardium. They lie immediately below the membrane and appear histologically as areas of free red cells with no obvious myonecrosis. Microangiopathy may be present and in most cases degeneration of the muscles may also be present (see Vitamin E).

Diagnosis

The heart lesions are characteristic. Oedema disease, *Actinobacillus pleuropneumoniae* and *Streptococcus suis* Type II infections may also cause sudden death with fluid or fibrin in body cavities. Death from the porcine stress syndrome usually follows exertion. The histopathology and liver Vitamin E analysis usually confirm.

Treatment and control

The use of high levels of Vitamin E (2-3 times the recommended levels) prevents the development of the condition and implies a Vitamin E deficiency. Parenteral Vitamin E alone or with selenium may be used to treat animals in affected groups. Vitamin E levels may be restored to normal within a few hours by injection but may take 2 weeks by feed supplementation.

References

Kirby, P.S. (1981). Steatitis in fattening pigs. Vet.Rec. **109**, 385.

Mortimer, D.T. (1983). Vitamin E/selenium deficiency syndrome in pigs. Vet.Rec. **112**, 278-279.

Pallares, F.J., Yaeger, M.J., Janke, B.H., Fernandez, G., Albur, P.G. (2002). Vitamin E and selenium concentrations in livers of pigs diagnosed with mulberry Herat disease. J.Vet. Diagn. Invest. **14**, 412-414.

Putnam, M.E. (1982). Vitamin E for pigs. Proc.Pig Vet.Soc. **9**, 178-183.

Vleet, J.F. van. (1982). Comparative efficacy of five supplementation procedures to control Vitamin E selenium deficiency in swine. Am.J.Vet.Res. **43**, 1180-1189.

Gritz, B.G.de (1995). Copper zinc dismutase (Cu Zn SOD) in antioxidanrt deficient pigs. J.Vet. Med. Ser. A. **42**, 561-573.

Vitamin K.

Clinical disease associated with deficiency of this vitamin has been recorded in 5-6 week old pigs 1-2 weeks after weaning. Pigs were fed on rations without added Vitamin K and in one case housed in a flat-deck. Antimicrobials, including sulphadimidine, were being fed at therapeutic levels. Sulphadimidine is a Vitamin K antagonist and flat-deck housing prevents the consumption of faeces containing Vitamin K2 synthesised by intestinal microflora. Affected pigs fail to grow and develop subcutaneous haematomas, prolonged bleeding times, lameness and swelling of joints. Some became pale and some died (to 20% mortality).

319

The condition can be reproduced experimentally by feeding weaned piglets a low Vitamin K diet containing sulphadimidine (with or without other antibiotics) and housing them on wire. Defects in coagulation appeared after 35 days and the condition after 64 days. Conditioned deficiencies may also occur in coumarol/warfarin poisoning, and calcium excess and the condition must also be distinguished from mycotoxicosis.

Treatment with oral and injectable Vitamin K (l0 g menadione bisulphite per tonne or one i/m injection of 20 mg Vitamin K1 per piglet) provide treatment or prophylaxis.

Reference

Newsholme, S.J., Cullen, J.S.C., Nel, P.W., Peyers, F. (1985). A haemorrhagic syndrome in recently weaned pigs ascribed to hypovitaminosis K. J.South African Vet.Ass. **56**, 101-102.

Water soluble vitamins

Thiamine (Vitamin B1) Deficiency

Not likely to occur under natural conditions as a single entity unless pigs are fed rations containing large amounts of heat-treated carbohydrate, e.g. bakery waste in swill to which no balancer has been added. Up to 47% of thiamine requirements are met by bacterial synthesis in the gut. Requirements may be increased by high ambient temperatures and reduced by high fat concentrations in the diet. Thiaminases from bracken fern (*Pteridium aquilinum*) fronds or rhizomes can cause death after sows have grazed infested pastures for 10 weeks but other thiaminases in food can cause disease.

Clinical signs include inappetence, poor growth rate, emaciation, a fall in temperature and respiratory rate resulting in death within 5 weeks from congestive cardiac failure in experimental conditions. There is cyanosis of the skin and mucous membranes. Sudden death, vomiting and depression have been reported in bracken poisoning. The post-mortem findings include enlargement of the heart, myocardial degeneration and fibrosis, pulmonary oedema, pleural effusion, pleurisy and pleural fibrosis. The thiamine status of pigs can be monitored by the levels of erythrocyte transketolase present. In deficiency they are low. Affected pigs may be treated with thiamine by injection.

References

Edwards, B.L. (1983). Poisoning .by *Pteridium aquilinum* in pregnant sows. Vet.Rec. **112**, 459-460.
Lund, L.J. (1985). Bracken poisoning in sows. Proc.Pig Vet.Soc. **13**, 96-97.
Gibson, D.M., Kenelly, J.J., Aherne, F.X. (1987). The thiamine status of pigs fed sulphur dioxide treated high moisture barley. Can. J.Anim.Sci. **67**, 841-854.

Riboflavin (Vitamin B2 Deficiency)

Clinical signs

Slow growth, some lameness, frequent diarrhoea, conjunctivitis, skin changes such as alopecia and matting of the hair with sebaceous secretions may be seen in growing pigs. Irregular oestrus, delayed oestrus and, eventually, anoestrus have been reported in deficiency in sows. Erythrocyte glutathione reductase levels appear to reflect riboflavin status and a 50% decline in active enzyme occurs before other deficiency signs appear. The birth of piglets with oedema of the forelegs has been recorded where sows have received deficient diets. Inclusion of 2.5g of riboflavin per tonne of feed prevents deficiency in finishers but 3.2-3.3 g/tonne may be required for pregnant sow rations.

Affected piglets should be killed humanely.

Niacin or Nicotinic Acid Deficiency

May occur when diets are fed in which maize, low in tryptophan (a nicotinamide precursor) and niacin itself, is the major ingredient.

In some cases the syndrome has been reported to result from the ingestion of antimetabolites such as 6 amino nicotinamide.

Clinical signs

These include inappetence, persistent diarrhoea and a dirty yellow skin with dermatitis, alopecia or coat abnormalities. Posterior paralysis in which swaying of the hindquarters, knuckling and even flaccid paralysis may occur has been described. Paralysed animals should be humanely destroyed.

Pathology

Haemorrhages in the walls of the stomach and duodenum may be seen, the mucosa of the small and large intestine may be swollen and friable and there may be ulceration of the large intestinal mucosa. Necrotic enteritis, resembling that seen in salmonellosis or intestinal adenomatosis, may be present. Histological lesions include a mucinous degeneration of the large intestinal mucosa differing from lesions of intestinal adenomatosis and focal lesions, especially destruction of glial cells may occur in the intermediate grey matter of the lumbar and cervical enlargements of the spinal cord. There may be widespread vacuolation of the white matter.

Treatment

Tryptophan supplementation of ration should be carried out to give 2.7 kg/tonne or nicotinic acid should be added to give 14-20 g/tonne.

Reference

O'Sullivan, B.M., Blakemore, W.F. (1980). Acute nicotinamide deficiency in pig induced by 6-aminonicotinamide. Vet. Pathology **7**, 748-758.

Pyridoxine (Vitamin B6)

Deficiency of this vitamin rarely occurs naturally. There is some suggestion that high fat diets may require supplementation and that supplementation may improve litter size in sows on maize and soya bean oilmeal. I.0 g/tonne additional pyridoxine is sufficient although 1.8 g/tonne has recently been suggested.

Reference

Easter, R.A., Anderson, P.A., Michel, E.J. and Corley, J.R. (1983). Response of gestating gilts and starter, grower and finisher swine to biotin, pyridoxine, folacin and thiamine additions to corn-soya bean meal diets. Nutrition Reports International. **28**, 945-954.

Pantothenic acid deficiency

Definition

Deficiency of pantothenic acid occurs in pigs fed bakery wastes and results in nervous signs including the characteristic goose-stepping.

Aetiology and pathogenesis

Pantothenic acid is a coenzyme in the metabolism and synthesis of fats, carbohydrates and proteins. It is present at low levels in flour products such as bakery waste and levels are particularly low in cooked swill made from such waste. Levels may be barely adequate in some other types of ration especially where high oil levels and added copper are present. Its absence leads to demyelination of nerves.

Clinical signs

In weaned pigs a faulty action of the hind legs results in a mincing gait and progresses to posterior paralysis and collapse. Another type of disturbance begins as a snatching movement of the hind limb and progresses to a "goose-stepping" action in which the hind limb is snatched up to the belly and returns with the hock near the ground to cause a waddling or duck-like progression. There may be alopecia and a diarrhoea which is rarely watery. At least one of an affected group may be seen goose-stepping. In sows and young litters, diarrhoea may occur in the sow and loss of hair occurs in the piglets.

Animals which are paralysed and recumbent do not recover readily and should be killed humanely.

Pathology

Oedema of the intestine, especially of the colon and degeneration of the peripheral nerves, posterior root ganglia and demyelination of the spinal cord are seen. The peroneal nerve is commonly affected.

Diagnosis

The goose-stepping is characteristic and further confirmation comes from the dietary history. Pathological findings are useful in confirmation and plasma pantothenate and dietary pantothenate levels can be determined by microbial assays. Dietary levels in deficiency are usually 4-10 mg/kg.

Treatment

Injection of individuals with multivitamins may be of value and the diet should be supplemented with 10-12 g/tonne of calcium pantothenate. In byproduct/swill fed units a specially formulated mineral and vitamin mixture (low in salt as byproducts may contain high levels) should be added after boiling and cooling. 10-12g calcium pantothenate per tonne will prevent the condition.

Biotin deficiency

Definition

A syndrome in which skin changes, hair loss and, in particular, hoof defects occurs in breeding herds. Reproductive performance is reduced.

Aetiology and Pathogenesis

Dietary biotin is normally present in adequate amounts in pig rations, although in feeds containing wheat or barley, the vitamin may be less readily available to pigs than in maize-based diets. Biotin is a cofactor in a number of enzymes especially carboxylation or transcarboxylation reactions. In growing pigs lipogenesis is affected through Acetyl CoA carboxylase. Deficiency in biotin on wheat and barley-based rations occurs quite commonly and at least 180 mg/tonne should be present for health.

Clinical signs

In field cases in the UK, the foot and skin lesions have been identified in sows. The foot lesions appear on the underside of the hoof and are only seen when the claw is cleaned. Others appear as longitudinal cracks on the wall originating in the coronary band. Heel and sole erosions and cracks also occur. High cull rates because of lameness, low numbers born, especially born alive and reared and long weaning to service intervals may also be seen. There may be alopecia and a dry scaly skin which may progress to give dermatitis with brownish crusts and petechial haemorrhages.

In the experimental syndrome, progressive hair loss occurs, the skin becomes dry and scaly and a white film and transverse grooves occur on the tongue. After 5-7 weeks on a deficient diet, claw defects occur. Erosion of the heel occurs first and is followed by cracking of the sole. Cracks appear in the now rubbery horn of the sole and the claw wall and result in lameness. Secondary infection may occur. Growth may be reduced in piglets receiving biotin-deficient diets although this is not described in maize diets and skin and hoof defects have been recorded. Reproductive effects measured over 4 parities indicate that l-1.4 pigs per sow per year are lost, that weaning to service intervals may be increased by up to 4 days and that conception to first service may be reduced by 9%.

Pathology

In addition to the gross changes described above, the skin and claw lesions appear as areas of necrosis in the stratum corneum of the epithelium of the skin, oral and oesophageal mucosa and in the claws.

Diagnosis

The foot lesions resemble those of swine vesicular disease and this condition must be discounted before a diagnosis of biotin deficiency can be reached. Diagnosis can be confirmed by analysing the biotin content of the ration (100-220 µg/kg is the normal range), and noting the response to biotin supplementation of the diet. The reproductive effects can be confirmed only by supplementation of the diet in controlled studies. Populations with plasma levels of 60 ng/100 ml benefit from supplementation. An ELISA has recently been developed for plasma biotin.

Treatment

Supplement the diet with 400 mg-1250 mg/tonne of d biotin in all sow rations. Biotin is available as Rovimix H (1% d biotin, Roche) 40g premix/tonne is necessary for most purposes, for growing gilts, and pregnant and lactating sows to prevent foot lesions and improve litter size. Levels up to 3,000 mg/tonne may be necessary to reverse hoof lesions.

References.

Brooks, P.H. (1982). Biotin in pig nutrition. Pig News and Information **3**, 29 -32.

Brooks, P.H., Smith, D.A., Irwin, V.C.R. (1977). Biotin supplementation of diets, the incidence of foot lesions and the reproductive performance of sows. Vet. Rec. **101**, 46-50.

Bryant, K.L., Kornegay, E.T., Knight, J.W., Webb, K.E., Notter, D.R. (1985). Supplemental biotin for swine: 1. Influence on feed lot performance, plasma biotin and toe lesions in young gilts. J.Anim.Sci. **60**, 136-144.

Bryant, K.L., Kornegay, E.T., Knight, J.W., Webb, K.E., Notter, D.R. (1985). Supplemental biotin for swine: 2. Influences of supplementation to corn and wheat-based diets on reproductive performance and various biochemical criteria of sows during four parities. J.Anim.Sci. **60**, 145-153.

Bryant, K.L., Kornegay, E.T., Knight, J.W., Veit, H.P., Notter, D.R. (1985). Supplemental biotin for swine. 3. Influence of supplementation to corn and wheat-based diets on the incidence and severity of toe lesions, hair and skin characteristics and structural soundness of sows housed in confinement during four parities. J.Anim.Sci. **60**, 154-162.

Penny, R.H.C., Cameron, R.D.A., Johnson, S., Kenyon, P.J., Smith, H.A., Bell, A.W.P., Cole, J.P.L., Taylor, J. (1981). Influence of biotin supplementation on sow reproductive efficiency. Vet. Rec. **109**, 00-01.

Penny, R.H.C. and others as above (1980). Foot rot of pigs ; the influence of biotin supplementation on foot lesions in sows. Vet. Rec. **107**, 350-351.

Simmins, P.H. and Brooks, P.H. (1983). Supplementary biotin for sows : effect on reproductive characteristics. Vet.Rec. **112**, 425-429.

Simmins, P.H., Brooks, P.H. (1988). Supplementary biotin for sows, effects on claw integrity. Vet.Rec. **122**, 431-435.

Webb, N.G., Penny, R.H.C. and Johnston, A.M. (1984). Effect of a dietary supplement of biotin on pig hoof horn strength and hardness. Vet.Rec. **114**, 185-189.

Folic Acid (Folacin)

Folacin compounds with folic acid activity are normally present in adequate quantities in the diet and are supplemented by bacterial synthesis in the gut. Folacin is involved in the synthesis of methyl groups, serine, purine and thymine and in some amino acid transformations. Deficiency in growing pigs can lead to slow weight gain, fading hair colour, anaemia, leucopaenia, thrombopaenia and reduced haematocrit and is chiefly associated with the long-term feeding of sulphonamides. Supplementation of sow rations suggests that the addition of folic acid (2-5mg/Kg) to diets can reduce embryonic mortality and improve numbers born alive and increase their post-natal survival. This effect appears to occur if feeding takes place from 7 days prior to fertilisation and for 17 days afterwards. 15mg/Kg is required to prevent the reduction in serum folate which occurs during pregnancy.

Cyanocobalamine (Vitamin B12)

Supplementation with this vitamin improves the rate of growth of pigs on diets composed largely of vegetable proteins but no specific deficiency syndromes have been identified. It is included in some piglet iron preparations, and such B12-supplemented products may improve growth rates of piglets. A suggestion that it may improve sow reproductive performance has been made.

Ascorbic acid (Vitamin C)

There is some evidence that Vitamin C supplementation of the diet may improve weight gain in young piglets and improve iron utilisation. Early-weaned pigs may benefit from feed supplementation at 75mg/Kg It has also been shown to improve navel bleeding in piglets in some cases when fed to sows and may improve the numbers born alive and numbers weaned when given at I g./kg feed from day

105 of gestation. Vitamin C deficiency may arise as a recessive hereditary condition when foetuses may develop multiple haemorrhages and numbers born be decreased.

References

Kristensen, B., Thomsen, P.D., Palludan, B., Wegger, I. (1986). Mitogen stimulation of lymphocytes in pigs with hereditary Vitamin C deficiency. Acta Vet.Scand. **27**, 486-496.
Wegger, I., Palludan, B. (1994). Vitamin C deficiency causes haematological and skeletal abnormalities during foetal development in swine. J. Nutr. **124**, 241-248.

Non-nutritive feed additives

These may be present in prepared diets and consist of:

(a)   Therapeutic antimicrobials or other medicines.
(b)   Growth promoters or "growth permitters" (not EU).
(c)   Probiotics.
(d)   Substrates for microorganisms (Prebiotics).
(e)   Enzymes.
(f)   Acidifying agents.
(g)   Flavourings.
(h)   Preservatives.
(i)   Oral vaccines
(j)   Inert carriers to improve the handling and dispersal of ingredients.

Labels of bags or specifications of bulk diets include additives (a) to (i) in EC countries. Inert carriers are detailed in the Summary of Product Characteristics (SPC) for medicinal additives.

(a) <u>Veterinary medicines</u> are only included upon prescription (a Medicated Feedingstuffs Prescription (MFS), UK) and can only be incorporated by someone registered under the Medicated Feedstuffs Regulations (UK). The medicines which may be incorporated have been mentioned in the text. A recent and unusual additive is zinc oxide which is included as an antidiarrhoeal agent for recently weaned pigs at levels of up to 3,100 g/tonne (2,400g zinc, PigZin, DSM Products).

(b) <u>Growth promoters</u> are antimicrobials or minerals such as copper included to improve daily liveweight gain and feed conversion efficiency by 5-10% or more. Their effect in S.P.F. pigs and in herds with a high health status is minimal. It appears, therefore, that they suppress subclinical bacterial disease. Antimicrobial and hormonal growth promoters are no longer used in the EU. In the UK, some hormonal effect is achieved by the use of uncastrated boars. Copper is still permitted to 170 ppm to 12 weeks of age and 25 ppm, the nutritional level from 12 weeks.
Growth promoters included inorganic compounds such as copper, and organic compounds such as antibiotics and synthetic antimicrobials. Some disadvantages of antimicrobial growth permitters have been:

1.   The development of resistance to the same antimicrobial or others of its class used for therapy in animals, e.g. tylosin.

2.   Interference with other antimicrobials, e.g. the interaction between salinomycin and tiamulin.

3. The reduction in natural B vitamin synthesis in the gut.

4. Overgrowth of elements of the 'normal' gut flora which occurred following withdrawal of a growth promoter to cause subclinical or clinical disease following recolonisation of a non-immune gut. This type of disease is poorly documented.

5. Resistance to antimicrobials such as avoparcin was selected in gut bacteria such as enterococci and caused concern that it contributed to the pool of vancomycin resistance in immunosuppressed humans and compromised therapy. These concerns led to the withdrawal of antimicrobial growth promoters in the EU.

6. Residues of medicines or additives might persist in carcase meat and in this case an age range is normally specified for their use and withdrawal times are given. Withdrawal times should be strictly observed and the widespread introduction of tests for residues in meat now ensures that this is done. Many growth promoters were not absorbed. Some, such as copper have been limited on environmental grounds.

(c) Probiotics are dried but still viable cultures of microorganisms such as lactobacilli, streptococci and yeasts which are said to colonise the intestine and prevent colonisation by disease causing agents. The main points in the pig's life where they are of theoretical value are in the neonate, after weaning and after antimicrobial treatment. Their value has not been demonstrated unequivocally by controlled scientific studies of the type which proved the efficacy of antimicrobial growth promoters, but they have been of value on individual farms. Probiotics may be killed by antimicrobial use.

(d) Substrates for microorganisms (prebiotics) such as fibre have been included in some rations for reasons mentioned above and with similar results.

(e) Enzymes such as proteases, phytases, xylanases and amylases are routinely included to liberate nutrients such as phosphorus and to aid digestion.

(f) Acidifying agents such as fumaric and citric acids or proprietary mixtures of organic acids lower gastric pH and inhibit microorganisms such as E.coli and salmonella in feed. There is experimental evidence to support an effect on performance.

(g) Flavourings may give a feed an unexpected smell or colour but the feed may be perfectly wholesome.

(h) Preservatives such as salt or formalin may be present in whey or skim and antioxidants such as ethoxyquin are used to preserve wet stored barley and are often present in many feeds. Propionic acid may be associated with low levels of Vitamin E and rapid destruction of fat soluble vitamins. Some labile constituents such as antimicrobials may be enteric coated.

(i) Bacterial antigens. Have been included in oral vaccines but are currently rarely used (EU)

(j) Inert carriers such as bentonite may be included to enable the successful mixing and dispersal of ingredients.

Processing

Heating destroys B Vitamins such as thiamine, drugs such as penicillin G and bacteria such as salmonellae. Heat is generated during pelleting and this should be taken into account when considering heat labile feed ingredients. The boiling of swill also affected heat-labile vitamins but this heat treatment may also increase the digestibility of some waste foods.

Storage

Feed should not be used after the expiry date printed on the label and should be protected from heat and moisture. Mould growth may occur in bins (see mycotoxins) and rodent and bird contamination may give rise to infections. Fodder mites may infest feed and make it unpalatable and they and their eggs may appear in faeces. Storage of premixes beyond their expiry date commonly leads to problems.

Food Chain Security

The Food and Feed Directives (EU) lay down regulations intended to ensure that animal feeds are clean and wholesome and provide regulations and Codes of Practice to ensure that feed is not re-contaminated after processing. This is particularly the case where salmonella control is involved but involves the entire food chain. The introduction of Food Chain Information at slaughter in the EU will involve considerable detail of the feeding of pigs being made available to the Official Veterinarian.

CONGENITAL AND HEREDITARY CONDITIONS

Introduction

A number of abnormalities may be seen in the newborn piglet or may appear shortly after birth. Such congenital conditions may be produced by one of the factors outlined below. Others are of genetic origin but do not become apparent until much later.

1. Spontaneous developmental abnormality
2. Heritable abnormalities
3. Infectious agents
4. Nutritional deficiency or poisoning
5. Unknown cause.

In investigating a problem involving congenital conditions, it is important to recognise those under genetic control, and those caused by infection, nutritional deficiency or poisoning as the methods of control used in each case are so different. Those which are expressed later like lymphosarcoma and the porcine stress syndrome must be differentiated from other conditions in older pigs.

1. Spontaneous developmental abnormality

This may occur sporadically in any pig herd but may be more common where late matings have occurred (old egg or sperm), or where old breeding stock are used. Hermaphroditism, some hernias, cardiovascular abnormalities, cleft palates, monsters, Siamese twins etc. may be spontaneous and not controlled by heritable genetic abnormalities, but in general, developmental abnormalities are relatively uncommon. Should they become so within a herd, a genetic, infectious or nutritional origin should be considered.

Cystic lymph nodes

Cysts in ileal mesenteric lymph nodes, caecocolic lymph nodes and colonic lymph nodes up to 2 cm in diameter may be found in otherwise normal pigs.

2. Heritable conditions

A number of congenital conditions in pigs are heritable or are predisposed to by genetic factors. These include a number of breed characteristics. Some of these conditions are described below. Where genetic factors are influenced in their expression by nutrition or other environmental factors such as infection this will be indicated. The molecular basis of the genes and pathways governing many of these characters is currently being determined

Hernias "Ruptures"

These are one of the commonest congenital defects of pigs (up to 1.5%, currently 0.3% UK) and may be inguinal, umbilical or diaphragmatic. Their production is familial, and in some cases of inguinal hernia, governed by a double recessive gene or is polygenic. The heritability of inguinal hernia has been shown to be 0.29-0.35 depending on breed. Inguinal hernias are usually unilateral and are only expressed in the male. Hernias cause problems in a number of ways:

a) by enlarging to such an extent that they touch the ground and ulcerate
b) by being damaged during fighting
c) at castration where surgical repair of both sides is required
d) by strangulation when intestines or omentum become trapped following peritonitis, Glasser's Disease, fighting and enteritis. Once intestines become trapped, animals show signs of abdominal pain and distension and the hernia becomes tense. The intestines present cannot be manipulated back into the peritoneal cavity and the skin over it becomes discoloured and necrotic.

When hernias reach the ground, ulcerate severely or become strangulated, the animal should be destroyed humanely unless surgical relief is to be carried out.

Treatment

Surgical reduction of inguinal hernias is required at castration but where castration is less common for economic and welfare reasons, surgical correction is unnecessary. The procedure must be of economic benefit to be carried out. The operation requires anaesthetic and involves the blunt dissection of the testis enclosed in its peritoneum, massaging the enclosed intestine back into the abdominal cavity and then securing the pouch at the inguinal ring using retaining stitches and finally removing the testicle. Both sides should be treated in the same way as the increased intra abdominal pressure may cause herniation on the intact side.

Control

Suggest the culling of sows giving rise to affected litters or boars whose progeny have a high incidence of the condition if the incidence is sufficiently high to make this an economic proposition. The frequency of inguinal hernias has been assessed by sire:son analysis in some boar studs. Animals with large hernias may require self-certification as casualties and be penned separately on transport for slaughter.

Hermaphrodites

True hermaphrodites have both testicular and ovarian tissue sometimes as an ovotestis. Hereditary, less common than male pseudohermaphroditism in which male gonads and karyotype (38 XY) are present but the reproductive tract has a number of female features such as fallopian tubes and uterus or reduced penis size. The external genitalia are generally female in form. Overall incidences of 0.09% have been recorded UK. Pregnancy has been recorded in hermaphrodites, also mosaicism. Animals may have the 38 XX karyotype, inherited as an autosomal recessive and expressed as true hermaphrodites to XX males with or without genital ambiguities, 38 XX XY mosaicism inherited as an autosomal recessive and testicular feminisation (38XY). 17-β-nortestosterone may be found in urine, fat and kidney in some of these animals, and may affect hormonal determination at meat inspection.

References

Pond, W.G. (1961). Cornell Vet. 51, 394.
Hunter, R.H.F. (1988). Intersexuality in domestic pigs. Proc.Pig Vet.Soc. 21, 135-139.
Hunter, R.H.F., Greve, T. (1996). Intersexuality in pigs-clinical, physiological and practical considerations. Acta vet. Scand. 37, 1-12.

329

Pailhoux, E., Parma, P., Sundstrom, J., Vigier, B., Servel, N., Kupio, T., Locatelli, A. Pelliniemi, L., Cotinot, C. (2001). Time course of female –to-male sex reversal in 38,XX fetal and postnatal pigs. Developmental Dynamics **222**, 328-340.
Pailhoux, E., Pelliniemi, L., Barbosa, A., Parma, P., Kuopio, T., Cotinot, C. (1997). Relevance of intersexuality to breeding and reproductive biotechnology programmes:XX sex reversal in pigs. Theriogenology **47**, 93-102.

Cystic kidneys

Inherited cysts of tubular origin in both Landrace and Large White pigs occur congenitally. Their production is governed by an autosomal dominant mode of inheritance but the actual numbers produced may be under polygenic control. Recruitment to the cyst population appears to occur throughout life. There appear to be no clinical consequences during normal adult life but kidney condemnations may reach 47.5% at slaughter in some populations

Piglets in affected herds may remain stunted after weaning and become pot-bellied. They should be killed humanely. At post-mortem examination polycystic kidneys with or without hydronephrosis may be found.

References

Wells, G.A.H., Hebert, C.N., Robins, B.C. (1980). Renal cysts in pigs : prevalence and pathology in slaughtered pigs from a single herd. Vet. Rec. **106**, 532-535.
Wijeratne, W.V.S. and Wells, G.A.H. (1980). Inherited renal cysts in pigs : results of breeding experiments. Vet. Rec. **107**, 484-488.

Hypoplastic kidney and renal agenesis

A condition in which small kidneys or no kidneys are found in piglets of up to 8 weeks of age. Governed by an autosomal recessive gene and often results in death. Ureters may be capped with undifferentiated mesenchyme.

Reference

Mason, R.W., Cooper, R. (1985). Congenital bilateral renal hypoplasia in Large White pigs. Aust.Vet.J. **62**, 413-414.

Polycystic disease

A familial polycystic disease with cysts in kidneys, bile ducts, epididymus, uterus and pancreas. Affected piglets die within 1-3 days.

Inverted nipples

More than one nipple may be affected in this simple recessive system. The mechanism of inversion appears to be due to proliferation of fibrous tissue at the base of the teat resulting from a lack of oestrogen receptors and is most common anterior to the umbilicus. It has been suggested that boars producing 4% or more affected female progeny in 40 litters should not be used for breeding and that there is a heritability of around 20%. Environmental damage may also cause inverted nipples.

Reference

Done, J. T. (1980). Teat deficiencies in pigs. Vet. Annual. **20**, 246-254.

Cryptorchidism

A sex-linked autosomal recessive character governed by 2 loci with a heredity of 0.057 (up to 0.22 in some breeds). The testicles may be at the inguinal ring or further into the peritoneal cavity. Not important unless boars are intended for breeding, in which case they should be rejected as there are associated sperm defects. May be associated with boar taint in countries where castration is routine, but both aromatase and oestrogen secretion by cryphorchid testes is lower than from scrotal testes. If slaughter is delayed boar taint may be a problem. An overall incidence of 0.24% has been recorded UK, but 2.26% in Germany and up to 8% by experimental breeding. The left testis is three times more likely to be affected than the right. The abdominal testes should be removed by laparotomy during castration in pigs intended as companion animals.

References

Rothschild, M.F., Christian, L.L., Blanchard, W. (1988). Evidence for multigene control of cryphorchidism in swine. J.Hered. **79**, 313-314.
Pinart, E., Camps, R., Briz, M.D., Bonet, S., Egozcue, B.J. (1998). Unilateral spontaneous cryptorchidism: structural and ultrstructural study of sperm morphology. Animal Repro. Sci. **49**, 247-268.

Atresia ani

A common condition in which the rectum fails to open to the exterior. A thin membrane or a considerable band of fibrous tissue may be present. Male pigs usually have swollen abdomens and die within 3 weeks of birth, but in females the rectum may open into the vagina and the animal survives in 50% of cases. The condition is definitely familial may be governed by a recessive gene, probably with incomplete (50%) penetrance and may not occur in more than 50% of an affected litter. It may also arise as a result of environmental or developmental abnormality. It may be present in 0.3% pigs in the UK. A heritability of 0.009% has been suggested.

Treatment

Mild cases may be treated surgically, badly affected piglets should be killed humanely.

Control

If a genetic mechanism is clearly involved in the outbreak in question do not breed from affected gilts or from the sibs of affected animals. Cull breeding stock if cost effective and do not use the same boar on the same sow.

Congenital meningoencephalocoele (Cranioschisis)

Recorded in Landrace and Large Whites and inherited. Affected pigs have exposed meninges protruding through incomplete fusion of parietal or frontal bones and the mortality rate is high. An autosomal recessive condition. If it becomes a problem, a cost benefit analysis will decide whether culling is worthwhile.

Reference

Wijeratne, W.V.S., Beaton, D., Cuthbertson, J.C. (1974). A field occurrence of congenital meningoencephalocoele in pigs. Vet. Rec. **95**, 81-84.

Hereditary dwarfism

A simple autosomal recessive causing dwarfism and chondrodysplasia has been reported from Denmark. Another type affecting the limbs only has been described from Czechoslovakia. Dwarfism is involved in the foundation of some breeds of minipigs widely used for research which have adult weights of less than 60kg. Clinically affected pigs require humane slaughter.

Reference

Jensen, P.T., Nielsen, D.H., Jensen, P. and Bille, N. (1984). Hereditary dwarfism in pigs Nord.Vet.Med. **36**, 32-37.
Kaman, J., Drabek, J., Zert, Z. (1991). Congenital dysproportional chondrodysplasia. Acta.vet.Brno. **60**, 237-251.

Inherited Thick Forelegs (Hyperostosis)

The forelegs are markedly enlarged below the elbows and the skin is tense and may be discoloured. Mortality due to crushing and starvation commonly occurs within 2-6 days, but affected animals have been reared to adulthood. A simple autosomal recessive character governs the condition which occurs in 1-3 piglets per affected litter and appears to operate by causing a periosteal detachment distal to the elbow with subsequent periosteal bone formation. It has been associated with localised hypertension.

References

Doize, B. and Martineau, G.P. (1984). Congenital hyperostosis in piglets : a consequence of a disorganisation of the perichondrial ossification groove of Ranvier. Canadian J.Comp.Med. **48**, 414-419.
Kay, M.M. (1962). Canad.J.Comp.Med. **26**, 218.
Roels, S., Simoens, P., Ducatelle, R. (1996). Localised arteriosclerotic changes in congenital hyperostosis in pigs. Vet. Rec. **139**, 446-447.

Crooked Tails or Kinky Tail

Absence or malformation of the tail occurs commonly in the Landrace and Large White breeds, is familial, and is thought to be inherited. May be dominant but with low penetrance. Incidence UK is 1.7%.

Legless Pigs

An autosomal recessive lethal factor leading to absence of leg bones.

Reference

Johnson, L.E. (1940). 'Streamlined pigs'. A new legless mutation. J. Hered. **31**, 239-242.

Cleft Palate

Affected piglets die of starvation after a few days as they cannot create sufficient vacuum in their mouths to suck milk. Affected piglets should be killed humanely. Governed by an autosomal recessive gene in most cases but can also result from chromosomal trisomy and poisoning by hemlock (*Conium maculatum*).

References

Koch-Weimar, P. and Neumuller-Jena, O. (1932). Dt. Tierarzte.Wschr. **40**, 353.
Painter, K.E., Keeler, R.F., Buck, W.B. (1985). Congenital skeletal malformations induced by maternal ingestion of *Conium maculatum* (poison hemlock) in newborn pigs. Am.J.Vet.Res. **46**, 1368-1371.

Syndactyly (mule-foot)

Dominant to normal cloven foot (autosomal dominant).

Reference

Detlefsen, J.A., Carmichael, W.J. (1921). Inheritance of syndactylism, black and dilution in swine. J.Agric.Res. **20**, 595-604.

Polydactyly (Supernumerary digits)

Inherited and appears to be an autosomal dominant which is lethal in the homozygote and expresses polydactyly in the heterozygote.

Reference

Malynicz, G.L. (1982). Complete polydactylism in Papua New Guinea village pigs with otocephalic homozygous monsters. Annals de Genetique et de selection Animale **14**, 415-420.

Arthrogryposis

Joints, usually of the limbs are fused. Affected piglets die after birth but may also delay farrowing. Arthrogryposis may result from a single autosomal recessive gene. A gene for arthrogriposis multiplex congenita (*amc*) has been mapped to chromosome 5 in Swiss Large White pigs. Arthrogriposis can also result from neural or muscular defects, has occurred in Menangle virus infection and has been attributed to poisoning with thorn apple (*Datura stramonium*), hemlock (*Conium maculatum*) or *Nicotiana* (tobacco). Affected pigs should be destroyed humanely.

References

Genini, S., Malek, M., Spilar, S., Trung thanh Nguyen Menetrey, F., Gebert, S., Hagger, C. Neuenschwander, S., Kadarmideen, H.N., Stanzinger, G., Vogeli, P. (2004). Arthrogriposis multiplex congenita (AMC), a hereditary disease in swine, maps to Chromosome 5 by linkage analysis. Mammalian Genome **15**, 935-941.
Lomo, O.D. (1985). Arthrogryposis and associated defects in pigs: indication of simple recessive inheritance. Acta Vet.Scand. **26** 419-422.

Hereditary Rickets

Identified in German Landrace as an autosomal recessive vitamin D dependent rickets type 1. Also in other breeds. Homozygotes grew slowly and developed hypocalcaemia with severe secondary hyperparathroidism and hypophosphataemia by 8 weeks of age. Cholecalciferol injections reverse the syndrome and it appears to be due to low 1, 25 dehydroxy Vitamin D3 levels in plasma caused by an inherited deficiency of the 1-hydrolase enzyme. The molecular mechanism has been described.

References

Chavez, L.S., Serda, R., Choe, S., Davidi, L., Harmeyer, J., Modal, J.L. (2003). Molecular basis for pseudos vitamin D-deficiency rickets in the Hannover pig. J.Nut. Biochem. **14**, 378-385.
Fox, J., Maunder, F M W , Randall, V.A., Care, A.D. (1985). Vitamin D dependent rickets type 1 in pigs. Clinical Science **69**, 541-548.

Skin conditions

Dermatosis vegetans

A relatively rare hereditary disease of young pigs characterised by lesions of the skin and hoof and a giant cell pneumonitis which is usually fatal. It is governed by a semi-lethal factor with recessive autosomal inheritance and has been seen in Landrace pigs in Britain which are descendants of an original carrier Swedish Landrace import.

Skin lesions. These may be present at birth or develop at 2-3 weeks of age from raised pink swellings on the abdomen or inside the thighs, spreading and passing through a pityriasis rosea-like stage, and, after 5-8 weeks become thickened and covered with greyish-brown or black crusts.

Foot lesions. "Clubfoot" are less common but are always present at birth with swelling and erythema in the coronary area of the hoof and the production of defective horn on the walls, sole and bulb of the foot.

Giant cell pneumonitis. This is the characteristic finding and essential to the diagnosis in older pigs. In pigs of more than 1 week of age, the giant cells may be demonstrated and nodules of them appear as firm red-brown bodies 13 mm in diameter throughout the lung. These may regress to leave alveolar fibrosis in pigs which survive until 1 year of age.

Course of the disease. A decline in growth appears after 5-6 weeks and most affected pigs are dead within 6 months. Affected pigs should be humanely destroyed.

Control

Breed affected sows with Large White boars.

References

Done, J.T., Loosmore, R.M. and Saunders, C.N. (1967). Dermatosis vegetans in pigs. Vet. Rec. **80**, 292-297.
Evensen, O., Bratberg, B. (1990). A sequential light microscopic study of the pulmonary lesions in porcine dermatosis vegetans. Res.Vet.Sci. **49**, 50-55.

Pityriasis rosea

A common condition of unknown aetiology, possibly governed by an autosomal dominant gene with incomplete penetrance and seen in young pigs. The condition is definitely familial, may be more common in Landrace and has recently been given the name porcine juvenile pustular psoriaform dermatitis.

Clinical signs

The condition may be seen in individual animals or whole litters, but usually only occurs in 2-3 pigs per litter. The lesions appear at 2-4 weeks of age as a few 2-3 cm hyperaemic patches on the flanks, groin or thighs and expand rapidly to form reddish rings with a normal centre. The normal area gradually expands as the condition continues. The condition is self-limiting with a course of about 2 months and resolves completely. Pruritis is not seen even at the height of the disease when the lesions may cover a large amount of the surface area. Weaners may be disfigured at sale time and may not command their true price.

Control

Change the boar if a large number of cases occur in a herd.

Reference

Corcoran, C.J. (1964). Pityriasis rosea in pigs. Vet. Rec. **76**, 1407-1409.

Epitheliogenesis imperfecta   (Congenital ectodermal defect)

This appears as raw patches with raised edges on the skin and may be mistaken for wounds. In Britain it has been recorded in Saddleback and Large White Pigs and is due to a single autosomal recessive character. Healing may occur or infection may result in death. Animals with large lesions should be humanely destroyed.

Reference

Parish, W.E. and Done, J.T., (1962). Seven apparently congenital non-infectious conditions of the skin resembling congenital defects in man. J. Comp. Path. **72**, 286-298.

Hairless Pigs

Hairlessness is dominant to normal coat with incomplete penetrance and so heterozygotes can be picked out. Iodine deficiency may also cause it.

Reference

Roberts, E. and Carroll, W.E. (1931). The inheritance of hairlessness in swine. J. Hered. **22**, 125-132.

Congenital Porphyria

An uncommon condition in which excess porphyrins are produced and discolour the bones and teeth and, in some cases the kidneys and lymph nodes. Porphyruria is difficult to demonstrate and there appear to be few effects upon health although anaemia has been described. Photosensitsation does not occur.

Autosomal dominant genes are involved. Has been identified in Duroc pigs in Japan where it may be recessive and in a Belgian Landrace where the pigment fluoresced red-brown and was due to uroporphyrinogen decarboxylase and uroporphyrogen-III-cosynthetase dysfunction.

References

Jorgensen, S.K. (1959). Congenital porphyria in pigs. Brit.Vet. J. **115**, 160-175.

Roels, S., Hassoun, A., Hoorens, J. (1995). Accumulation of protoporphyrin isomers I and III and multiple decarboxylation products of isoporphyrin in a case of porphyria in a slaughtered pig. J.Vet. Med. Ser A **42**, 145-151.

Muscular Conditions

Congenital splay leg (Myofibrillar hypoplasia)

This important (up to 1.5 per cent) condition occurs as an additive polygenic trait with no clear evidence of dominance, especially in Pietrain, Landrace and Welsh pigs. It appears to occur twice as frequently in males and a maternal effect has been identified, apparently mediated through larger litters which have more affected piglets and a shorter (0.9 day) gestation period. There are too few Type I myofibrils in the fibres of muscles of the foreleg, lumbar group and, most important, the hindleg. The condition appears to represent a failure of muscle fibres to mature in sufficient numbers to provide adequate support at birth. The semitendinosus muscle is most severely affected in the hindlimb.

Affected piglets are unable to stand, and are often found with a hindlimb extended anteriorly along the axis of the body with the opposite member abducted. If not killed by crushing and if able to feed, affected piglets become normal within 10 days of birth. Affected piglets may develop sores on the perineum and erosion of the base of the tail. Up to 50% of affected piglets may die if not assisted. They are particularly prone to chilling.

The condition becomes apparent 2-3 hours after birth and 2-3 piglets may be affected in each litter. Affected piglets may be kept warm and reared artificially for 2-3 days and returned to the sow. Non-slip floors and the use of elastic bands on the hindlimbs may improve viability. Crossing Landrace or Welsh sows with Large White boars reduces the incidence. The use of physostigmine has been suggested as an aid to recovery in piglets 12 hours or more of age. Repeated massage of the hindlimbs improves survival dramatically.

Humane killing may be appropriate where severely affected animals, or those with extensive ulceration, lose condition and cannot be nursed.

The incidence of splayleg may increase when PRRS outbreaks occur, in zearalenone poisoning and following the induction of farrowing before day 113.

References

Blackburn, P.W. (1988). Splayleg piglets : treatment. Proc.Pig.Vet.Soc. **21**, 185-186.

Bradley, R., Ward, P.S., Bailey, J. (1980). The ultrastructural morphology of the skeletal muscles of normal pigs and pigs with splayleg from birth to one week of age. J.Comp.Path. **90**, 433-466.

Thurley, D.C., Gilbert, F.R. and Done, J.T. (1967). Congenital splayleg of piglets : myofibrillar hypoplasia. Vet. Rec. **80**, 302-304.

Ward, P.S. (1978). The splayleg syndrome in new-born pigs : a review I. Vet. Bull. **48**, 279-295.

Ward, P.S. (1978). The splayleg syndrome in new-born pigs : a review II. Vet.Bull. **48**, 381-399.

Pietrain creeper syndrome

A progressive, familial myopathy of Pietrain pigs has been described in one herd in Britain, features of it have been detected in another and also in Landrace pigs. The onset of the disease occurs in pigs of either sex at 2-3 weeks of age in up to 30% of an affected litter. Tremor of the hindquarters appears and within a few days occurs in the forequarters. The limbs become partly flexed and a "tip-toe" gait is adopted. Reluctance to stand becomes progressively more common and affected piglets walk on permanently flexed carpal joints and on the digits of the flexed hindlimbs. Creeping continues until around 65 days after the onset when permanent recumbency develops and the pigs must be destroyed. They remain alert and feed and grow normally.

Muscle cells in the proximal limb muscles vary greatly in size, may have internal nuclei and many are degenerating. The condition appears to be inherited as an autosomal recessive.

References

Wells, G.A.H., Pinsent, P.J.N. and Todd, J.N. (1980). A progressive familial myopathy of the Pietrain pig : the clinical syndrome. Vet Rec. **106**, 556-558.
Bradley, R., and Wells, G.A.H. The Pietrain 'creeper' pig: a primary myopathy. In Animal models of neurological disease, eds. Rose, F.C. and Behan, P.O. Pitman Medical (1980) 34.

The Porcine Stress Syndrome (P.S.S.)
Pale Soft Exudative (P.S.E.) Muscle and Malignant Hyperthermia

Definition

A complex of conditions associated with an autosomal recessive gene of variable penetrance. Animals of well muscled strains may die suddenly during transport (P.S.S.), give rise to pale, watery pork at slaughter (P.S.E.) and develop malignant hyperthermia when exposed to halothane anaesthesia. Back muscle necrosis may also develop.

Incidence

The incidence of this condition may be based on the number of clinical cases, usually deaths in transport, the number of animals which have tested positive for the homozygous or heterozygous forms by phenotypic assessment (principally the halothane test) and most recently and accurately, figures produced since 1991 for the distribution of homozygous and heterozygous carriers of the gene in the pig populations in a breed or an area. Examples of the incidence of clinical disease include figures from the Netherlands, where deaths in pigs transported to slaughter reached 0.7% in 1980 and P.S.E. occurred in up to 30% of carcases. In Britain, deaths during transport were fewer, 0.08% in 1974. Phenotype testing suggests that the condition occurred in the Dutch, West German (68%) and Belgian (86%), Landrace, the prevalence of the condition was about 11% (1980).

Figures obtained for the presence of the gene give a definitive picture of prevalence. Tests in the US, Canada and UK (1993) showed that 97% Pietrain, 35% Landrace, 15% Duroc, 19% Large White, 14% Hampshire, 19% Yorkshire and 16% Crossbred pigs carried the gene with gene frequencies of from 0.72 (Pietrain) to 0.07 (Hampshire). 1% of pigs were homozygous and 20% pigs tested were carriers. In a French study the French Landrace animals tested were completely free from the gene. Positive steps to eliminate the condition have lowered the incidence.

Aetiology

The cause of the condition is the substitution of cytosine (C) for thymidine (T) at position 1843 on the ryr 1 gene on chromosome 6 P11 921. The gene codes for ryanodine, responsible for gating (controlling) the calcium (Ca^{++}) channel in the sarcoplasmic reticulum of skeletal muscle. The point mutation of C for T results in the replacement of the aminoacid arginine at position 615 in the ryanodine peptide with cysteine, thus altering its function. The altered protein facilitates the opening of the calcium channel and inhibits its closure. The flow of calcium ions stimulates contracture of the muscle and sets in train all the other consequences described below. The altered channel can be stimulated by lower concentrations of Ca^{++}, ATP and caffeine in muscle of genotype MHnn (Malignant Hypothermia homozygote) than in normal animals (MHNN). Inhibition of gating by Ca^{++} and Mg^{++} is also damped down, so responses continue longer. Anaesthetics such as halothane and stress raise Ca^{++} and ATP levels so that further Ca^{++} release occurs and the muscle becomes unresponsive to inhibition. The heterozygote MHNn is intermediate between the two homozygotes in terms of Ca^{++} flows.

The mutation appears to have arisen once and to have spread to all affected breeds. The ryr 1 gene was previously designated for halothane sensitivity n for sensitive i.e., affected pigs were Hal nn, normals Hal NN and is transmitted as an autosomal recessive with high or complete penetrance.

The homozygote Hal NN and the heterozygote Hal Nn are both resistant to the effects of simple halothane anaesthesia. The Hal (MH) gene is linked to a series of other characters, some of which have been used to identify stress susceptibility. They are as follows in apparent order of linkage. S (the suppressor gene of the AO blood group), Phi (phospho-hexoisomerase), Hal MH (the halothane susceptibility gene), H (a blood group) Po2 (serum post albumin protein 2) and Pgd (6 phosphogluconate dehydrogenase. The linkage can be expressed S(AO)-Phi-Hal-Po2-Pgd. Possession of the gene is associated with heavily muscled or lean breeds and the selection of pigs for meatiness and carcase conformation has aided spread by selection and by the use of breeds with a high prevalence of the gene such as Pietrains as sires for slaughter pigs.

Pathogenesis

The condition occurs as a result of a switch of energy utilisation in the muscles of susceptible pigs from aerobic to anaerobic metabolism resulting from the increased Ca^{++} flux in the calcium channel of the sarcoplasmic reticulum and the prolonged activity which follows. An enormous increase in lactate production, an increase in body heat production and poor production of A.T.P. result. Body temperature rises partly due to a peripheral vasoconstriction and accumulation of lactate. Muscle damage leads to increases in plasma creatine phosphokinase and, in some cases, potassium ions. Calcium uptake and release from the sarcoplasmic reticulum appears to be critical in the pathogenesis of the condition. Noradrenaline levels are high and it appears to be metabolised less quickly than in normal pigs. High cortisone levels and an increased rate of thyroxine and triiodothyronine utilisation also occur in affected pigs. Triggering of the mechanism can result from stress of movement, some anaesthetic agents and slaughter when anaerobic glycolysis also develops.

The possession of the halothane susceptible gene leads to an increase of carcase lean, a slower growth rate and, in sows, 1.16 fewer births and 1.76 fewer weaned pigs per litter than in resistant litters. Heterozygotes are economically superior to either homozygote.

Clinical signs

Pigs of 9 weeks of age or more and especially heavy hogs or adults, are affected. Early signs of stress include muscle and tail tremor which progress to dyspnoea, blotched red and pale skin, an increase in body temperature to more than 41.5°C. followed by collapse, muscle rigidity and death. Some of these changes may be induced by anaesthesia. The condition is more common when the environmental temperature rises above 22°C. The changes are so rapid that humane slaughter is rarely an option.

Pathology

Few changes are seen, but there is some oedema and collapse of the lung. Rapid development of rigor mortis occurs. Pale, soft exudative muscle develops in 60-70% of stress-susceptible pigs within 15 minutes of death and can be seen as pale areas contrasting with the deeper red unaffected muscle bundles when the longissimus dorsi or ham muscles are cut in section. Muscle pH falls to pH 6.0 or less within 45 minutes of death. There may be some necrosis and change in cardiac muscle. Histological lesions include the presence of degenerating and regenerating muscle fibres, but these may represent previous episodes of the condition.

Diagnosis

The clinical signs of blanching of the skin and rigidity following stimulus are suggestive if seen. The rigid carcase and the presence of pale soft exudative lumbar or ham muscles with a low pH may also suggest the condition. The body conformation, breed, a history of stress or high ambient temperatures are often helpful. Other causes of sudden death in large pigs such as anthrax, twisted bowel, bloody gut, gastric torsion, electrocution, vegetative endocarditis etc. should be ruled out. Susceptible pigs can be identified in life by the polymerase chain reaction for the normal and altered genes in blood or tissue. This test is available commercially and animals which have been screened and found to be negative may bear a tag N 1843. Heterozygotes and homozygotes for the MHn gene are also identified. Extraction methods and PCR techniques developed for meat use may also be used on tissue at post mortem to confirm the presence of genetic susceptibility.

Where this test is not available, the phenotype can be determined by older tests such as the halothane test, using halothane 3 or 5% for 3-5 minutes in young pigs 9 weeks of age. Affected pigs become rigid and sometimes develop raised rectal temperatures. Anaesthesia should be discontinued or death will result. This test reliably detects susceptible homozygotes but a repeat test for 3 minutes coupled with succinylcholine at 0.75 mg/kg may reveal heterozygotes amongst apparently negative animals. Intravenous halothane and the use of halothane anaesthesia on adult pigs induced using barbiturate may also be used. Raised plasma levels of creatinine phosphokinase or pyruvate kinase may also be helpful, also the detection of Phi B,, Pgd B, the absence of the AO blood groups and the presence of the Ha/Ha blood groups may also be helpful. The use of caffeine solutions on the contractibility of isolated biopsied muscle specimens has also been used. The use of carcase meat conductivity and pH measurements may also be useful at slaughter. 45 minutes after slaughter reactors may have a meat pH of 5.9 or less. New DNA hybridisation tests are being developed and one for Phi has been described.

Treatment

Pigs which develop malignant hyperthermia under anaesthesia may be treated successfully if the condition is recognised early (for instance by a rise in end expiratory pCO_2) by hyperventilating with oxygen, use of metamizol β blockers, bicarbonate and cooling or with Dantrolene at 7mg/kg. Some muscle damage may occur.

Control

Clinically affected animals or those prone to stress should be given adequate ventilation, cooled with water drips or sprayed in hot weather, starved for 12 hours before transport and not transported at environmental temperatures exceeding 22°C (72°F). Tail lifts help reduce transport stress. Any mixing likely to result in fighting should be avoided. Access to sugar solutions in the lairage may prevent P.S.E. Pentobarbitone anaesthesia should be used in stress-susceptible pigs. Stress can be reduced by the use of azaperone or carazalol prior to movement.

As selection programmes for lean carcases and large hams tend to increase the prevalence of stress in susceptible pigs, some countries and companies have adopted a policy of testing for and eliminating stress susceptible animals. Others have used homozygous stress susceptible sire lines on resistant dam lines to combine the economic advantages, carcase quality and prolificacy of the heterozygote. The success of companies and countries in reducing the incidence of the gene in individual lines has now been confirmed using PCR gene testing and a number of breeds and lines are now free from the gene. Both sow and boar lines which combine the meaty phenotype with the MHNN (stress free) genotype are now commercially available and the presence of stress susceptible animals (MHnn) in a herd is now unnecessary.

References

Allen, W.M. Harding, J.D.J. and Patterson, D.S.P. (1970). Experimentally induced acute stress syndrome in Pietrain pigs. Vet. Rec. 87, 64-69.

Fujii, J., Otsu, K., Zorzato, F., DeLeon, S., Khanna, V.K., Weiler J.E., O'Brien, P.J., MacLennan, D.H. (1991). Identification of a mutation in porcine ryanodine receptor associated with malignant hyperthermia. Science 253, 440-451.

Gregory, N.G. and Wilkins, L.J. (1984). The intravenous halothane test as an experimental model for quantifying stress sensitivity in pigs. J.Science of Food and Agriculture 35, 147-153.

Lambert, A.J., Houde, A., Drolet, R., D'Allaire, S. (1996). Determination of halothene gene mutation associated with malignant hyperthermia in sows dead of cardiac failure. J.Vet. Diagn. Invest. 8, 513-515.

Mabry, J.W., Christian, L.L., Kuhlers, D.L. and Rasmussen, B.A. (1983). Prediction of susceptibility to the porcine stress syndrome. J.Heredity 74, 23-26.

MacLennan, D.H., Duff, C., Zorzato, F., Fujii, J., Phillips, M., Korneluk, R.G., Frodis, W., Britt, B., Worton, R.G. (1990). Ryanodine gene is a candidate for predisposition to malignant hyperthermia. Nature 343, 559-560.

O'Brien, P.J., Shen, H., Cory, C.R., Zhang, X. (1993). Use of a DNA-based test for the mutation associated with porcine stress syndrome (malignant hyperthermia) in 10,000 breeding swine. J.Am.Vet.Med.Ass. 203, 842-851.

Associated conditions

a)   Back Muscle Necrosis

Necrosis of the longissimus dorsi is a sporadic condition of sudden onset in pigs of more than 50 kg in bodyweight. Pain and difficulty in movement, pyrexia and unilateral or bilateral swelling of the back occur. A proportion of pigs die in the acute stage from lactic acidosis and cardiac insufficiency. The condition appears in herds in which the porcine stress syndrome occurs.

Lesions include discolouration of the skin over the affected area, generalised congestion and some petechiation. Ruptures, areas of pallor and haemorrhage are present in the back muscles. The pH of affected muscle is

340

lower than that of adjacent unaffected muscle. Local haemorrhage, loss of myofibrillar material and calcified muscle cells and other degenerative changes were seen in histological sections.

Diagnosis is based on the clinical signs, and should be supported by measurements of plasma creatinine phosphokinase levels which are raised. Post-mortem findings are confirmatory but both longitudinal and transverse sections of the affected muscle mass should be carried out.

Reference

Bradley, R., Wells, G.A.H. and Gray, L.J. (1979). Back muscle necrosis of pigs. Vet.Rec. **104**, 183-188.

b) Malignant hyperthermia

This occurs during halothane anaesthesia of stress-susceptible pigs or when the ambient temperature rises above 28°C. Beyond this temperature heat loss cannot occur in the absence of water and body temperatures climb to 41.5°C or beyond and death results. Water cooling and tranquillisers may reduce mortality.

c) Pale soft exudative muscle (P.S.E.)

This results from excessive glycolysis in stress-susceptible pig muscle at slaughter and causes low pH (less than 6) and high temperature (41°C or more) 45 minutes after slaughter. There is excessive drip and taste is impaired.

Asymmetric hindquarter syndrome

A disparity of the size of one hindleg in which fat and muscle cell distribution in the muscles of the posterior thigh are abnormal. Careful examination and dissection are required for diagnosis. Appears at 2-3 months of age, is familial and may be of genetic origin.

Reference

Done, J.T., Allen, W.M., Bailey, J., De Gruchy, P.H., Curran, M.K. (1975). Asymmetric hindquarter syndrome (AHQS) in the pig. Vet. Rec. **96**, 482-485.

Nervous Conditions

Congenital Tremor

Three of the types of tremor present in piglets are known to be heritable. They are:

Congenital Tremor AIII
(Congenital cerebrospinal hypomyelinogenesis)

A severe, coarse tremor of the head and forequarters with side to side undulation of the hindquarters sometimes accompanied by squealing may be seen in male Landrace piglets at birth. The clinical signs disappear when the animal is asleep, and are accentuated by stress such as cold or the ingestion of cold liquids, or being made to walk backwards.

The condition is governed by a sex-linked recessive gene carried by the sow and is due to a deficiency in the number of oligodendrocytes and a resulting inability to myelinate CNS nerve fibres. A low proportion of litters are affected, and in these, 25% of piglets show signs. The condition recurs in successive litters of the same parents.

Affected piglets are prone to starvation and crushing and a high proportion of affected piglets die. The condition may be seen as a faint shimmer of movement of the head and shoulders in adult Landrace boars, especially when they are forced to walk backwards.

Control

Mate Landrace sows with Large White boars or unaffected Landrace boars.

Reference

Harding, J.D.J., Done, J.T., Harbourne, J.F., Randall, C.T., Gilbert, F.R. (1973). Congenital tremor type A III in pigs: an hereditary sex-linked cerebrospinal hypomyelinogenesis. Vet. Rec. **92**, 527-529.

Congenital Tremor AIV

A hereditary tremor seen in a low proportion of litters in British Saddleback pigs and occurring in 25% of the litter. The condition is recessive but not sex-linked and is due to a defect in the lipid metabolism of the CNS (possibly due to an isoform of the proteolipid protein gene) which results in demyelination and remyelination. Not common. The condition causes high mortality in affected piglets and recurs in subsequent litters of the same parents.

Saddleback X Large White Tremor

A monogenic autosomal recessive tremor has been recorded in Large White X Saddleback mating and is distinct from AIV. There is ataxia, dysmetria, perverse movement and a loss of righting reflex. It is a progressive cerebellar disorder.

Reference

Kidd, A.R.M., Done, J.T., Wrathall, A.E., Pampligione, G., Sweesey, D. (1986). A new genetically-determined congenital nervous disorder in pigs. Br.Vet.J. **142**, 275-285.

Circulatory disorders

von Willebrand's disease

A haemophilia-like condition has been described and occurs in both sexes. Factor VIII is reduced and platelets are more stable than normal. Clotting times are 15 minutes or more. Autosomal recessive. Other conditions may also occur.

Reference

Thiele, G.L., Rempel, W.E., Fass, D.N., Bowie, E.J.W., Stewart, M., Zoecklein, L. (1986). Inheritance of a new bleeding disease in a herd of swine with Willebrand's disease. J.Heredity **77**, 179-182.

Thrombocytopaenic purpura and Haemolytic Disease of the Newborn.

Definition

Thrombocytopaenic purpura is a disease of young piglets characterised by multiple haemorrhages and death of the whole or part of a litter 3 or 14-30 days of age after they have ingested colostrum containing antibodies to their platelets.

Incidence

Low, less than 1%.

Aetiology

Thrombocytopaenic purpura is caused by the formation of antibodies to foetal thrombocyte antigens in the sow by isoimmunisation. the ingestion of these antibodies in the colostrum and their absorption by the piglets results in a fall in the circulating levels of thrombocytes to about $200 \times 10^9/l$ at 2 days of age (normally higher, 250-300). Recovery takes place to $400 \times l0^9/l$ at 5 days and from the 9th day onwards declines to a level of $50 \times l0^9/l$ when purpura appears. Megakaryocytes and other cells in the bone marrow are affected and replacement of circulating thrombocytes does not occur. Pigs which die from purpura frequently have no circulating thrombocytes.

The uneven effect of the condition in a litter appears to be related to growth and the ingestion of colostrum, well-grown piglets which have sucked most colostrum being most severely affected. In order for the disease to occur, the thrombocyte type of the boar must differ from that of the sow and she must have had at least one previous litter to a boar of that thrombocyte type.

Clinical signs

The disease appears in piglets of 14-30 days of age with a lesser peak at 3 days of age. In most cases only a quarter of the litter is affected. Most affected piglets die. Death may occur without clinical signs but affected piglets are often pale and listless with an increased respiratory rate. A blotchy, purple skin, haemorrhages, mainly on the belly, and vivid scratch marks may be seen. m e mucous membranes are usually pale and the faeces may be blood stained. There is no fever.

Pathology

Affected pigs are in good bodily condition. Haemorrhages of varying sizes are seen in the epicardium, myocardium, pleura, joints and skeletal muscles. All lymph nodes are engorged with blood.

No megakaryocytes are present in the bone marrow. Platelets are low in numbers ($50 \times l0/l$ or less) or absent from the blood of affected pigs.

Epidemiology

The condition is not uncommon and affects the second and subsequent litters of sensitised sows bred to the same boar. It has been recorded most frequently in Large White and Landrace pigs and is particularly common when a Large White boar is used on a Landrace sow.

343

Diagnosis

The characteristic clinical and post-mortem picture may be confirmed by platelet counts. Septicaemic conditions should be ruled out.

Treatment and prevention

Affected piglets should be kept warm and offered fluid replacer, given multivitamins and antimicrobials for 3 or 4 days as supportive treatment. The use of Vitamin K has not been reported. When a sow has been bred to the same boar after having a litter of affected piglets, they too will be affected. The condition can be prevented by transferring the litter to another sow for 24 hours or until the colostrum containing the antibody is used up. Artificial feeding can also be practised. The same boar should not be used on sows which have had affected litters and, if the problem is widespread in a herd it may be economic to change the boar to one of a different breed.

References

Saunders, C.N., Kinch, D.A. (1968). Thrombocytopaenic purpura of pigs. J. Comp. Path. 78, 513-523.
Saunders, C.N., Kinch, D.A., and Imlah, P. (1966). Vet.Rec. 79, 549.

Haemolytic disease of the newborn

A condition in which isoantibodies produced by the sow to foetal red cells are absorbed by the piglets in the colostrum, causing intravascular haemolysis which results in jaundice and, sometimes, death in piglets aged 2-3 days. This condition resembles thrombocytopaenic purpura in its aetiology and pathogenesis and frequently occurs with it. It may be differentiated from thrombocytopaenic purpura by the early deaths (2-3 days of age), the presence of jaundice and by the demonstration of low red cell counts in the blood of the affected piglets.

Control in the same way as thrombocytopaenic purpura.

Reference

Hall, S.A., Rest, J.R., Linklater, K.A. and McTaggart, H.S. (1972). Concurrent haemolytic disease of the newborn and thrombocytopaenic purpura in piglets without artificial immunisation of the dam. Vet. Rec. 91, 677.

Porcine membranoproliferative glomerulonephritis type II

An autosomal recessive deficiency of Factor H with complete penetrance occurred in Norwegian Yorkshire pigs. Deficiency of Factor H, a protein regulating complement, resulted in reduction in levels of complement, accumulation of dense deposits of complement fraction C3 in the glomeruli leading to thickening of the glomerular capillary walls and proliferation of the mesangial cells. Lowered levels of complement are first detectable at one week of age, renal failure becomes noticeable at 3-4 weeks and death occurs at 5 weeks of age. The condition was eradicated by assaying the plasma of potential carriers for lowered factor H levels and removing the 13.5% positive animals from the breeding population.

References

Hogasen, K., Jansen, J.H., Harboe, M. (1997). Eradication of porcine factor H deficiency in Norway. Vet. Rec. **140**, 392-395.
Jansen, J.H., Hogasen, K., Grondahl, A.M. (1995). Porcine membranoproliferative glomerulonephritis type II: an autosomal recessive deficiency of Factor H. Vet. Rec. **137**, 240-244.

Hereditary scurvy. Vitamin C or ascorbic acid deficiency

Described as an autosomal recessive (the *od*, osteogenic disorder gene) in Denmark. Affected pigs lack the ability to synthesise ascorbic acid possibly because of the absence of gluconolactone oxidase in the acid liver. Piglets are born normal but, after weaning, plasma hydroxyproline and alkaline phosphatase levels fall. These plasma changes are followed by inappetence and reluctance to move. Subperiosteal haemorrhages and lesions of the metaphyses of the bones are seen When sows are deprived of Vitamin C the changes noted above occur *in utero* and piglets may be born with them. A DNA based test has been developed.

References

Hasan, L., Vogeli, P., Stoli, P., Kramer, S.S., Stranzinger, G., Neuenschwander, S. (2004). Intragenic deletion in the gene encoding L-gulonolactone oxidase causes vitamin C deficiency in pigs. Mammalian Genome **14**, 323-333.
Thode Jensen, P. *et al.*, (1983). Acta Vet.Scand. **24**, 392-402
Wegger, I., Palludan, B. (1994). Vitamin C deficiency causes haematological and skeletal abnormalities during foetal abnormalities in swine. J.Nutrition. **124**, 241-248.

Hereditary Lymphosarcoma

Hereditary lymphosarcoma has occurred at least once in a Large White herd in which it appears to be produced as an autosomal recessive gene. The condition occurs in 25% of the progeny of carriers. Affected piglets become stunted and pot-bellied with enlarged peripheral lymph nodes. They become affected by 6 months of age and do not survive beyond 15 months of age, never reaching sexual maturity. Circulating lymphocyte levels may be raised and blast cells may occur in the circulating blood.

The pathological findings are of a multicentric lymphosarcoma with enlargement of all lymph nodes, especially those of the alimentary tract and bronchus. 5 mm foci of tumour may be seen in peripheral nodes. The liver may be enlarged with white focal lesions as is the spleen. The thymus is involuted. diagnosis of a lymphosarcoma can be reached on pathological grounds, but the involvement of a genetic component requires breeding studies or studies of the incidence of the condition.

Reference

Head, K.W., Campbell J.G., Imlah, P., Laing, A.H., Linklater, K.A., MacTaggart, H.S. (1974). Hereditary lymphosarcoma in a herd of pigs. Vet. Rec. **95**, 523-526.

Barking Piglets (Respiratory distress syndrome)

A syndrome in which piglets are born with features of immaturity, including domed heads, sparse erect hair, failure to develop normal respiration (a barking grunt occurs) and soon die. Inadequate lung expansion is present with an absence of surfactant and the thyroid is small and functions poorly. An autosomal recessive.

References

Gibson, E.A., Blackmore, R.J.J., Wijeratne, W.V.S., Wrathall, A.E. (1976). The 'barker' (neonatal respiratory distress) syndrome in the pig. Its occurrence in the field. Vet. Rec. 98, 476-479.
Wrathall, A.E., Bailey, J., Wells, D.E., Herbert, C.N. (1977). Studies on the barker neonatal respiratory distress syndrome in the pig. Cornell Vet. 67, 543-598.

Inherited congenital goitre

Piglets are born hairless and swollen with enlarged thyroid glands. Autosomal recessive.

Reference

Welchman, D.B. de, Cranwell, M.P., Wrathall, A.E., Christensen, P. (1994). An inherited congenital goitre in pigs. Vet. Rec. 135, 589-593.

3. Congenital defects resulting from infectious conditions

Congenital Tremor AI. (Myoclonia congenita)

This results from infection of the sow by swine fever (hog cholera) virus either of high virulence, low virulence or sometimes, vaccine strains at 10-50 days' gestation and was responsible for 12% of all outbreaks of trembling in piglets seen between 1963 and 1965 in the U.K. A high proportion of the litters are affected, more than 40% of pigs within a litter are affected and mortality may be medium or high. Piglets of both sexes and dams from any breed are affected. It does not recur in successive litters from the same parents. Affected piglets show various degrees of muscular tremor, ataxia and inability to stand and suck. When placed on their feet, they may collapse. The tremor is still noticeable after 2-3 weeks. Outbreaks may last up to 4 months.

At post-mortem examination, the cerebellum is abnormally small with almost complete absence of the vermis. This cerebellar hypoplasia may only be obvious in mildly affected animals after comparing the cerebellum:brain weight ratios (0.04-0.08 if affected). Spinal cord changes are most repeatably seen at the level of the third cervical vertebra. There are fewer myelinated axons than in unaffected piglets, apparently because of subnormal or delayed myelination. Maternal antibodies to swine fever can be detected and in some animals (see swine fever) virus may be isolated.

Diagnosis

It is important to differentiate this type of congenital tremor from other causes. The high proportion of litters affected, the high mortality and the presence of the condition in piglets of both sexes born to sows of any breed are useful characters. The presence of cerebellar hypoplasia at post-mortem examination distinguishes it from all but AII and AV. In the latter there is usually a

346

history of organophosphorus treatment and the outbreak lasts for only a month, in AII mortality is low. Virus isolation or demonstration or antibody studies will confirm Swine Fever.

Control

Notifiable and controlled as Swine Fever.

References

Bradley, R., Done, J.T., Hebert, C.N., Overby, E., Askaa, J., Basse, A. and Bloch, B. (1985). J.Comp.Path **93**, 43-59.
Harding, J.D.J., Done, J.T. and Derbyshire, J.B. (1966). Congenital tremors in pigs and their relation to swine fever. Vet. Rec. **79**, 388-390.

Congenital Tremor AII (Myoclonia congenita)

Other infections or unknown conditions in the dam may give rise to congenital tremor. A fairly clearly-defined infectious condition occurs in most pigkeeping areas of the world. Infection in adults is asymptomatic except for the production of affected litters. A high proportion of litters are affected and more than 80% of the piglets within these litters are born with tremor but little mortality occurs (a difference from AI). Piglets of both sexes may be affected, and affected litters may be born to dams of any breed. The condition does not recur in successive litters from the same parents and the outbreak lasts about 4 months. Affected piglets which suck usually survive and have only slight tremor by 6-8 weeks of age. The disease can be reproduced by infecting pregnant sows with brain suspension from affected piglets at day 30. Circovirus type II is associated with some cases of the condition, but the direct evidence for this virus as a cause is still equivocal.

Cerebellar hypoplasia may occur and varying degrees of hypomyelinogenesis are found. Circovirus type II has been demonstrated in infectious brain tissue. Antibody to Swine Fever and Bovine Viral Diarrhoea is absent. The condition may otherwise be difficult to distinguish from AI. Control may involve the exposure of non-pregnant sows and gilts to infected piglets in an attempt to reduce the length of an outbreak. Trembling in neonatal piglets may be associated with Aujeszky's disease and may not necessarily be congenital.

Reference

Done, J.T., Wooley, J., Upcott, D.H. and Hebert, C.N. (1986). Porcine congenital tremor Type AII: spinal cord morphometry. Br.vet.J. **142**, 145-150.
Vanderkerckhove, P., Maenhout, D., Curvers, P., Hoorens, J., Ducatelle R. (1989). Type A2 congenital tremors in pigs. J.Vet.Med. (A). **36**, 763-771.

Weak piglets

A number of infectious conditions can lead to the birth of weak piglets. These include leptospirosis, Brucella (not UK), enterovirus and PRRS infections and possibly, parvovirus infections. Premature farrowing or late abortion due to a number of infectious agents may also lead to the birth of weak piglets. These may be born early as a result of direct infection of the foetus (toxoplasmosis) or due to fever e.g. erysipelas. In utero infections may also cause stunting, reduce birthweight and thus liveability.

Stillborn animals often accompany litters of weak pigs.

4. Congenital conditions attributable to nutritional deficiencies or poisoning

Congenital Tremor AV

Exposure of the dam to Trichlorfon or Neguvon between days 45 and 79 (especially 75-79) of gestation can result in the birth of a high proportion of litters containing trembling piglets. 90-100% of piglets of both sexes within affected litters may be born with rhythmic tremor, may stumble and fall and have difficulty in sucking. The mortality rate is high. Outbreaks may last about a month, but where the chemical is applied routinely (in some mange treatments), it may occur for longer periods. Severity of the tremor is dose-related.

The most consistent pathological features are cerebellar hypoplasia (cerebellum:whole brain ratio often 4%), reduced spinal cord size and hypomyelinogenesis. History will separate AV from AI and AII.

Reference

Wells, G.A.H. (1977). Haloxon neurotoxicity. Pig Farming **25**,73-76.

Pope, A.M. et al. (1986) Trichlorfon-induced cerebellar hypoplasia in neonatal pigs. J.Am.Vet.Med.Assn. **189**, 781-783.

Mulberry Heart Disease

Mulberry heart disease may be found in young piglets and has been seen in piglets *in utero*. It has been described in more detail under Vitamin E deficiency. The hereditary form has been identified in Danish pigs and is non-responsive to vitamin E and selenium therapy.

Cleft palate

Cleft palate may result from Hemlock poisoning (*Conium maculatum*). See also arthrogryposis

Splayleg

Splayleg may result from Fusarium intoxication in the sow as a result of eating mouldy rations.

Weak piglets

These may result from a deficiency of vitamins such as Vitamin A (accompanied by microphthalmia and generalised oedema with herniation of the cerebellum through the foramen magnum and abnormalities such as cleft palate). Vitamin E (weak with some splayleg) and pantothenic acid deficiency. There may also be weak piglets in litters affected by zearalenone and ergot poisoning. The use of prostaglandins in herds with improperly recorded service dates may lead to the birth of premature, weak piglets.

Hairless pigs may result from iodine deficiency.

5. Conditions present at birth but of unknown cause

Congenital Tremor Type B

Congenital tremors of unknown cause with no consistent gross or microscopic lesions are assigned to Group B. At least three types appear to exist. One may have cerebellar hypoplasia and lowered levels of cerebroside and lipid in the spinal cord, another has none of these features and yet others have few if any distinctive changes at all. It seems likely that more aetiological agents and conditions will be distinguished in this area. At least one of these types may be due to a virus as it appears to be transmissible.

The bleeding navel syndrome

This has occurred in a few pig herds. Affected piglets bleed to death as a result of failure of closure of the umbilicus or relaxation of previously closed vessels 2-6 hours after birth. Large, pale piglets, often covered with blood are found. There may be an underlying immaturity of collagen. Attendance at farrowings and ligation of the umbilicus with Holliston baby navel clamps can reduce mortality but recent studies have shown the condition may be prevented in some cases by feeding ascorbic acid (1-5 g per sow per day) to sows for at least six days prior to farrowing. Vitamin K injections given to sows have also been reported to have some effect.

Reference

Sandholm, M., Honkanen-Buzalski, T. and Rasi, V. (1979). Prevention of navel bleeding in piglets by preparturient administration of ascorbic acid. Vet. Rec. 104, 337-338.

THE INVESTIGATION AND CONTROL OF CONGENITAL DISORDERS

Congenital abnormalities occur in about 1-5% of all pigs born. Obvious abnormalities or those which cause death e.g. atresia ani tend not to be passed on as such animals are not selected for breeding. There is thus a tendency for abnormal pigs to be eliminated and for any inherited component of the condition to be eliminated as well.

Dominant genetic traits are rapidly seen and eliminated as they are expressed in all animals carrying them (AA).

Recessive genetic traits will only be expressed by homozygotes (aa) but not by heterozygotes (Aa). An incidence of 1% of recessive trait indicates that 18% of the population are heterozygotes.

Sex linked conditions are only expressed in males but if mated with a carrier, females homozygous for the trait may express it.

Recessive genetic traits may be identified by the familial pattern recorded in an existing closed herd but are less easily identified where breeding stock of unknown carrier status is regularly introduced. A repeatable incidence of 25% of the progeny in successive matings of the same boar and sow would indicate a recessive genetic trait. In a few conditions such as PSS or pityriasis rosea this may happen, but in other conditions such as atresia ani the results are less clear-cut and a genetic influence can only be determined because of a high incidence of the trait following carrier matings or mating carriers with recessives.

Chromosomal or developmental abnormalities appear spontaneously and, unless associated with genetic transmission or a particular environmental cause will be sporadic.

Environmental factors such as nutrition, infection and poisoning may be distinguished by history of disease in sows at the relevant stage of gestation e.g. swine fever.

They may also occur in sows of different breeds on the same farm and the abnormality may fail to reappear in any sow mated with the same boar on a subsequent occasion. Some congenital abnormalities of infectious origin may only occur in the litters of recently-introduced gilts. In some cases the condition responsible can be identified and in others transmission can be proved experimentally. Nutritional deficiencies such as Vitamin A deficiency or excesses such as selenium toxicity can be identified by analysis of the ration if they continue. Toxins and poisonings are usually associated with exposure of sows to a toxin such as trichlorphos at the appropriate stage of gestation and either fail to recur in subsequent litters or occur in animals on other farms receiving the same treatment or food.

Control

This should rely on the correction of environmental factors such as nutrition, toxin exposure and infection whenever possible.

Where a genetic component is suspected, it is

(1)   Common practice not to retain affected individuals for breeding unless, as in P.S.S., there is an economic advantage.

(2)   Culling of the affected individual, its sibs and, possibly, its parents may also be commonly practiced if the incidence of the trait is less than 3% particularly if this will have no effect on genetic progress.

(3)   When the incidence of the trait is more than 3%, full sib culling may be carried out, but only if advantageous.

(4)   Test mating of possible carriers with homozygous recessives can be carried out with subsequent elimination but to reduce the frequency of a recessive gene from 0.5% to 0.25% would require 6 generations of selection solely against that gene.

(5)   The identification of carriers by means other than test mating leaves decisions as to control to be based solely on economics and the genetic advantages to be gained by retaining or eliminating the gene e.g. the use of PSS-resistant sire lines and PSS-sensitive dam lines. Examples of such detection and elimination schemes include PSS (halothane testing and now PCR to detect affected and carrier animals).

References

Bampton, P.R. (1994). The investigation of genetic and hereditary disorders of pigs. Pig J. **32**, 68-82.

Nicholas, F.W. (1998). Genetics of morphological traits and inherited disorders, in The Genetics of the Pig, Eds Rothschild, M.F. and Ruvinsky, A., CAB International, Chapter 4, 71-104.

Online Mendelian Inheritance in Man (OMIM) at http://www.ncbi.nlm.nih.gov:/omim/-

Online Mendelian Inheritance in Animals (OMIA) at http://www.angis.org.au/-

Steane, D.E. (1985). Congenital abnormalities. Proc.Pig Vet.Soc. **12**, 38-49.

Wrathall, A.E. (1988). The boar and congenital problems. Proc.Pig Vet.Soc. **21**, 116-134.

MISCELLANEOUS CONDITIONS

Mastitis in sows

Mastitis in sows may be localised to a single gland or may involve more than one to cause fever, depression and death. Losses due to piglet mortality may be considerable. Coliform mastitis and the sporadic chronic mastitis affecting single glands are described separately as is agalactia.

a) Coliform mastitis

Definition

Coliform mastitis may be caused by any enterobacterial organism. Infection may be localised to a single gland or may involve more than one to cause fever, depression and death. Agalactia is common and piglet mortality and growth depression in the litter may be considerable.

Incidence

Worldwide. May be a major cause of loss in affected herds.

Aetiology

The acute and severe forms of this condition are often associated with *Klebsiella spp.* and may occur in outbreaks of fatal disease often associated with the trauma of a particular type of sawdust bedding. A wide variety of *E.coli* serotypes and RAPD types may be isolated, often differing from gland to gland. Other coliform organisms may be identified. Recent studies suggest that the *E.coli* types all possess fimbriae and can adhere to epithelial surfaces and that 95% are serum resistant.

Pathogenesis

In many cases, traumatic injury resulting from unclipped piglet teeth, sawdust bedding (particularly important in Klebsiella mastitis), or poor quality flooring is a contributory factor in initiating infection. One, or both glands supplying a single teat may be infected. Infection usually enters via the teat canal following teat contamination and bacteria multiply in the gland. In some cases, infection may be transient, producing an endotoxin-mediated cellular response and a shift to the left in blood white cell counts and in others, colonisation, multiplication and acute mastitis with systemic signs and agalactia apparently caused by the effect of *E.coli* endotoxin on prolactin production. Introduction of either endotoxin or interleukin I to the mammary gland will cause mastitis and agalactia and endotoxin can be detected in the blood in mastitis.

Clinical signs

Acutely affected sows are usually depressed, inappetent and pyrexic (temperatures of 40.5-42°C (105-107°F) are not uncommon). The udder is usually swollen and oedematous, often with massive congestion. Any secretion that may be obtained after oxytocin injection is purulent. Pain in the udder may lead to restlessness in the sow when piglets attempt to suck. The litter rapidly loses

condition. The condition occurs within 1-3 days of parturition in most cases and death frequently results. Coliform mastitis appears to regress within 3-4 days although in severe cases the lactation may cease entirely if death does not occur. Subacute infection or infection in one or more glands occurs much more commonly than the acute syndrome and may be recognised by the increased hardness of one or more glands and, in its early stages, by a square area of reddening of the skin over the affected gland. The litter loses condition and in subclinical *E.coli* mastitis this loss of condition may draw attention to its presence. Secretion may appear grossly normal in subacute or subclinical infection but raised cell counts (>10^6/ml) can be demonstrated by cytology.
Evidence is emerging that mastitis may reduce fertility at the next mating.

Euthanasia is only indicated in acute disease when the body temperature falls below normal, the animal can no longer rise and respiratory distress develops.

Pathology

At post-mortem examination of acute cases, the carcase muscle and the liver may be pale and the subcutaneous tissue over the affected mammae is oedematous. The cut surface of affected mammae is diffusely or focally reddened. An acute inflammatory reaction and necrosis of the alveolar epithelium is present. *E.coli, Klebsiella* spp. or other coliform organisms may be isolated from the affected glands, although in many cases the organisms have already been eliminated. Sows with subacute or subclinical mastitis rarely die. Lesions are restricted to the few glands affected. Often only one of the two glands supplying 1 teat is reddened and engorged with milk.

Epidemiology

Outbreaks occur on individual farms and are frequently associated with faecal contamination or wetness of bedding. In the case of Klebsiella mastitis, infected sawdust may be associated with the outbreak. There appears to have been a reduction in the acute form of the disease causing death in recent years. The environmental origin of the causal organisms is underlined by their disparate nature.

Diagnosis

Acute mastitis is easily recognisable. Subclinical mastitis may be palpated, but the exact identity of the affected gland may only be detected after cell counts on expressed milk. Cell counts in infected glands may reach 2.0 x 10^8/ml with 75% polymorphs but levels of 4.0 x 10^7/ml may be found in involuting unsucked normal glands. Normal milk contains 1 x 10^6 cells/ml. Chronic mastitis is easily palpable upon inspection during lactation and easily seen in dry sows. Isolation of bacteria from milk confirms the presence of mastitis and can aid the selection of treatment.

Treatment and control

Acutely ill sows may be saved by parenteral treatment with antibiotics such as neomycin, tetracyclines, ampicillin, amoxycillin, streptomycin, fluoroquinolone and ceftiofur or by the use of trimethoprim: sulphonamide injections for 2-4 days. Oxytocin should also be given. In some cases treatment is effective. The litter should be fostered or reared artificially. After recovery it may be necessary to cull the sow. In severely affected cases the prognosis is poor but rehydration with saline given intravenously by flutter valve may cause a dramatic improvement in moribund animals. Other supportive treatment should be given and recent studies suggest that anti-inflammatory drugs such as flunixin meglumine (Finadyne, Schering Plough) and meloxicam (Metacam, Boehringer Ingelheim) may have some value. In subacute cases, rehydration is not necessary.

Control depends upon the use of hygiene, use of soft bedding other than sawdust, clipping piglets' teeth, early treatment and, possibly, the use of commercial *E.coli* vaccines may reduce the incidence if the condition is due to *E.coli*. Prophylactic treatment with trimethoprim:sulphonamide at 15 mg/kg given in the feed from day 112 of gestation to day 1 post-partum may prevent the condition as may feed medication with other agents. Animals which have had severe or repeated bouts of mastitis should be culled.

References

Hulten, F., Persson, A., Eliasson-Selling, L., Heldmer, E., Lindberg, M., Sjogren, U., Kugelberg, C., Ehlorsson, C.J. (2004). Evaluation of environmental and management-related risk factors associated with chronic mastitis in sows. Am. J.Vet. Res.65, 1398-1403.

Jones, J.E.T. (1979). Acute coliform mastitis in the sow. Vet. Annual, 19, 97.

Martineau, G.P., Smith, B.B., Douze, B. (1992). Pathogenesis, prevention and treatment of lactational insufficiency in sows. Veterinary Clinics of North America: Food Animal Practice : Swine Reproduction 8, 661-684.

Persson, A., Morner, A.P., Kuhl, W. (1996). A long term study on the health status and performance of sows on different feed allowances during late pregnancy III E. coli and other bacteria, total cell content, polymorphonuclear leucocytes and pH in colostrum and milk during the first 3 weeks of lactation. Acta Vet. Scand. 37, 293-313.

Smith, B.B. and Wagner, W.C. (1985). Effect of *E.coli* endotoxin and thyrotropin-releasing hormone on prolactin in lactating sows. Am.J.Vet.Res. 46, 175-180.

Wegmann, P. and Bertschinger, H.U. (1984). Sequential cytological and bacteriological examination of the secretions from sucked and unsucked mammary glands in and without mastitis. Proc.Int.Pig Vet.Soc. 8, 287

b) Sporadic or chronic mastitis

Definition

Mastitis may affect single glands particularly in older sows to result in abscess formation and loss of the individual gland often with few systemic clinical signs.

Incidence

In one UK survey 18.8% of culled sows were affected. Only one gland was infected in 60% of affected sows.

Aetiology and Pathogenesis

A.pyogenes, *Actinomyces suimastitidis*, streptococci, staphylococci, *Bacteroides* spp. fusobacteria and clostridia may all be isolated. The organisms enter the gland as does *E.coli* but do not usually cause the systemic reaction seen in coliform mastitis.

Clinical signs

Often noted only when an affected gland fails to return to normal after weaning. It may be noted as local inflammation and pain over that portion of the udder during lactation and pus may be expressed. As oedema may spread over more than one gland, the exact location of the affected gland may not be identifiable. There is often teat injury. Assessment at weaning confirms that teat injury is common (present in 60% sows regardless of lactation number), especially in the thoracic and anterior abdominal pairs. Palpable lesions are present in 15% pigs following weaning of the first litter, in 30% after two litters and in 60% in subsequent litters, but most changes disappear within 7 days of weaning. Culling should be carried out when multiple abscesses or ulceration are present but humane slaughter is rarely indicated.

Pathology

Abscessation and fibrosis, often coupled with physical damage to the teat or its end may be found. The bacteria listed above may be isolated.

Epidemiology

Bedding and unclipped teeth and flooring such as perforated metal which predispose to teat damage may all allow organisms to colonise the udder and cause the condition.

Diagnosis

Clinical signs as above, confirmed by expression of pus and isolation of organisms. Milk of mastitic glands contains raised numbers of somatic cells (total cell count, TCC 17.76×10^6/ml, normal 12.17×10^6/ml).

Treatment and control

Parenteral antimicrobials including penicillin if staphylococci or streptococci are involved. Oxytocin administration may be of value. Control can be established by improving husbandry. Affected sows should only be retained if they have sufficient functioning teats.

References

Delgado, J.A. and Jones, J.E.T. (1981). An abattoir survey of mammary gland lesions in sows with special reference to the bacterial flora of mammary abscesses Br. Vet. J. **137**, 639-643.
Persson, A. (1997). Clinical assessment of udder health status of sows at time of weaning with special reference to bacteriology and cytology of milk. J.Vet. Med. Ser. A **44**, 143-158.

The Post Partum Dysgalactia Syndrome (PPDS), Mastitis. Metritis, Agalactia Complex (M.M.A.), Periparturient Hypogalactia Syndrome (P.H.S.)

Definition

A complex syndrome in which hypogalactia or agalactia occur within 12-72 hours of parturition. Fever, anorexia, vulval discharge and mastitis may all accompany the basic change and the growth rate and survival of the litter are usually affected.

Incidence

Recent surveys suggest that the most severe forms are becoming less common.

Aetiology

Bacterial invasion of the mammae and subsequent production of endotoxins which are absorbed, cause the systemic signs. A similar syndrome can be reproduced experimentally, in some cases, by the intravenous injection of endotoxin into sows. Endotoxin cannot, however, always be demonstrated in the plasma of affected animals, neither can bacteria or mastitis be identified in the mammary glands and the timing of such an event in relation to farrowing may be important. Bacteria in the gut or in endometritis may be the source of endotoxin. ß-haemolytic streptococci and coliforms have been associated with the condition and in many cases mastitis may be present in one or more glands.

Hormonal causes have been suggested as levels of a number of hormones may be depressed following parturition. If so, the initiating factors have not been identified. Hormones involved in lactation include insulin, cortisone and prolactin, oxytocin, oestrogen and progesterone and changes in the levels of all these have been demonstrated in pigs with agalactia. Levels of oxytocin are often half those in normal sows. Prolactin levels may be dramatically reduced by small volumes of endotoxin and recent studies suggest that the inhibition of prostaglandin F2 alpha production in the uterus (possibly by infection) may remove an important stimulus to prolactin secretion. Management and nutrition appear to be important in the aetiology and low exercise, high nutrient density rations, overfeeding and poor hygiene all appear to predispose to the condition. The importance of water intake and stress or disturbance during parturition is not yet clear.

Clinical signs

The syndrome usually occurs within 12 hours - 3 days of parturition. Inappetence is commonly the first sign to be noted, followed by depression, restlessness when being suckled and loss of condition in the litter. Affected sows may have a slight fever, 39.5-41°C if mastitis is present. Vulvar discharge and constipation are frequently with associated with this condition but neither may be present. The disease lasts for a minimum of 3 days and then resolves spontaneously. By this time the litter may have been lost. The condition may be preceded by delays in parturition (>5 hours) and may vary in its intensity. In mild cases of hypogalactia unaccompanied by mastitis or other elements of the complex, depressed daily liveweight gain in piglets (<105 g/day, normal 125 g/day) may be the only indication of the problem.

Affected sows recover, but hypoglycaemic piglets which do not respond to treatment may require euthanasia in extremis.

Pathology

Neither mastitis nor metritis is a constant finding. Where mastitis occurs, it appears to be patchy within a gland and of an acute catarrhal nature. Oedema of the subcutaneous tissue and inflammatory changes in the draining lymph nodes occur where mastitis is present. Histologically the glands of affected pigs often resemble those of sows at 110 days' gestation.

Epidemiology

The condition sometimes occurs in batches It is particularly common where hygiene is poor and where sows are fat.

Diagnosis

Clinical signs are the main method of diagnosis. Confirmation of bacterial mastitis may be made by the examination of milk samples. Disease in the litter, such as diarrhoea, septicaemia or hypothermia, may lead to decreased intake of milk and overstocking of the udder. When fever is present, other disease (e.g. erysipelas) may be the cause. A history of difficulty in farrowing, or small litters or incomplete cleansing, may indicate retention of a foetus or placentae. Examination per vagina, if within 24 hours of parturition, will establish this. In some cases mycotoxins such as trichoethecenes may be involved.

Treatment

Affected sows should be given frequent doses of oxytocin. Parenteral broad spectrum antimicrobial may be given and is advisable when mastitis, metritis or fever are present. Ampicillin, tetracyclines, trimethoprim sulphonamide or enrofloxacin may be given. Anti-inflammatory drugs such as flunixin meglumine and meloxicam have been reported to improve recovery. The value of corticosteroids is equivocal. The litter should be given supplementary feeding and left with the sow.

Control

Hygiene, and exercise of sows prior to farrowing and during the early stages of lactation may help. Restriction of the feed for the last two or three days before farrowing and partial replacement with bran, may help reduce the incidence. Reduction of feed intake to 1 kg/day from 100 days gestation and use of vegetable protein has reduced the incidence of hypogalactia in some cases.

The use by farmers of oxytocin in early cases of agalactia may be helpful and reduce the need for veterinary involvement. Treatment should begin when sow body temperature is 39.4°C 12-18 hours post farrowing. Routine injections of antibiotic and oxytocin post farrowing have been shown not to be helpful. Recent studies have indicated that treatment with trimethoprim: sulphonamide in the feed at 15 mg/kg bodyweight from day 112 of gestation to day 1 *post partum,* reduces the incidence of the disease markedly as may in-feed medication with other sulphonamides or tetracyclines. The use of long acting tetracycline (Terramycin LA, Pfizer) injections given 1 day before farrowing has been shown to be beneficial in some herds. Recently some studies have shown significant decreases in agalactia in sows which have farrowed early as a result of prostaglandin use, but this may not apply at 111 days' gestation. Other studies have found no difference.

References

Goransson, L. (1989). The effect of feed allowance in late pregnancy on the occurrence of agalactia *post partum* in the sow. J.Vet.Med. Series A **36**, 505-513.

Kensinger, R.S., Collier R.J., Bazer, F.W. (1986). Ultrastructural changes in porcine mammary tissue during lactogenesis. J. Anat. **145**,49-59.

Liptrap, R.M. (1987). Lactational failure in the sow. Veterinary Annual **27**, 134-138.
Martineau, G.P., Smith, B.B., Douze, B. (1992). Pathogenesis, prevention and treatment of lactational insufficency in sows. Veterinary Clinics of North America : Food Animal Practice : Swine Reproduction **8**, 661-684.
Peter, A.T., Huether, P., Doble, E., Liptrap, R.M. (1985). Prostaglandin F2 alpha and prolactin in experimental hypogalactia in sows. Res.vet.Sci. **39**, 221-229.

"Actinomycosis" of the Udder

Chronic mastitis may sometimes involve more than one teat and spread along the udder to cause a large swelling which is hard to the touch and may touch the ground. It is frequently ulcerated. *Actinomyces sp.*especially *A. suimastitidis*, may be isolated from fewer than 50% of cases but a variety of other organisms are present. Amyloidosis may be found in the kidneys of affected animals. Affected animals should be culled, but severely affected animals with lesions too large for transport should be destroyed humanely.

Vulval Discharges

Discharges from the vulva may be physiological when they occur immediately post-partum, as when semen leaks post service, but may also be pathological. They may originate from the uterus in endometritis, from the vagina in vaginitis, from the vulva itself or from the urinary tract in cystitis and pyelonephritis. Vulval discharge is not always apparent in these three underlying syndromes and apparently unaffected animals may prove to be affected upon further investigation. Cystitis and pyelonephritis have been considered under bacterial disease, post-partum and post-service vulval discharges and endometritis are considered below.

Post-partum Vulval and Vaginal Discharges
(Post-farrowing vulval discharges, PFD)

Definition

Discharges from the vulva occur in sows after farrowing. They are often copious and may then be linked with depression of production parameters such as performance of the litter and subsequent productivity. They may indicate the presence of metritis.

Incidence

Extremely common worldwide (92% farms Australia). Also present in a high proportion of some farms (to 60%).

Aetiology

A number of bacterial species including ß-haemolytic streptococci of Groups G and L, *A.pyogenes, Actinobacillus suis, Bacteroides spp. Clostridium spp.* and *Haemophilus spp.* may be isolated. Coliforms may also be present as may be staphylococci. The bacteria appear to colonise the physiologically-disturbed uterus and vagina. The exact predisposing factors are not yet clear, but the incidence may be reduced by antimicrobial cover from before farrowing and by hygiene.

357

Pathogenesis

Some of these bacteria are present or identifiable prior to farrowing but with the normal post-parturient flow of materials from the involuting uterus, they increase in numbers and give rise to histological evidence of inflammation in the walls of the vagina and/or give rise to endometritis. The discharge eventually resolves but may be accompanied by mild cystitis or by metritis. The mechanism of infection is not yet clear but infection is probably ascending and often follows interference at farrowing.

Clinical signs

Post parturient vulval discharge occurs initially (12-36 hours) as a clear mucoid, serous or bloody discharge and may in normal circumstances dry up. In some cases (up to 60-70% of sows in a herd) it may persist for 5-7 days. For some days after this pus may be seen during urination or may be found on the floor behind the sow. When post-parturient vulval discharge is prolonged, extended weaning to service intervals may be recorded although recovery is apparently complete before weaning. Subsequent fertility may be reduced by 10% in animals recovered from discharge.

Direct inspection by endoscope can distinguish between endometritis, vaginitis and vulvitis. In endometritis, the onset may be early (1.6 days), discharge volume high (100 ml) and the discharge may be white-yellow in colour. Systemic signs of metritis include rectal temperature >40°C, (104°F), inappetance and agalactia in severe cases. Death (5%) may occur and the farrowing rate may be half that of unaffected sows.

Vaginitis is twice as common as metritis, has a later onset (day 4) and produces less discharge (11-30 ml) less inappetance, no deaths and little effect on subsequent fertility. Vulvitis represents only 10-72% of all discharges, appears on day 3, produces the least volume (scant-6 ml) lasting for 2 days and is least likely to affect appetite and has little effect on fertility.

Humane slaughter is only indicated in recumbent animals with metritis which have not responded to treatment or are unable to rise.

Pathology

Pus may be found in the vagina and may originate from the uterus in metritis or from vaginitis alone. Larger than normal numbers of neutrophils may be seen migrating through the vaginal wall in histological sections. Endometritis may be found and appreciable volumes of pus may be present in the uterine lumen.

Epidemiology

The condition appears to be present in individual herds and to occur in cycles.

Diagnosis

Easily seen in the early stages, a speculum or endoscope may be required to see pus or inflammation later in the disease and it is relatively easily distinguished from cystitis. In early cases, incomplete parturition should be considered. Late cases or those with a closed endometritis may only be suspected when systemic signs develop. Swabs for bacteriological examination should be guarded or a speculum used to reduce vulval contamination.

Treatment and control

Antimicrobial therapy may be given parenterally, locally by irrigation of the vagina or placement of pessaries or by the inclusion of antimicrobial at therapeutic level in the feed over the period of farrowing and for 7 days afterwards. Control of the problem has been achieved by routine antimicrobial injection at farrowing. Antimicrobials used include tetracyclines, ampicillin, ceftiofur and trimethoprim sulphonamide.

Hygiene is important in prevention. Faecal accumulations behind sows should be removed before and after farrowing, all interference at farrowing should be carried out using clean hands and antimicrobial treatment should be considered immediatey interference has been carried out. Sows with endometritis should be culled at the next opportunity after confirmation.

References

Bara, M.R., Cameron, R.D.A. (1994). A study of the incidence, characterisation, effect on reproductive performance and predisposing factors associated with post-farrowing vulval discharges. Proc.IPVS. **13**, 400.

Madec, F., Miquet, J.M., Leon, E. (1993). La pathologie de la parturition chez la triue. Etude epidemiologique dans cinq elevages. Rec.Vet.Med. **168**, 341-349.

Taylor, D.J. (1984). Clinical and bacteriological effects of antimicrobial therapy on naturally-occurring post-partum vulval discharge in sows following service. Proc.Int.Pig Vet.Soc. **8**, 151.

Vulval Discharges after Weaning (Post Mating Discharge, PMD)

Definition

Vulval discharges of vaginal or uterine origin occur from 7 days post-service onwards and may be copious. They are associated with a high rate of return to service.

Incidence

Worldwide, 24% of herds affected. In a UK survey 1980-85, individual cases could occur in almost any herd. 28% Australia 1994.

Aetiology and pathogenesis

Bacteria such as *E.coli, Proteus* spp., *streptococci, Staphylococcus hyicus. Actinomyces hyovaginalis* and *A.pyogenes* can be isolated from the discharges, although only *E. coli* at high numbers (10^9 organisms) and *S. hyicus* are capable of initiating the syndrome experimentally following intrauterine inoculation. The source of infection may be faecal or slurry contamination of the vulva, existing cystitis or uterine infection or service by individual boars kept under poor hygienic conditions. Vulval discharge increases markedly when multiple services are carried out under unhygienic conditions and results from a combination of vulval damage, exposure to infection from the poor hygiene and rising levels of progesterone as the animal enters metoestrus towards the end of the service period. Vaginitis may result or infection may progress to endometritis. Uterine infection may result in death of the eggs or developing embryos and delayed return to service. *A.pyogenes* has been shown to be capable of this.

Clinical signs

Vulval discharge appears first as tacky mucus on the vulval lips 15-20 days post-service. A creamy discharge then develops and may persist until at least 80 days post-service. Returns to service usually follow. Discharge is more common in older sows and rare in gilts or first parity animals. Endometritis, vaginitis and cystitis may all occur and may be distinguished by endoscopy. Volumes of discharge are usually highest (90 ml), fertility is lowest (farrowing rate 14%) and depression of appetite are most severe in endometritis. Vaginitis occurs in fewer cases of PMD than with endometritis, has a later onset (12-30 days) produces lower volumes of discharge (14-26 ml) has a 70% farrowing rate and is not fatal.

Pathology

Vaginitis and endometritis alone or together may be present in culled sow Necrotic embryos may be present.

Epidemiology

Frequently associated with poor hygiene and poor crate design. Individual boars, boars kept in dirty conditions or purchased from several sources may be strongly associated with tho condition.

Diagnosis

Based on inspection. The presence of blood or mucus in the discharge indicates cystitis or pyelonephritis. Frequently found during investigation of high rates of return. Discharge may be visible only on the underside of the tail, on faeces or on the backplate of the crate in stalled sows. It is difficult to detect in loose-housed sows. Discharge may pool in the anterior vagina and be visible through a speculum or endoscope. Bacteria may be isolated. Levels of 2% post mating discharge are acceptable on a herd basis, but levels of 3-5% require interference.

Treatment and control

Sows can be treated parenterally with antimicrobial such as long-acting oxytetracycline at the first signs of discharge but this may not save the pregnancy or cure the problem. Prevention involves injection at weaning followed by feed medication with oxytetracycline at therapeutic level for 21 days. The placement of antimicrobial in the anterior vagina (but not in the cervix) immediately post service may also have a beneficial effect. Boars should be treated by washing the preputial sac and instilling an antibiotic solution daily for 5 days. Treatment should be accompanied by rigorous cleaning and disinfection of sow and boar accommodation and consideration should be given to lowering slurry levels in dry sow houses and to altering the back plates of stalls in countries where these are still in use. The poor farrowing rate of endometritis-affected sows makes culling advisable.

References

Bara, M.R., Cameron, R.D.A. (1994). A study of the incidence, characterisation, effect on reproductive performance and predisposing factors associated with post-mating vulval discharge (PMD). Proc. IPVS. **13**, 399.
Jana, B., Kucharski, J., Ziecik, A.J. (2004). Effect of intrauterine infusion of *E. coli* on hormonal patterns in gilts during the oestrus cycle. Reproduction, Nutrition, Development **44**, 37-48.

MacLachlan, N.J. and Dial, G.D. (1987). An epizootic of endometritis in gilts. Veterinary Pathology **24**, 92-94.

Muirhead, M.R. (1986). Epidemiology and control of vaginal discharges in the sow. Vet.Rec. **119**, 233-235.

Muirhead, M.R. (1998). Vulval discharges and endometritis in sows-a new technique for control and prevention. Proc IPVS **15**, 228.

Winter, P.J.J.de, Verdonck, M., Kruif, A.de, DeVriese, L.A., Haesebrouck, F. (1995). Bacterial endometritis and vaginal discharge in the sow: prevalence of different bacterial species and experimental reproduction of the syndrome. Animal Repro. Sci. **37**, 325-335.

Endometritis in Sows with no vulval discharge

Organisms found in metritis include *E.coli, Bacteroides spp,* clostridia, streptococci especially *S dysgalactiae equisimilis, A.pyogenes,* arcobacters, sporolactobacilli and staphylococci. In many cases the organisms enter at farrowing or service, reach high levels and are then eliminated but some remain, particularly after difficult farrowings. Where vulval discharges are absent, returns to service may indicate endometritis or pyometra. The latter may be detected by ultrasound. Metritis is present in approximately 30% of sows culled for infertility and its prevention may only be feasible if a programme such as that described above is adopted or if strategic antibiotic injections are given over farrowing and service. The economics of this practice have to be considered for each individual herd.

References

Berner, H. (1984). Pathogenesis, clinical signs and bacteriology. Proc.Int.Pig Vet.Soc. **8**, 284.

Muirhead, M.R. (1984). The investigation and control of a production problem in pigs: low litter size, vaginitis and endometritis. Vet.Annual **24**, 118-126.

Seasonal Infertility (Summer Infertility)

Seasonal infertility occurs mainly in summer and results from a combination of the effects of day length (a putative residual effect remaining from the ancestral wild boar) and high temperature. Effects are most obvious in the female, but high temperature may also have an effect on semen quality and libido in the boar. Sows may be seasonally infertile, becoming anoestrus for a period of 19 weeks (range 11-30), but cycling throughout this period without demonstrating oestrus. In addition, there may be reduced conception during the summer.

These effects may be overcome in part by boar stimulation and shading of the mating area, cooling of the boar and sow using wallows or sprays and mating early in the morning when temperatures are lowest. Melatonin has been evaluated as a means of overcoming the effect in sows, but was not completely effective, but the provision of additional roughage was useful in one study and there may be a satiety effect. The addition of 4 units of oxytocin to semen doses improved farrowing to first service in summer to levels found at other times of the year. Lighting programmes have been used where total confinement is practised, but is not feasible in outdoor situations.

References

Bassett, J.M., Bray, C.J., Sharpe, C.E. (1996). Summer infertility in outdoor sows: lessons from studies on "seasonally-barren" sows. Pig J. **36**, 65-85.

Pena, F.J., Dominguez, J.C., Carbajo, M., Ariel, L., Alegre, B. (1998). Treatment of swine summer infertility syndrome by means of oxytocin under field conditions. Theriogenology **49**, 829-836.

Tast, A., Halli, O., Virolainen, J.V., Oravainen, J., Heinonen, M., Peltoniemi, O.A.T. (2005). Investigation of a simplified artificial lighting programme to improve the fertility of sows in commercial piggeries. Vet. Rec. **156**, 702-705.

Preputial Ulceration and Disease in Boars

Ulcers and inflammation of the preputial diverticulum may occur and lead to pain and swelling. There may be enlargement of the superficial lymph nodes and it may be possible to detect the inflamed organ. Eversion of the sac under anaesthetic will confirm. It may be excised surgically or the animal may be treated.

Porcine Dermatitis and Nephropathy Syndrome (PDNS)

Definition

A syndrome in which circular or irregular red or purple macules and papules develop on the skin of grower and finisher pigs. Affected pigs are depressed, may be lame anda high percentage die. Haemorrhagic lymph nodes and enlarged, pale, petechiated kidneys are present at post mortem examination.

Incidence

Described in Chile in 1976 and since 1987 in the UK as a sporadic condition, the syndrome has now been reported from many countries where PMWS is present. In 2003, at least 10% of UK holdings with more than 50 pigs.had experienced the disease. It was absent from Northern Ireland and uncommon in Scotland.

Aetiology

The aetiology is currently uncertain. The original sporadic cases frequently yielded a particular strain of *Pasteurella multocida*, but the epidemic disease is firmly associated with PMWS, and PCV2 can be demonstrated in the tissues of most, if not all, cases. As the disease commonly occurs in older pigs than PMWS (6-8 weeks of age), in pigs aged 11-14 weeks and affected animals have high levels of antibody to PCV2, it has been postulated that the vasculitis and immune glomerulonephritis of PDNS are associated with or caused by the continued immune reaction to that virus. Other agents such as PRRSV have been suggested as contributing to the condition, but the evidence for their involvement is not consistent.

Pathogenesis

Not yet described in detail. A systemic necrotic vasculitis and an immune glomerulonephritis underlie the lesions and are progressive.

Clinical signs

Affected pigs are often aged 11-14 weeks but can be up to 22 weeks in age and become depressed, fevered and anorectic. The disease may be of sudden onset or occur in pigs which have had PMWS. Affected animals first develop irregular red or purple patches over the hindquarters and back and discoloured swellings may occur on the lower limbs. The macules may coalesce to form irregular patches, develop crusts and finally fade, sometimes leaving scars. They are found on the margins of the ears, dependent parts of the abdomen and thorax, on the perineal area and the limbs. Affected animals may recover or die of renal failure within a few days of the appearance of the skin lesions.
Badly-affected animals which are dull, unable to rise and have leg lesions, severe ulceration or renal failure (high blood urea) should be killed humanely.

Pathological Findings

Gross lesions include those of the skin, macroscopic lesions of pneumonia and general lymphadenopathy. There may be gross enlargement of the kidneys which are whitish and petechiated and the swollen lymph nodes may be haemorrhagic. There can be haemorrhages on serous surfaces and ulceration of the ileocaecocolic junction. There may be joint lesions. The underlying lesions in the acute phase consist of a necrotising leucocytoclastic vasculitis of small arteries in the dermis and in various extracutaneous areas such as the renal pelvis and synovial membranes. There is an interstitial pneumonia and perivascular cuffing. Immunoglobulin and complement can be demonstrated around necrotic vesels in the skin in early lesions and PCV2 virus can be demonstrated in macrophages in the same areas. There are lesions of immune glomerulonephritis in the kidney. Some accounts describe the presence of streptococcal antigens in these lesions.

Epidemiology

The sporadic form of PMWS occurring in the UK pre-1999 was not associated with any other syndrome and had a low mortality ().5%). The current, epidemic, form is strongly associated with PMWS, may follow it in an individual herd and has a high mortality rate (60-80% of cases early in an outbreak) and the post-weaning mortality may rise to 20% in an affected herd where PMWS is also present. The two conditions can occur separately or together.

Diagnosis

The clinical signs suggest PDNS but cannot be distinguished with certainty from those of the swine fevers, and advice from the state veterinary service should be sought at the beginning of an outbreak or when a case is discovered at abattoir for the first time from a farm. The pathological findings of the skin lesions, enlarged kidneys and haemorrhagic lymph nodes provide confirmation of PDNS, but are not sufficient to rule out the swine fevers, but laboratory testing for those viruses is negative and PCV2 will be present. Histopathology may be helpful as the immune glomerulonephritis is less likely in the swine fevers.

Treatment and Control

363

There is no specific treatment. Some affected animals will recover and should be supported and secondary bacterial infections controlled, but they should not be sent for slaughter until the skin lesions have disappeared, as lesions become more prominent after scalding and dehairing.

There are no specific control measures, and, as with PMWS, the outbreak will peak and then begin to decline after about 8-10 months. If management measures can control underlying PMWS (all in, all out management, use of immune sows, vaccination against respiratory disease), then the outbreak may be controlled earlier than if there is a constant supply of susceptible pigs.

References

Gresham, A., Cook, A.J.C., Thomson, J.R., Kennedy, S. (2003). Survey of veterinary practitioners on PMWS and PDNS in the UK. Vet. Rec. 153, 400-402.Segales, J., Piella, J., Marco, E., Mateu de Antonio, E.M., Espuna, E., Domingo, M. (1998). Porcine dermatitis and nephropathy syndrome in Spain. Vet. Rec. 142, 483-488.
Thibault, S., Drolet, R., Germain, M.C., D'Allaire, S., LaRochelle, R., Magar, R. (1998). Cutaneous and systematic necrotising vasculitis in swine. Vet. Path. 35, 108-116.
Wellenberg, G.J., Stockhofe-Zurwieden, N., Jong, M.F. de, Boersma, W.J.A., Elbers, A.R.W. (2004). Excessive porcine circovirus type 2 antibody titres may trigger the development of porcine dermatitis and nephropathy syndrome: a case control study. Vet. Microbiol. 99, 203-214.

Rotting Prepuce Syndrome

This may be a form of transit erythema occurring on wheat straw or a form of the porcine dermatitis and nephropathy syndrome and occurs in uncastrated boars of 50-75 kg The ventral prepuce becomes abraded, erythematous, oedematous and exudative and may heal or progress within 48-72 hours to necrosis of prepuce and the adjacent abdominal wall. Lesions may reach 30 cm in length. Affected pigs may die and should be sent for slaughter or killed humanely.

Reference

Marriott, D.W. (1993). The rotting prepuce syndrome. Pig.Vet.J. 31, 152-159.

Stomach ulcers/Gastric Ulceration

Ulceration occurs in the pars oesophagea of the stomach to give a clearly-defined syndrome of major importance in the pig industry. It also occurs in the glandular part of the stomach where its significance is not yet clear.

1.   Gastric ulceration (Ulceration of the pars oesophagea)

Definition

Gastric ulcers of the pars oesophagea are common in pigs kept under modern husbandry conditions and may cause clinical disease or death when haemorrhage or perforation occurs. In the majority of cases, they are an incidental finding at slaughter but may reduce growth rate and feed conversion rates.

Incidence

Gastric ulceration has been identified in most pig-rearing countries. The incidence found at slaughter may vary between 2% and 60% although it may be higher in individual herds. Figures for incidence are complicated by the influence of pre-slaughter handling where increased holding time increases lesions and recording of changes as true ulceration (5.9%) erosions (11.4%) hyperkeratosis (36.7% Minnesota 1994 figures). Healed ulcers indicate a higher incidence if recorded. The mortality from the condition may reach 10% in outbreaks in fattening pigs and farrowing sows.

Aetiology

The aetiology of gastric ulceration in pigs is unknown. A number of factors have been shown to influence their development, but the condition appears to be one of multiple aetiology in which more than one factor is involved. The aetiology does not appear to be connected with age as pigs of all ages are affected. No evidence of breed incidence or hereditary transmission has been found although an association with litter has been identified within farms.

a) Infection

Infection of the gastric mucosa with two separate types of infectious agents has recently been associated with gastric ulceration. Study of the effects of acid on the stratified squamous epithelium of the pars oesophagea confirms that organic acids such as acetic acid can initiate lesions which can progress, with the assistance of hydrochloric acid to erosion and ulceration. These events are less likely with hydrochloric acid alone. Experimental studies in gnotobiotic pigs reproduced these results with cultures of lactobacilli and *Bacillus spp* and a carbohydrate rich diet. The other infectious agents are the helicobacters and arcobacters, *especially H. heilmannii*. Experimental infection with H. heilmannii has not reproduced gastric ulceration, it does not colonise the epithelium of the pars oesophagea specifically and is most common in the glandular portions of the stomach. An unnamed Helicobacter-like organism from the gastric mucosa of the pig has now been shown to colonise the stomach of gnotobiotic pigs and cause gastrooesophageal ulceration and may be the cause or important in the disease.
Ulceration of the gastric fundus has been observed in a number of infectious conditions, e.g. swine fever, T.G.E. and *S.choleraesuis* infection. Studies of the organisms associated with the bases of ulcers have shown that staphylococci, streptococci and *Candida albicans* are present in many cases. Pneumonia has been associated with gastric ulceration.
Ulceration of the glandular portion of the stomach has also been associated with infection by Hyostrongylus rubidus and may occur following achlorhydria in chronic enteric disease.

b) Toxicity

Copper toxicity was once considered as contributing to gastric ulcer
c)   Nutrition

A number of attempts have been made to protect pigs from gastric ulceration by the addition of vitamins, etc., to the feed. Some success has been claimed when selenium, alpha tocopherol, cystine or methionine supplements are given or when the proportion of unsaturated fatty acids in the diet is lowered. High levels of oxidised unsaturated fatty acids may play some part in the aetiology of the condition. It has been suggested that zinc supplementation may reduce the incidence. There are clear associations between the use of wheat in feeds and the occurrence of the condition.

d) Feed processing

Studies of the effects of the particle size of feeds and their fibre content have shown that finely-ground pelleted feeds may predispose to gastric ulceration. It has been suggested that the increased moisture content of the stomach contents of pigs fed on finely-ground feed may allow better mixing of the enzymes and closer contact of ingesta and the epithelium of the oesophageal area. Pepsin levels are higher in the stomachs of pigs fed on finely-ground and pelleted feeds, and the pars oesophagea is exposed to lower pH and more bile salts in such conditions. The critical feed particle sizes used to demonstrate these effects are 550 μm as the fine particle and 750 μm for the coarse particle. These particle sizes may not be associated with the initiation of the condition, but play a major part in the maintenance and exacerbation of the lesions.

e) Season

Seasonal changes in incidence have been observed.

f) Stress

Gastric function has long been known to be affected by stress and 'stresses' such as transport, starvation, mixing, overcrowding, increase the incidence of gastric ulceration in pigs. Ulceration appears more common in pigs of middle social rank. The exact mechanism whereby stress produces or enhances gastric ulceration is not clear, but may be concerned with the increased secretion of hydrochloric acid and digestive enzymes during stress. Experiments which provide chronic stress alone do not result in ulceration.

g) Starvation

Starvation for 24 hours can cause early changes to the epithelium of the pars oesophagea which appear to be exacerbated or reduced by diet and other factors. Many of the conditions listed above cause reduction in food intake (major infectious diseases, transport, stress of mixing, pneumonia) and their association with ulceration may result from reduction in food intake

Pathogenesis

Hyperkeratosis of the pars oesophagea proceeds to erosion and then to ulceration. Ulcers may remain open and blood vessels may rupture. Healing may occur at any stage but is accompanied by scarring if ulceration has occurred.

Clinical signs

The disease may vary from peracute to subclinical. Peracute cases are often found dead in good condition. Animals of any age may be affected, but sows before and after parturition and rapidly growing pigs between 20 and 40 kg are most commonly affected. Animals which survive the acute intragastric haemorrhage become recumbent, breathe rapidly and may grind their teeth in pain. They refuse to eat or drink, the body temperature is low and all visible mucous membranes are cold and pale. Affected pigs may vomit and stand with a rigid back. Pain can be elicited by pressure at the xiphisternum. Subacute cases may show intermittent melaena, passing dark, dry faeces, with anorexia and a reduced growth rate. The subclinical form is most commonly seen at slaughter. Affected pigs grow significantly more slowly than unaffected animals especially when cicatrisation of the oesophagus has occurred.

Pathological findings

Stomach ulcers occur most commonly in the oesophageal area surrounding the cardia which is covered with stratified squamous epithelium. There may also be ulcers or gastritis in mucus and acid-secreting regions. There may be linear, raised parakeratotic lesions of the eosophageal epithelium.

Normal epithelium in this area is pearly white and has been scored 0 in numerical scoring systems. Changes ranging from thickened, hardened, rough yellow-brown epithelium (score 1) through slight, light brown superficial erosions and sloughing (score 2) to ulcerations reaching the deeper layers (score 3) may all be seen. The bases of the ulcers may be covered with necrotic material and clotted blood may be seen adhering to exposed blood vessels. Chronic ulcers may appear as craters floored by the smooth muscle. Scarring may reduce the size of the cardiac sphincter.

Pigs which have died as a result of haemorrhage from an ulcer are pale, the stomach is often distended with clotted blood and the intestines are filled with blood which may be altered. The haemorrhage may be traced to the edge or floor of an acute ulcer or to the sides of a chronic one. Perforation may also occur.

Ulcers may also heal with scarring. Histological sections of early lesions show inflammation of the lamina propria, swelling of the cells of the epithelium and extension of the rete pegs into the lamina propria. The bases of ulcers are usually infiltrated with eosinophils, mononuclear cells and neutrophils. In chronic ulcers, fibrosis of the base may occur. Fibrinonecrotic membranes containing bacteria may be present. Healing ulcers become covered with epithelium and are fibrotic.

Diagnosis

Gastric ulceration is difficult to diagnose in the live pig without recourse to endoscopy. The presence of tarry blood in the faeces for 3-8 days without the presence of fever or other signs and pallor of the mucous membranes or white parts of the animal, and raised plasma pepsinogens (5.15 affected 1.5 normal), are suggestive of gastric ulceration. In younger pigs, proliferative haemorrhagic enteropathy produces similar signs. Gastric ulceration must be differentiated from swine dysentery which normally affects all the pigs in a group. The faeces of pigs affected with swine dysentery normally contain mucus and fresh blood and when the blood-stained intestine is rinsed, the mucosa appears congested and inflamed. In gastric ulceration, clotted blood washes off. Salmonellosis is usually associated with fever and a putrid diarrhoea.

Anaesthesia followed by endoscopy can allow the cardia to be inspected. Ulceration can be clearly seen, but hyperkeratosis may not be detectable. The procedure may take as little as 8 minutes per pig. Ulceration detected by endoscopy may not appear as severe at postmortem examination.

Treatment and control

Treatment by blood transfusion or i.v. fluid therapy can relieve the clinical signs and ranitidine syrup may be given orally at 300 mg/sow/day. Antimicrobial cover may also assist the recovery of valuable individual animals. Gastric ulceration may be reduced by removing stress, relieving overcrowding, using proper ventilation and also by reducing the growth rate of young stock by omitting growth promoters from the rations and by increasing fibre levels in the diet, particularly by the use of oats or sugar beet pulp. Zinc, selenium and Vitamin E levels should be supplemented if inadequate. Specific measures shown to reduce ulceration include the use of melatonin 5mg/Kg in feed, methionine supplementation and the inclusion of straw . The most important preventive measure is to increase the particle size of the ration to 750 μm for a three week period after events likely to cause the early lesions and ensuring that the ration is fed as meal rather than pellet. Even developed ulcers may resolve if this feeding regime is adopted. Particle size in pellets may also be increased. The pH of whey should be checked and very acid whey should not be fed.

References

Argenzio, R.A., Eisemann, J. (1996). Mechanisms of acid injury in porcine gastro-oesophageal mucosa. Am.J.Vet.Res. **57**, 564-573.

Ayles, H.L., Friendship, R.M., Ball, R.O. (1996). Effect of dietary particle size on gastric ulcers assessed by endoscopic examination and relationship between ulcer severity and growth performance of individually-fed pigs. Swine health and Production **4**, 211-216.

Davies, P.R., Grass, J.J., Marsh, W.E., Bahnson, P.B., Dial, G.D. (1994). Time of slaughter affects prevalence of lesions of the pars oesophagea of pigs. Proc.IPVS **13**, 471.

Kavanagh, N. (1994). Gastric ulcers in pigs. In Practice **16**, 209-213.

Krakowka, S., Eaton, K.A., Rings, D.M., Argenzio, R.A. (1998). Production of gastro-oesophageal erosions and ulcers in gnotobiotic swine monoinfected with fermentative commensal bacteria and fed high carbohydrate diet. Vet. Path. **35**, 274-282.

Krakowka, S., Rings, D.M., Ellis, J.A. (2005). Experimental Induction of bacterial gastritis and gastric ulcer disease in gnotobiotic swine inoculated with porcine *Helicobacter*-like species. A.J.Vet.Res. **66**, 945-952.

Mackin, A.J., Friendship, R.M., Ball, R.O., Ayles, H.L. (1997). Development and evaluation of an endoscopic technique permitting rapid visualisation of the cardiac region of the porcine stomach. Can. J.Vet. Res. **61**, 121-127.

2. Ulceration of the glandular parts

Ulceration of the fundes, pylonis and cardia occurs in a number of specific infectious diseases such as T.G.E. *S.cholerae suis* infection and swine fever. Gastritis occurs as a result of *H.rubidus* infection in the stomachs of adults and gastritis of varying degrees of severity follows the achlorhydria associated with diarrhoeic disease. *Helicobacter* heilmannii (spiral organisms long known from the crypts and ulceration of this part of the stomach) may not be important. Clinical signs, pathogenesis and economic importance (if any) of this widespread condition have not yet been evaluated.

Gastric Torsion in Sows

A condition in which sudden death from gastric torsion follows feeding. The condition occurs most commonly following once-daily feeding and can be prevented by feeding twice daily, preferably rapidly, using automatic feeders. In one survey in the UK it was responsible for up to 12% of sow deaths with intestinal torsions.

Affected pigs are found to have stomachs grossly distended with food and twisted about the mesenteric axis. Splenic torsion and, sometimes, associated splenic rupture, may also be present. It is thought that rapid ingestion of feed, possibly coupled with fermentation of the food mass, leads to dilatation and, in conditions of excitement, to torsion. If pigs are seen at the dilated stage, exercise may prove beneficial.

Retroversion of the Bladder (in Sows)

Detected at farrowing when exhausted sows may be found to have a mass occluding the anterior vagina. This is the bladder which has been reflected. If the sow is made to stand, the bladder can be manipulated out of the way. Death may otherwise occur.

The Intestinal Haemorrhage Syndrome
"Bloody Gut"/Whey Bloat

Definition

A syndrome in which large pigs 35 kg - adult become pale, have distended abdomens and die suddenly. At post-mortem examination, the small intestine is distended with blood-stained fluid and there may be gaseous distension of the colon. Volvulus may be present and there is usually blood-stained fluid in the abdomen. The carcase is pale.

Aetiology

a) Whey. In whey-fed pigs, an anticlockwise torsion of the whole intestinal mass allows the caecum to point cranially. The large and small intestines are involved and the twist occurs at the root of the mesentery and does not involve the duodenum. Affected pigs may be seen live. Some appear bloated and recover, others die. Excessive gas production from whey reaching the colon has been suggested as a cause of this condition (Whey bloat or Colonic bloat).

b) Manipulation. Animals turned when anaesthetised have developed the condition.

c) Allergy. Allergy to milk protein or some other component of the diet has been suggested as a cause. The evidence for this view is the presence of large numbers of eosinophils in the lesions.

d) Non whey fed pigs. A similar syndrome may be seen in pigs fed on skim milk, or wet or dry meal. Volvulus may or may not be present and in some cases there is no gas in the caecum. The aetiology is unknown.

e) Infection. *Lawsonia intracellularis* has been suggested as a contributory cause in cases in which no volvulus occurs and enteropathogenic *E.coli*,

C.perfringens type C and enterotoxigenic *Clostridium perfringens* Type A may be involved in some An enterotoxin may be involved in some.

Clinical signs

Found dead or seen with abdominal colic, a mild rise in body temperature and, sometimes, pallor of the body.

Pathology

The gross pathological changes are described above. The small intestine is almost always autolytic but in animals seen to die there is massive inflammatory change with shedding of the small intestinal villous epithelium, loss of villi and migration of inflammatory cells into both the lamina propria and the lumen which is filled with cells, red cells and bacteria.

A wide variety of clostridia can be isolated from these lesions including both sporulating and vegetative *C.perfringens* Type A and *C.perfringens* enterotoxin has also been demonstrated.

Epidemiology

In whey fed units, deaths occur more commonly as the whey concentration rises. Elsewhere deaths occur sporadically, usually with one or two pigs dying in any one pen.

Diagnosis

Based on characteristic post-mortem findings.

Treatment

As deaths occur suddenly, treatment can rarely be given. A spasmolytic may be of value and may be accompanied by injection of an antibiotic. Trimethoprim:sulphonamide was used successfully on one farm where the problem occurred frequently. Change of diet may be preventative. Reduction in the whey concentration can reduce mortality but also reduces growth rate.

References

Todd J.N., Jones T.D., Morgan T.L., Francis P.G., Hewitt S.G. (1977). Intestinal haemorrhage and volvulus in whey fed pigs. Vet. Rec. **100**, 11.

Noyes, E., Pijoan C., Ruth, G., Raffe, M. (1988). Intestinal torsions in swine under anaesthesia. Vet.Rec. **122**, 47-48.

Colitis

Definition

A diarrhoea of weaned pigs of any age from weaning to slaughter (but particularly from weaning to 40kg), the cause of which is not immediately apparent and which may result in loss of performance.

Incidence

Present in 8% of herds in the UK (1997-8). Identified in France, Belgium, Denmark, The Netherlands, Canada, the U.S. and Eire.

Aetiology and pathogenesis

The syndrome is currently poorly defined and the aetiology and pathogenesis is unknown at present. In many cases described in the literature, agents known to cause disease in this age group have not been sought. Two main areas have been considered important, nutrition and infection.

Nutrition has been considered relevant because field observations suggest that the syndrome occurs on a particular feed and that when that feed is changed the disease disappears. In many cases the use of this 'suspect' feed on other farms is not associated with the syndrome. Firmer evidence comes from studies in which the same diet was fed as pellets, meal and as ground pellets. Disease occurred on the pelletised ration and not on the meal. Pigs fed ground pellets were intermediate between the groups. Pelleting may caramelise carbohydrates, alter particle size, destroy micronutrients or growth promoters and involve the use of pelleting agents or binders.

Both nutrition and infection can have the same final common pathway in the production of visible diarrhoea. Visible diarrhoea results when there is a failure of absorption in the large intestine. In colitis this can result from delivery of undigested feed components to the colon as a result of the poor digestibility of the feed (oligosaccharides and poorly-digestible proteins), the presence of antinutritional factors such as antitryptic agents, intestinal hurry, and the presence of villous atrophy resulting from infection. The undigested food components provide a substrate for fermentation. This can be one component contributing to failure of the large intestinal mucosa to absorb water, but specific infections of the mucosa can reduce or abolish its ability to absorb water and cause the diarrhoea or pasty faeces which are features of the disease. Nutritional factors known to affect digestion include the presence of trypsin inhibitors in peas, beans and raw soya and the effects of poor quality fat. Infection may also be important, and colitis occurs after lactogenic immunity to enteric pathogens and 'normal' flora is withdrawn at weaning although passive serum antibody to some pathogens may persist until 6-10 weeks of age. Exposure of pigs to colonisation or infection with a wide range of agents occurs from that time onward at a rate which depends upon exposure to the agent and the immune status of the individual pig. Enteric pathogens suppressed by antimicrobial treatment and the mixing which occurrs when housing is changed enhance the spread of agents to which immunity is lacking. The age of onset of specific infections may be affected by these management practices.

Infection of the small intestine of the growing pig with rotaviruses, epidemic diarrhoea and enteroviruses is common and may cause residual villous atrophy. T.G.E. may also occur in immune herds at this period. Bacterial diseases such as classic enterotoxigenic *E.coli* enteritis and attaching and effacing *E.coli* enteritis, salmonellosis and *Lawsonia intracellularis* infection of the small intestine, cryptosporidiosis and some *Eimeria* infections may all reduce small intestinal digestion. Torovirus, enterovirus and some degree of rotavirus infection may all infect the colon at this stage. Primary bacterial pathogens of the large intestine include *B. hyodysenteriae*, *B. pilosicoli*, other enteric spirochaetes, *L.intracellularis*, salmonellae, *Yersinia enterocolitica* or *Y. pseudotuberculosis* and secondary infections include campylobacters. Studies with *C.perfringens* type A have shown that this organism can initiate a syndrome resembling some forms of "colitis" and *Bacteroides fragilis* strains have also been shown to be capable of causing diarrhoea in weaned pigs.

Parasites such as Oesophagostomum and *Trichuris suis* may also damage the large intestinal mucosa and some *Eimeria* species may also affect the large intestine. Cryptosporidia are often present in the intestines of affected pigs. Both *Balantidium coli* and *Tritrichomonas spp.* may colonise lesions caused by other agents.

These infectious agents must be considered when studying the aetiology and pathogenesis of the syndrome. They may be solely responsible for the 'colitis' (a recent Scottish study failed to identify one of the above agents in only 8/98 affected farms) interact with nutrition by lowering the absorptive capacity of the small intestine by causing villous atrophy and allowing nutirents to reach the large intestine or by reducing the absorptive capacity of the large intestine.

Clinical signs

Softening of the faeces and the occasional passage of mucus. Diarrhoea can also develop. Individual pigs may be affected for 3-20 days and appear hollow-flanked, dirty and restless. Growth rates may be depressed and feed conversion may be affected. The syndrome is most common in the 8-10 week age group but can occur later. The faeces of affected pigs may froth and bubble immediately after taking from the rectum.

Pathology

In classic 'colitis' only the large intestine is affected. The contents are fluid, contain bubbles and sometimes have an oily sheen. In early cases the mucosa appears to be normal even histologically, and on scanning electron microscopy. Local loss of microvilli from colonic epithelial cells may occur. In some cases there may be more obvious colonic lesions.

Epidemiology

Present within individual farms, transfer from farm to farm may occur with breeding stock. The condition may be present more commonly under unhygienic conditions. There may be an association with feed type.

Diagnosis

Diagnosis is based on the clinical signs and the absence of the comprehensive list of agents listed above. The small intestine should be examined post-mortem and the respiratory tract should be examined where poor growth rate is a problem, to confirm that pneumonic conditions are not contributing to the poor productivity.

Treatment and control

Specific causes of mild diarrhoea and colitis such as spirochaetal diarrhoea should be identified and treated or controlled. In cases where spirochaetal diarrhoea has been identified, tiamulin, valnemulin, lincomycin or tylosin have been used successfully. Where *C.perfringens* type A is important, avoparcin inclusion as the growth promoter had dramatic effects , but amoxycillin or trimethoprim sulphonamide may be of value. Where *L. intracellularis* or *Y.enterocolitica* is present, tetracyclines may be of value. Accommodation should be cleaned and all-in, all-out housing adopted.

Nutritional colitis can be eliminated in some cases by changing pelleted feed for meal (but not for reground pellets) or by using a diet specifically formulated to prevent the condition. Such diets have been formulated to eliminate or reduce antitryptic factors (for example by inactivating thoroughly those present in soya meal) and indigestible carbohydrates. The use of some varieties of wheats or peas may be avoided. These diets are available commercially in the UK, but may not be available in all countries. It may be difficult to prepare them where home mixing is practised.

Other diseases such as pleuropneumonia, which contribute to growth depression in this age group should be eliminated and other enteric diseases identified should be treated and controlled.

References

Jestin, A., Popoff, M.R., Mahe, S. (1985). Epizootiogic investigations of a diarrhoeic syndrome in fattening pigs. Am. J. Vet. Res. **46**, 2149-2151.
Smith, W.J. and Nelson, E.P. (1987). Grower Scour/non-specific colitis. Vet. Rec. **121**, 334.
Thomson, J.R., Smith, W.J., Murray, B.P., Murray, D., Dick, J.E., Sumption, K.J. (2001). Porcine enteric spirochaete infections in the UK: surveillance data and preliminary investigation of atypical isolates. Anim.Health.Res.Rev.**2**, 31-36.

Rectal Stricture Syndrome

Definition

A syndrome in which the rectum of growing and finishing pigs becomes fibrosed and the animal dies with megacolon.

Incidence

The condition occurs worldwide in outbreaks affecting up to 10% of growing or finishing pigs, but is sporadic.

Aetiology and pathogenesis

The aetiology is unknown, but it often follows untreated rectal prolapse in which sloughing has occurred and may follow any enteritis in which excoriation of the rectal mucosa and the associated mucocutaneous junction is a feature. This area has a blood supply from the posterior haemorrhoidal artery and from the perineal arteries but mucosal ulceration or arteriolar thrombosis at the interface may cause damage to the mucosa and result in scarring. In male pigs the presence of the retractor penis muscle lying across the rectum at this point may exacerbate changes. The circulatory and inflammatory changes are commonly due to salmonella infections but in the UK this is not always the case. In some cases the syndrome follows the use of an antimicrobial such as tylosin and it has been said to result from overgrowth by *Candida spp.* and other yeasts which may be isolated from affected colons. Another site at the brim of the pubis may be inflamed in the chronic stage of enteric disease. Bacteria such as *Selenomonas* appear to be associated with the lesions and chlamydia and *Lawsonia intracellularis* may be present.

The condition often develops within 10 days of a dietary change and is often preceded by stickiness and erythema at the mucocutaneous junction accompanied by a marked reluctance to defaecate.

Clinical signs

Affected pigs become dull, depressed, anorexic and cease to grow. The abdomen becomes grossly distended and the outline of the swollen colon may be seen. In some cases the partially occluded rectum allows the passage of soft ribbon-like motions.

Humane slaughter should be carried out when complete rectal stricture is present and when two successive weighings one week apart show no growth.

Pathology

A grossly distended large intestine is seen. A band of fibrous tissue, sometimes with abscessation on its dorsal side, may be found at the anus, 3-4 cm proximal to it or at the brim of the pubis up to 10 cm cranial to the anus.

Diagnosis

The presence of a pig aged 5 weeks or more with a distended abdomen depressed and standing in the corner of a pen is suggestive and the diagnosis can be confirmed by the insertion of a thermometer or gloved finger into the rectum when an obstruction will be met 2-4 cm into the rectum. Post-mortem examination will confirm.

Treatment and control

It is technically possible to exteriorise the constricted rectum dorsal to the anus while the pig is anaesthetised. The rectum can be cut proximal to the obstruction and sewn in to the perineum to form a new anus. A rubber ring can be used to exteriorise the caecum or mid-colon in a colostomy. Surgically treated pigs may grow rapidly to gain market weight or may develop fresh strictures. Animals which fail to gain weight for the first three weeks post-operation should be destroyed. The syndrome may be reduced in incidence by the prompt repair of rectal prolapses (see below) and the treatment of outbreaks of chronic diarrhoea in animals at risk may eliminate the early inflammatory lesions of the rectal wall and prevent the disease.

Rectal Prolapse

Rectal prolapse may occur in pigs of any age but is more common in males aged 14-16 weeks. In male piglets it may follow straining resulting from the impaction of phosphate crystals in the urethra. In weaned pigs it may follow medication with tylosin and to a lesser extent other antimicrobials and is often accompanied by soft faeces and by coughing. The condition has been reported to follow the inclusion of 20% excess lysine in the diet. The rectal mucosa protrudes visibly and can be damaged when pigs are mixed and fight as a result of the raised abdominal pressure of the alarm calls. The hyperoestrogenism associated with zearalenone may predispose to the condition in sows but most commonly it is a consequence of tethering heavily gravid sows with the hindquarters lower than the body or hanging over a drop in countries where tethering is still permitted..

The consequences are similar in all cases. The prolapsed rectum may become reduced naturally, become strangulated, necrotic and drop off or be bitten off by the other pigs. Rectal stricture, death from loss of blood or peritonitis may all occur. Animals may recover if separated from their fellows, the prolapse may be reduced under anaesthetic and secured by a purse-string suture or amputated surgically. Animals may be treated in their groups by the insertion of an 18-20 cm helical corrugated plastic tube of 1.5 cm diameter for weaners and fatteners and 2-3 cm diameter for sows into the prolapse. Heavy duty rubber bands are placed over the prolapse near the anal ring. Tube and prolapse drop off after 5-7 days.

Affected animals of slaughter weight may be penned separately and transported for slaughter but extensively and irreparably-damaged animals should be slaughtered humanely.

References

Amass, S.F., Schinckel, A.P., Clark, L.K. (1995). Increased prevalence of rectal prolapse in growing/finishing swine fed a diet containing excess lysine. Vet. Rec. **137**, 519-520.

Douglas, R.G.A. (1985). A simple method for correcting rectal prolapse in pigs. Vet.Rec. **117**, 129.

Gardner, I.A., Hird, D.W., Franti, C.E., Glenn, J. (1988). Patterns and determinants of rectal prolapse in a herd of pigs. Vet.Rec. **123**, 222-225.

Uterine and Vaginal Prolapse

Similar in the sow to rectal prolapse but may also follow parturition, damage at service or the intake of zearalenone. May be reduced and secured under anaesthetic or amputated if necrotic. Uterine prolapse reduction is so traumatic that humane slaughter should be considered, but one series reported surgical success in 23/33 cases.

Heat Stroke

As environmental temperatures increase from 22°C to 40-41°C, pigs seek shade, water, mud or slurry in order to wallow and cool themselves. Animals in transit, stressed and unable to cool themselves - in sow stalls, farrowing crates or in full sun become dyspnoeic, salivate, breathe with difficulty and become restless. They may later become frenzied, cyanotic and die. A body temperature of 41°C (106°F) - 43°C (110 F) may be recorded. Pathological findings include blood-stained foam in the nostrils and trachea, congestion and haemorrhage in the carcase and some oedema, particularly in the lungs. Productivity may be depressed as may be feed intake. Diagnosis is based on history of high temperature and absence of other causes of death.

Treatment involves tranquillising affected pigs, e.g. with azaperone, cooling the limbs and belly with water and injecting a corticosteroid. Prevention: increase ventilation or, in hot countries, provide cold running water or sprinklers in each pen. N.B. The porcine stress syndrome may develop in environmental temperatures of 22°C+.

References

McGlone, J.J., Stansbury, W.F., Tribble, L.F. (1987). Effects of heat and social stressors on young pig performance. J.Animal Science 65, 456-462.
McGlone, J.J., Stansbury, W.F., Tribble L.F. (1988). Management of lactating sows during heat stress. J.Anim. Sci. 66, 885-891.

Sunburn

A cause of dermatitis in White pigs outdoors.   Reddening, oedema and then crusting and peeling occur. Affected pigs may be very hot to the touch. Shade (from protective nets if necessary) or wallows are sufficient to prevent and cure. Vesicles may result from contact with celery or parsnip leaves and exposure to the sun.

Frostbite

Occurs following exclusion of sows from shelter by other sows of the group. Deaths from chilling have recently been recorded in Vietnamese Pot Bellied pigs housed outdoors in winter in the UK.

Electrocution

This occurs when electrical wiring is directly available to pigs or when faulty electrical connections result in current passing through metal cage fittings. It may be caused by lightning strike in outdoor animals. Some affected pigs are found dead and may have burn marks at the point of contact. Survivors may be found in a dog-sitting position with posterior paresis, lame and unwilling to feed.

Carcases are congested and there may be froth on the lips. There is froth in the trachea and oedema of the lungs. Blood splashing of the heart and musculature is common. Examination of the skeleton frequently reveals fractures of vertebrae, particularly in the thoracic region, of the humerus and especially of the neck of the scapula, the pelvis and the neck of the femur. In some cases the fractures are of the body of vertebra L7, resulting in severance of the spinal cord and nerves and displacement of the sacrum. Decomposition often occurs rapidly following death by electrocution.

The skeletal damage, any burn marks and proximity to electric wiring differentiate sudden death from this cause from many other causes of sudden death including cardiac failure, septicaemias such as anthrax and erysipelas. Bacteriology or classic gross lesions distinguish the condition from the bacterial septicaemias, gastric torsion, gastric ulceration, vegetative endocarditis, the porcine stress syndrome, heatstroke and C.novyi infection.

When electrocution is suspected ensure that all metalwork and dead pigs are no longer live before investigation. In view of the fractures, animals unable to walk or rise should be killed humanely on site and not transported for slaughter.

Reference:

Alstine, W.G.van, Widmer, W.R. (2003). Lightning injury in an outdoor swine herd. J.Vet. Diagn. Invest. 15, 289-291.

Salt Poisoning

Salt poisoning is usually due to water deprivation and has been dealt with under that heading.

Carbon Monoxide Poisoning

Dramatic increases in the stillbirth rate may accompany the use of faulty gas heaters in poorly ventilated farrowing accommodation. Stillbirth rates up to 53% have been recorded. 50 ppm carbon monoxide is the acceptable upper limit and at levels of 120-150 ppm abortion and stillbirth occur. At 150-200 ppm, foetal blood reaches carboxy haemoglobin saturation point within 24-48 hours and the foetus dies. Affected piglets' tissues are cherry-red, there are serosanguineous pleural effusions, hypoxic leuco-encephalopathy and extramedullary haemopoiesis. Levels of 200-300 ppm impair the growth and activity of newborn piglets. No changes are seen in the sow. 200 ppm. does not appear to affect weaners but 200-300 ppm. may reduce performance.

Carbon monoxide can affect man and should be cleared before investigation of the accommodation is carried out.

References

Dominick, M.A. and Carson, T.L. (1983). Effects of carbon monoxide exposure on pregnant sows and their foetuses. Am.J.Vet.Res. **44**, 35-40.
Jennings, D.S. (2001). Chronic carbon monoxide poisoning in weaners. Pig J. **48**, 150-151.
Morris, G.L. Curtis S.E., Simon, J. (1985). Perinatal piglets under sublethal concentrations of atmospheric carbon monoxide. J.Anim.Sci. **61**, 1070-1079.
Morris, G.L., Curtis, S.E., Widowski, T.M. (1985). Weanling pigs under sublethal concentrations of atmospheric carbon monoxide. J.Animal Science **61**, 1080-1087.

Ammonia

Reduction in growth rate and feed conversion rate of up to 24% can result when atmospheric ammonia levels reach 150 ppm. Changes in the nasal mucosa may occur at levels as low as 25ppm.

Nitrate and Nitrite Poisoning

Definition

The ingestion of nitrate or nitrite results in gastroenteritis and dyspnoea, weakness, cyanosis and death.

Incidence

Occurs as outbreaks in finishing pigs on whey diets and where pigs have access to nitrates or more commonly, nitrites.

Aetiology and pathogenesis

Nitrate in straw and ammonia in slurry can be converted to nitrite by microbial action. Nitrite is available to the pig in drainage water and in water of condensation in badly-ventilated accommodation where concentrations may reach 8-10,000 ppm. Nitrites in whey can result from cheese-making. The lethal dose of potassium nitrite appears to be 22 mg/kg and for sodium nitrite is 88 mg/kg. Nitrogen dioxide may also be produced by other farm processes such as silage making. Ingested nitrate may be turned to nitrite in the gut, nitrite is absorbed and causes methaemoglobinaemia. When 75-90% of the haemoglobin is converted to methaemoglobin, deaths occur. The clinical signs and pathology are largely due to anoxia.

Clinical signs

Affected pigs have a raised respiratory rate with a rapid, weak pulse. Salivation, passage of large amounts of urine, dilated pupils, convulsions and opisthotonus all occur. Weakness and then cyanosis develop shortly before death.

Methaemoglobin can be detected in the blood, but samples need to be analysed by spectrophotometry or using the diphenylamine blue test. Recumbent animals which cannot be treated should be slaughtered humanely.

Pathology

The carcase may be brownish in colour and a brownish discolouration of the blood may be noted. Petechiae may be present on serous surfaces and oedema and emphysema of the lungs may be seen. The gastric and intestinal mucosa may be haemorrhagic and if care is taken upon opening the stomach, brown nitrogen dioxide gas may be seen.

Diagnosis

The afebrile nature of the condition and a history of whey feeding or poor ventilation, coupled with the post-mortem findings, may suggest this condition. It must be distinguished from the intestinal haemorrhage syndrome which may occur under similar conditions. Samples of gut contents or urine for nitrite determinations should be mixed with chloroform to arrest microbial nitrite production.

Treatment

Methylene blue i.v. 1-2 mg/kg bodyweight will improve affected animals. Good ventilation, removal of the source of nitrite and access to unlimited fresh water will all be beneficial.

Reference

McLoughlin, M.F., McMurray, C.H., Dodds, H.M., Evans, R.T. (1985). Nitrogen dioxide (silo gas) poisoning in pigs. Vet.Rec. **116**, 119-121.

Phenol or Coaltar Poisoning

Skin lesions: Phenols (in disinfectants) may cause teat necrosis and coronary band ulceration in piglets and cause pimples and weals on the skin when pigs are put into pens still wet with concentrated disinfectant.

Poisoning: Ingestion of phenols, cresols and coaltar products such as tarred paper and clay pigeon fragments (outdoor pigs) can cause sudden death, sometimes preceeded by weakness, depression, inappetence, abdominal tenderness and, occasionally, pallor and icterus of visible mucous membranes. Icteric or collapsed pigs should be slaughtered humanely.

Dead pigs have enlarged, friable red and yellow mottled livers. Excess fluid may be present in the body cavities, the kidneys may be enlarged and the lymph nodes haemorrhagic. Centrilobular necrosis and haemorrhage into the lobules are the most striking histological changes.

Treatment

Little or none; skin poisoning cases should be washed.

Reference

Wilkinson, J.D. (1994). Sudden deaths on an outdoor pig unit-a diagnostic exercise. Pig J. **32**, 123-128.

Warfarin Poisoning (Coumarin poisoning)

This occurs occasionally in pigs and may present as lameness, weakness and anaemia with subcutaneous haemorrhages and bleeding from all orifices, especially those of the head and anus.

Low red cell counts and prolonged clotting times may be found in blood samples and haemorrhages into the carcase are found at post-mortem examination.Treat with Vitamin K preparations, e.g. Menadione. Recovery is often complete, particularly if treatment can begin after ingestion of the poison.

Monensin poisoning

Monensin levels of 20 mg/kg-50 mg/kg body weight given orally cause anorexia, diarrhoea, ataxia, lethargy, dyspnoea, myoglobinuria and death. Electrocardiographic abnormalities are observed. Serum aspartate aminotransferase and creatine kinase levels are raised at the time that muscle and myocardial damage occurs. Pigs which have died from monensin toxicity have bilaterally-symmetrical pale areas in the diaphragm, thigh muscles, triceps, intercostal and longissimus muscles. Left atrial damage is seen in the heart, there is necrosis followed by degeneration of muscle cells and subsequent lysis and phagocytosis of cells. In damaged skeletal muscle there is hyaline necrosis, macrophage infiltration and eventually regeneration of fibres and their function. The urine is reddish-brown.

Monensin poisoning occurs in pigs given excess monensin (maximum therapeutic level 100 ppm not registered EU) or when other ionophores such as salinomycin are included at levels such as 166 ppm (8 mg/kg) and when tiamulin is included at therapeutic levels of 150-200 ppm in feed containing monensin. Similar toxicity may be seen with salinomycin, narasin and maduromycin.

Affected pigs may be killed humanely if recumbent and convulsing, but animals with posterior paresis normally recover within 10-20 days..

References

Plumlee, K.H., Johnson, B., Galey, F.D. (1995). Acute salinomycin toxicosis in pigs. J.Vet. Diagn. Invest. **7**, 419-420.

Tobin, F. (1994). Salinomycin toxicity in pigs. Pig J. **32**, 103-106.

Umemara, T., Kawaminami, A., Goryo, M., Itakura, C.(1985). Enhanced myotoxicity and involvement of both Type I and Type II fibres in tiamulin:monensin toxicosis in pigs. Vet.Pathology **22**, 409-414.

Vleet J.F. van, Amstutz H.E., Weirich, W.E., Rebar, R.H., Ferrans, V.J. (1983). Clinical, clinicopathologic and pathologic alterations of monensin toxicosis in swine. Int.J.Vet.Res. **44**, 1469-1475.

Arsanilic acid poisoning

This occurred in pigs receiving organic arsenicals when water was not freely available e.g. cold, interrupted supplies etc. Signs of toxicity include tremor of the head and incoordination later progressing to paralysis. Blindness may occur and death may result. Withdrawal of the drug and provision of unlimited fresh water normally allows recovery. Humane slaughter is advised for pigs which remain recumbent 2-3 days after withdrawal of drug.

Furazolidone toxicity

Furazolidone given at 70 mg/kg in the feed caused pigs to develop ataxia, paresis and signs of thrombocytopaenia. Higher levels caused vomiting, slight ataxia and feed refusal.

Carbadox toxicity

Three times the recommended levels (150 ppm) for 5 weeks resulted in dry faeces, reduced abdominal volume, reduced feed intake and loss of condition with altered hair coat. The colon is reduced in size with dry contents and there were adrenal and renal lesions.

Olaquindox toxicity

Ten times the recommended rate (500 ppm) resulted in inappetence, episodic paralysis and reduction in growth rate. Affected pigs were hairy. Lesions occur in the zona glomerulosa of the adrenal.

Reference

Newsholme, S.J., Walton, J.R., Elliot, G. (1986). Poor growth, episodic paralysis and adrenocortical injury in swine after accidental olaquindox overdosage. Vet.Rec. **119**, 554-555.

Reaction to Tiamulin

Reddening of the skin and, in severe cases, death may occur rarely when large pigs housed in deep manure or dirty conditions are treated for chronic swine dysentery with tiamulin at 150-200 ppm in feed. The reaction develops within 72 hours of first feeding and affects areas of faecal or manure contact. Dead pigs may have cardiac haemorrhages and the skin lesions consist of inflammation and necrosis of the epidermis. Removal of medicated feed, washing with water and provision of clean bedding cures the condition.

Reaction to Penicillin

Injections of procaine penicillin may cause an immediate reaction. Pigs may vomit, shiver and tremble and become depressed. Rarely they die.

Osteochondrosis, Degenerative Joint Disease and Epiphyseolysis

Definition

Osteochondrosis is a generalised skeletal disease with leg weakness occurring in animals less than 18 months of age. Changes are seen in the ossification process, particularly in the medial femoral condyle of the knee, the distal growth plate of the ulna and the 6th-8th costochondral junctions. The changes eventually lead to erosion of the articular cartilage and to painful osteoarthrosis of the joint. When the changes occur in the proximal growth plate of the femur the femoral head may be lost in epiphyseolysis and when they occur on the articular surfaces of joints, the condition is known as Degenerative Joint Disease

Incidence

Some degree of change may be present in up to 80% of pigs, particularly in meaty breeds such as Dutch Landrace or Swedish Landrace or Duroc.

Aetiology and pathogenesis

The aetiology is not known but histological lesions have been demonstrated in piglets 1 day of age and may therefore be congenital. Many of the traits found in osteochondrosis complex are heritable and abnormalities of the elbow joint surface are the best marker (h^2 =0.22). They become more obvious with age, although developing and healing lesions may occur at any one time. Areas of inadequately ossified cartilage remain in bone developing from the cartilaginous physis or growth plate separating epiphyseal and metaphyseal bone and at the epiphyseal-articular surface. These cartilaginous areas in bone lead to structural weakness and fracture or distortion of the bone, the separation of the cartilage from the underlying bone and to clefts in the epiphyseal plate. The underlying cause appears to be a defect in the chondrocytes which do not undergo normal hypertrophic maturation, but accumulate rough endoplasmic reticulum, lipid droplets and mitochondria. The surrounding matrix contains deposits of electron-dense material which may prevent normal vascularisation and thus ossification. A local disruption of the cartilage canal blood supply between cartilage and bone appears to be responsible for the subsequent necrosis and may be due to microfractures. The lesions may eventually heal and ossify. Growth rate and heredity appear to affect their development, but diet or flooring type appear to have no effect.

These changes lead to abnormal growth and change in the shape of bones and joints, including the vertebrae. One of the commonest sequelae identified in the UK is epiphyseolysis in which the head of the femur is shed in rapidly growing animals giving rise to leg weakness in animals approaching puberty.

Clinical signs

These include shortening of the step, knock and buck knees and swaying of the forelimbs. In the hindlimb the feet may be positioned too far forward, and pigs stand with their legs apart and show weakness at the pastern and swaying of the hindquarters. Changes increase with age. Epiphyseolysis may lead to sudden hindlimb lameness and pain at the hip but not necessarily at the stifle or hock. The affected leg is shorter than the unaffected one, but the thickness of the muscle mass makes palpation difficult. Animals may be unable to rise, adopt a dog-sitting position and resent movement. It occurs commonly in young gilts when first delivered or at service.

Osteochondrosis is a common cause of leg weakness and lameness in young breeding stock and may progress to arthrosis and deformation of affected bones or resolve completely by 6-9 months of age. Kyphosis may also develop as animals attempt to spare affected limbs. Animals unable to rise should be humanely slaughtered on the spot.

Pathology

The thickening of the cartilage with separation from underlying bone is the most prominent feature and in joints, flakes of cartilage may become 'joint mice' and give rise to synovitis. Deformation may take place at affected points in long bones or even fracture (femoral head). The microscopic changes have been described above.

Epidemiology

Common in heavy rapidly growing meaty pigs on hard flooring, but still present even in animals reared on grass or deep litter and has been recorded in wild boar. Forelimb weakness is obvious in some Duroc boars.

Diagnosis

The clinical signs are suggestive. The condition can be confirmed by radiography from 42 days in the distal humerus and from 63 days in the femur. They are readily identifiable at 100 days + and can be found at slaughter. Must be separated from inflammatory joint conditions such as erysipelas and mycoplasmal arthritis. Joint ill is usually confined to smaller pigs and foot lesions such as vesicular diseases and laminitis should be obvious. Epiphyseolysis may be confused with fracture of the femur especially pathological fracture in hypocalcaemic gilts.

Control

The growth rate of breeding stock can be reduced and it has been suggested that calcium and phosphorus levels of high nutrient density diets may need to be increased in order to supply adequate levels of these minerals in the rapidly-growing pig. Exercise may be beneficial and gilts intended for breeding may be kept in straw yards. It is much less common in Large White than in Landrace pigs and genetic studies with Duroc boars suggest that it can be selected against.

References

Blowey, R.W. (1994). Trochanter fracture and patellar osteochondrosis as causes of lameness in pigs. Vet.Rec. 134, 601-603.

Farnum, C.E., Wilsman, N.J. and Hilley, H.D. (1984). An ultrastructural analysis of osteochondritic growth plate cartilage in growing swine. Vet.Path. 21, 141-151.

Hill, M.A. (1998). Locomotory disorders of swine. Proc IPVS 15 (1) 181-194.

Hill, M.A., Ruth, G.R., Hilley, H.D. and Hansgen, D.C. (1984). Dyschondroplasias, including osteochondrosis in pigs between 29 and 150 days of age. Histological changes. Am.J.Vet.Res. 45, 903-916.

Hill, M.A., Hilley, H.D., Feeney, D.A., Ruth, G.R., Hunsgen, D.C. (1984). Dyschondroplasia, including osteochondrosis in boars between 25 and 169 day of age. Radiologic changes. Am.J.Vet.Res. 45, 917-925.

Hill, M.A., Ruth, G.R., Hilley, H.D., Torrison, J.L., Bagent, J.K. and Leman, A.D. (1985). Dyschondroplasias of growth cartilages (osteochondrosis) in cross-bred commercial pigs at 1 and 15 days of age. Vet.Rec. 116, 40-47.

Jorgenson, B., Nielsen, B. (2005). Genetic parameters for osteochondrosis traits in elbow joints of crossbred pigs and relationships with production traits. Animal Science, 81, 319-324.

Ytrehus, B., Ekman, S., Carlson, C.S., Teige, J., Reinholt, F.P. (2004). Focal changes in blood supply during normal epiphyseal growth are central in the pathogenesis of osteochondrosis in pigs. Bone (New York) 35, 1294-1306.

Proliferative osteitis

Proliferative osteitis of the femoral greater trochanter and the humeral medial condyle may cause lameness in sows. Sows with greater trochanter osteitis are usually first parity gilts after weaning, and found in the dog-sitting position and only rise with pain and discomfort Those with humeral medial epicondylar lesions are often recumbent and when made to rise do so with reluctance and have a marked forelimb lameness. There is a hard enlargement medial and proximal to the distal humerus.

Lesions of the greater trochanter appear as a haemorrhagic mass in the surrounding muscle 1-3 cm laterally and caudally from the trochanter which is covered with osteophytes and may be relatively radiolucent. The proximal end of the humerus has similar roughening of the medial condyle and in late cases extensive enlargement and damage to the elbow joint may occur, and fractures may develop.

Affected animals should be assessed as to their ability to be transported for slaughter and slaughtered humanely on site if unable to rise or to put weight on all four feet.

The condition may be reduced in its severity by care with the management of recently-weaned gilts which should not be penned on slippery floors with older animals or in large groups. Calcium and phosphorus intake during lactation should be maintained.

Reference

Blowey, R.W. (1992). Proliferative osteitis of the femoral greater trochanter and humeral medial epicondyle as a cause of lameness in sows. Vet.Rec.131, 312-315.

Hump Backed Pigs (Kyphosis)

In this condition pigs of all ages have a pronounced dip just behind the shoulders. Affected animals may mature normally, but some severely affected animals fail to grow normally and some die suddenly. The condition may be postural in some cases as the spine straightens at slaughter, whilst in others the spine does not straighten and skeletal changes may be present. These include narrowing of the vertebral canal and in some cases, the presence of hemivertebrae and fused/forked ribs. Death may occur when the spinal arteries rupture into the vertebral canal following trauma or excessive movement. Evidence for Talfan disease was found in one affected herd, but the condition also appears to be familial in some cases. Differentiate from back muscle necrosis.

Paralysed pigs should be humanely destroyed.

Foot Lesions

Foot lesions are an important cause of debility in pigs and occur in a number of systemic and nutritional conditions. In addition, foot lesions of the baby pig occur in response to the quality of the flooring and, in the adult, poor quality slatted flooring causes a posture leading to compression of the spinal nerves and eventual paralysis.

Foot Lesions in Baby Pigs

Erosion of the sole, bruising on the heels and of the accessory digits and erosion of the knees can all occur in sucking piglets when expanded metal flooring of the wrong mesh size or eroded concrete are used as flooring. Once the skin has been eroded, infection enters and can give rise to septic arthritis of the pedal joints or to synovitis and permanent lameness. Such conditions have a marked effect on growth rate and may impair it permanently if not treated.

All the lesions with the exception of tenosynovitis, are transient. Bruising of the sole occurs within 24 hours of birth, reaches a peak at 6-8 days of age and disappears by 14 days of age. Erosion of the sole reaches a peak at 5-7 days. Bruising and erosion of the heels/heel flap also disappear by 14 days of age as do accessory digit injuries which reach peak incidence at 7-8 days. Necrotic skin lesions are also transient.

Prevention depends on re-laying concrete, painting it with resin or rubber paint and on the use of mats. Plastic coating can be put on floors or they should be replaced with a perforated floor with a gap size of 10 mm or less.

Infected foot lesions do not respond completely to antimicrobial treatment in all cases. Where lesions have not resolved by weaning, the condition of the pig should be assessed and animals which are thin or unable to stand should be killed humanely.

Foot abscess (tenosynovitis) is more common in the piglets of multiparous sows with disease. Prompt control of sow disease and routine antimicrobial injection of piglets with tetracycline 100 mg at birth may reduce incidence.

References

Gardner, I.A., Hird, D.W., Sullivan, N.M., Pierce, R.J. (1990). Clinical, pathologic and microbiologic findings of foot abscess in neonatal pigs. J.Am.Vet.Med.Ass. **196**, 1791-1794.

Gardner, I.A., Hird, D.W. (1994). Risk factors for development of foot abscess in neonatal pigs. J.Am.Vet.Med.Ass. **204**, 1062-1067.

Foot Lesions in Older Pigs

One third of all sows culled in the U.K. are culled because of lameness and recent studies (1997) confirm that foot lesions are present in 93.8% finishing pigs in South Western England. The following conditions may be present.

1.   Foot-rot.

A term used to describe a variety of septic conditions affecting the claws of pigs of all ages. The primary lesion is some form of defect or penetration of wall or bearing surface of hoof which provides point of entry for secondary bacterial invasion. These include erosions of sole, heel and toe, fissures in the wall (sandcrack) and separation of wall from sole at the white line. Infection spreads in the hoof in 3 possible ways - a deep necrotic ulcer may develop involving the laminae and coronary band, necrotic tracks may reach the coronary band and form ulcers, or infection may penetrate deeply and involve the deep digital flexor tendon, or phalangeal bones or joints. When abscesses burst at the coronet, the condition is known as "bush-foot". Abrasive and chemical effects of newly-laid concrete contribute to the production of hoof defects. Wet, unhygienic conditions and poor bedding also contribute to what is often a herd problem. Bacteria such as *F.necrophorum, A.pyogenes* and spirochaetes may infect the lesions.

Clinical signs

Lameness depends on the number of feet involved. Affected animals tend to walk on tip-toe, with "paddling" or "goose-stepping" gait, and are reluctant to rise and move and may sit on their haunches. Lateral claws, especially of hind feet, are most commonly affected. The affected claw is warm, painful and the primary lesion is usually apparent. Severe pain occurs when abscesses develop at the coronary band and the leg is often held off the ground. Cellulitis may occur in the limb and reach the carpus or the hock. The heel and coronary band become swollen and blue-black in colour, with multiple sinus formation. Septicaemia and bacteraemia can occur and secondary abscesses may occur elsewhere, e.g. in brain, spine and liver. Bone and joint involvement may be seen. Rarefaction of the third phalangeal bone may occur. Alteration in joint spaces and new bone formation may also be noted.

Affected sows should be assessed for humane slaughter. Those too lame to transport, unable to bear weight on the limb or recumbent, should be humanely destroyed on the spot.

Treatment

Improve hygiene and management. In particular, ensure that slats have pencil edges and are at least 100 mm wide. Pigs should be run through foot baths containing 5-10% formalin (2-3 times a week). Paring septic hoof lesions, poulticing, and bandaging help, but are rarely economic. Amputation of the affected claw may be carried out. Inject with antibiotic such as tetracycline, ampicillin and use of a spray, e.g. tetracycline on local lesion. Ensure that biotin level of ration is adequate, particularly in the gilts of the herd.

2.   Laminitis.

Occurs mainly in boars and heavily pregnant or recently farrowed sows. Sometimes associated with post-parturient fever, the signs of which can mask the laminitis.

Clinical signs

Stiffness, reluctance to move, affected animals walk on the front of carpi, and are recumbent for long periods. Claws are warm and tender. Pulsation of digital arteries is prominent.

Treatment

Corticosteroids, anti-histamines, non steroidal anti-inflammatories. Reduce feed and, if fever, give a broad-spectrum antibiotic parenterally.

3.   Overgrowth and deformity of claws

Claws are not identical in size or shape. The lateral claws are slightly larger and broader. This is especially evident in the hind feet of pigs over 6 months of age. The toe is curved in the lateral, and pointed in the medial claw. Overgrowth is mainly seen in pigs over 1 year. The commonest causes are keeping pigs on muddy ground or on very deep litter with insufficient exercise. Boars, especially those kept in small pens, are often affected. Generally it only affects the main claws, but sometimes the accessory claws may also be affected. When a single claw is overgrown, it often results from a change in weight bearing secondary to some painful lesion. Gross deformity is less common and is usually congenital and may occur in one or a number of claws in the same pigs.

4.   Erosive foot lesions

These account for many of the foot lesions present in finishing pigs. In one English study, toe erosion was present in 33.0%, sole erosion in 62.1%, heel erosion in 13% and heel flaps in 14.4%. False sandcrack was present in 23.9% and wall separation in 11.5%.

References

Kornegay, E.T., Bryant, K.L., Notter, D.R. (1990). Toe lesion development in gilts and sows housed in confinement as influenced by two size and location. Applied Agri.Res. 5, 327-334.

Mouttotou, N., Hatchell, F.M., Lundervold, M., Greene, L.E. (1997). Prevalence and distribution of foot lesions in finishing pigs in South West England. Vet. Rec. 141, 115-120.

Wells, G.A.H. (1984). Locomotor disorders of the pig. In Practice 6, 43-53.

Adventitious Bursitis

Bursitis is common on the hocks of pigs which have been reared on hard floors from birth and may be present on up to 85% of pigs at slaughter. Bursae which are soft and fluctuating may give rise to pain and lameness. They occur most frequently on the lateroplantar, plantar, medial and point of the hock in white pigs. They are associated with lesions of the claws but not with infection. Trimming may be required at slaughter and up to 0.5 kg may be lost by growth depression and adverse effects on growth and carcase conformation..

The condition can be prevented by bedding on deep straw or sawdust and some types of slat such as polypropylene slats appear not to cause them.

References

386

Mouttotou, N., Hatchell, F.M., Greene, L.E. (1998). Adventitious bursitis of the hock in finishing pigs: prevalence, distribution and association with floor type and foot lesions. Vet. Rec. **142**, 109-114.
Smith, W.J., Smith, M. (1990). Adventitious bursitis of the hock, results of a study examining the epidemiology and development. Proc. IPVS. **11**, 300.

Teat necrosis

Teat necrosis may occur in neonatal pigs, appears as a black scab on each necrotic teat and affected piglets may reach 20% in some affected herds. It results from floor abrasion and is greatest on heated concrete floors with no bedding. A genetic predisposition has been identified. Teats which were necrotic in neonates may not develop in pubertal and farrowing gilts. Prevention involves using rubber matting or bedding in farrowing pens or placing bandage or plastic skin on the undersides of neonatal gilts.

Teat damage

May result from piglet biting, and if so, piglet's teeth may be clipped. Ends of teats may be cut off by sharp expanded metal floors.

Vulval damage

Vulvas may be damaged in neonates by being cut off in perforated floors and in sows during farrowing through normal tears or by damage against farrowing crate bars. Recently damage by rats which bite the vulvas of tethered sows has been seen. Animals are found with eroded vulvas and pools of blood. Vulva biting in sows has become a problem where loose housing is practised. It occurs when there is queueing for food or when heavily-pregnant sows on restricted rations are mixed in large groups. Increases in the number of times such sows are fed daily, inclusion of roughage in the diet, reduction of group size to 10 and stabilisation of groups may reduce it.

Other injuries

Fighting may lead to severe scratching and cuts, sharp fittings may also lead to cuts and kennelled sows may push through narrow doors and damage their shoulders. Pressure sores may develop when thin sows are penned on concrete and localised abscesses may occur on the skin particularly at injection sites and over the tail head and shoulder. Lesions in the backs of sows housed outdoors may be caused by crows or magpies which peck them.

Ear. Flank. Tail Biting and Penis Sucking

These vices all occur as a result of poor husbandry conditions and can be prevented by improving ventilation and especially reducing mean air speed, reducing humidity, reducing group size and the size variation within a group and by providing straw bedding, play chains, propellers, increased trough or feeder space or by using single space feeders.

Once these vices have begun, affected pigs may have to be removed from a group or, conversely, the animal carrying out the damage may have to be removed. These conditions may occur even under apparently ideal conditions.

Ear biting can lead to the loss of the whole ear or to necrotic crumbling lesions, particularly on the lower part of the pinna. They should be distinguished from the necrosis found in salmonellosis and other septicaemic diseases. Cervical lymph node enlargement may occur.

Flank biting must be distinguished from lesions of pig pox, trauma from rough pen fittings, and exudative epidermitis. As these lesions often contain S. hyicus, this organism has been suggested as a possible cause.

Tail biting is the most common and potentially the most serious of the vices. The tail may be chowed to the root and pigs may excavate a cavity in the perineum. Death frequently follows. Less severe damage frequently leads to local infection and to pyaemia with abscess formation, endocarditis and paralysis from spinal abscesses. A.pyogenes is the organism most frequently incriminated. A consequence of these injuries and the presence of infection is the requirement to inspect carcases more closely at abattoir.

Affected pigs should be assessed, penned separately if injuries are not severe, treated with parenteral antimicrobial, the lesions sprayed with a bitter disinfectant or antimicrobial spray and sent for slaughter as soon as possible, having notified the abattoir of the injuries and penned the animal separately. Paralysed pigs or those with extensive lesions should be killed humanely.

The condition can be prevented to a large extent by docking the tails of piglets. This produces a neuroma and renders the tail sensitive to biting. The pig responsible may be removed and the light may be lowered. Tail biting is further reduced by ensuring the absence of draughts. Straw bedding may help, but is no guarantee that tail biting will be prevented.

References

Done,S.H., Guise, J., Chennells, D. (2003). Tail Biting and Tail Docking in pigs. Pig J. **51**, 136-154.
Hunter, E.J., Jones, T.A., Guise, H.J., Penny, R.H.C., Hoste, S. (1999). Tail biting in pigs 1. the prevalence at six UK abattoirs and the relationship of tail biting with docking, sex and other carcase damage. Pig J. **43**, 18-32.

Penis sucking Also belly sucking/nuzzling. Least serious vice, results in a pendulous prepuce and may result from premature weaning or failure to adapt to drinkers.

GUIDE TO THE DIFFERENTIAL DIAGNOSIS OF PIG DISEASES

This section is intended as a guide to the notes on individual conditions. It is in the form of a list of the more common conditions seen in particular age groups of pig and takes no account of the conditions most likely to occur in individual husbandry systems. Conditions which are common will be marked thus*.

Disease of young piglets (Neonatal Morbidity and mortality) 0-7 days

Unless 24 hour weaning is practised, the piglet is nearly always on the sow at this point in its life.

1.   **Dead at birth "born dead"**

                                                                                                          Page

     a)   **Aborted. (Born before term)**

*Fever in sows caused by infectious disease**	
Enterovirus*	22
Aujeszky's Disease	72
Parvovirus	18
Fusarium	251
Erysipelas	223
Leptospirosis	110
Carbon monoxide	376
Brucellosis	117
Toxoplasmosis	283
PRRS*	60

     b)   **Born at term**

Mummified piglets	
SMEDI	25
Parvovirus*	18
Aujeszky's	72
PRRS*	60
Freshly dead	
Delays in parturition* (in membranes, non-expanded lungs)	
Congenital abnormality*	327
*Fever in the Sow**	
Fusarium poisoning	251
Carbon monoxide poisoning	376
Vitamin A deficiency	312
Toxoplasmosis	283
Leptospirosis	110
Aujeszky's Disease	72
Inclusion body rhinitis	55
Parvovirus*	18
Chlamydia	245
PRRS*	60

2. Dead after cleaning membranes

3. Weak piglets

Weak piglets may subsequently die. Conditions which contribute to weakness and cause death directly or by an inability to suck and thus death from hypoglycaemia are listed below.

(a) Nervous signs

(b) Respiratory disease

Thrombocytopaenic purpura		345
PRRS		60

(g) Skin lesions

Trauma*		
Exudative epidermitis*		220
Epitheliogenesis imperfecta		334
Vulval swelling		251
Coal tar or abrasive necrosis of teats and tails		378
Hairless pigs		334
		348

Disease of piglets 7 days - weaning

The age of weaning varies, but is commonly 21 days or more. Some of the conditions which appear in this age group may also occur in weaned pigs, especially those weaned at less than 21 days of age.

Page

(a) Nervous signs

Congenital tremor AII	346
Congenital tremor AIII	340
Congenital tremor AV	347
Aujeszky's disease	72
Vitamin A deficiency	312
Talfan, Teschen etc.	23
Tetanus	128
Leptospirosis	110
Actinobacillosis	115
Listeriosis	119
Haemophilus parasuis meningitis*	214
Streptococcal meningitis*	228
Middle ear infection	
Hypoglycaemia	299
Swine fever	82
African swine fever	90
Copper deficiency myelopathy (Copper deficiency)	309

(b) Respiratory signs

Inclusion body rhinitis*	55
Bordetella infection*	192
Atrophic rhinitis*	197
Reovirus	57
Adenovirus	46
Haemophilus infection*	214
Streptococcal infections*	228
Pneumocystis carinii	285
Enzootic pneumonia	178
Pasteurella infection	204
PRRS*	60

Diseases of Weaned Pigs

A number of conditions occur most frequently after weaning or are seen in their most characteristic form in the recently-weaned pig up to slaughter weight.

(d) Lameness and locomotor distrubance

(e) Systemic states with fever, sudden death

Diseases of Adult Animals

These will depend very much on the husbandry conditions and type of enterprise. An adult animal is considered as one which is retained for breeding or has been bred from.

(d) Lameness and locomotor disturbance

(e) Systemic states with fever and sudden death associated with fever

Page

(f)   Systemic states without fever, sudden deaths

Clostridium novyi (*oedematiens*)	129
Proliferative haemorrhagic enteropathy	170
Endocarditis from erysipelas etc.*	223
Porcine stress syndrome*	336
Mulberry heart disease	317
Hertztod	317
Gastric Ulceration	363
Intestinal Haemorrhage Syndrome*	368
Twists and intestinal accidents	
Heat stroke	374
Nitrate and Nitrite poisoning	376
Electrocution	375
Obstetrical accidents, dystocia*	
Cystitis (*E. coli*)*	241
Cystitis (*Actinobaculum suis*)	239
Others	

(g)   Skin conditions

Swine pox	58
Swine fever	82
Swine vesicular disease	95
Foot and Mouth disease	99
Actinobacillosis	115
Salmonellosis	150
Swine erysipelas*	223
Ringworm	249
Vulvovaginitis	251
Ergot	256
Lice*	287
Mange*	288
Mammary abscesses	352
Sunburn	375
Trauma - galls from crates, rubbed elbows, etc.*	
Fighting	
Vulva biting	386
Bird injuries	
Infections and local abscesses from trauma*	
Burns	
Ulcerative dermatitis	

(h)   Reproductive conditions

Parvovirus*	18
S.M.E.D.I.	25
PRRS*	60
Aujeszky's disease	72
Swine fever	82
Leptospirosis*	110
Brucellosis	117
Listeriosis	119

400

INDEX

403

Page

Page